Case Studies in Rheumatology

Case Studies in Rheumatology

Editor: Finley Cooper

AMERICAN
MEDICAL PUBLISHERS
www.americanmedicalpublishers.com

AMERICAN
MEDICAL PUBLISHERS
www.americanmedicalpublishers.com

Cataloging-in-Publication Data

Case studies in rheumatology / edited by Finley Cooper.
p. cm.
Includes bibliographical references and index.
ISBN 979-8-88740-615-2
1. Rheumatology. 2. Rheumatism. 3. Joints--Diseases.
4. Connective tissues--Diseases. I. Cooper, Finley
RC927 .R44 2023
616.723--dc23

American Medical Publishers,
41 Flatbush Avenue,
1st Floor, New York,
NY 11217, USA

ISBN 979-8-88740-615-2 (Hardback)

Contents

Preface

Every book is a source of knowledge and this one is no exception. The idea that led to the conceptualization of this book was the fact that the world is advancing rapidly; which makes it crucial to document the progress in every field. I am aware that a lot of data is already available, yet, there is a lot more to learn. Hence, I accepted the responsibility of editing this book and contributing my knowledge to the community.

Rheumatology is a medical specialty that focuses on the diagnosis and treatment of conditions affecting the musculoskeletal system, especially the conditions related to the joints, muscles, and connective tissues. Some of the rheumatic diseases which are treated within this field are inflammatory arthritis (such as rheumatoid arthritis), osteoarthritis, lupus, gout, fibromyalgia and vasculitis. These conditions can significantly impact a person's quality of life by causing pain, stiffness, swelling and limiting joint mobility. Treatment approaches in rheumatology may involve a combination of medications, lifestyle modifications, physical therapy and patient education. It also offers ongoing support and monitoring to optimize treatment outcomes and minimize the impact of rheumatic diseases on daily life. This book explores all the important aspects of rheumatology in the present day scenario. It will serve as a reference to a broad spectrum of readers.

While editing this book, I had multiple visions for it. Then I finally narrowed down to make every chapter a sole standing text explaining a particular topic, so that they can be used independently. However, the umbrella subject sinews them into a common theme. This makes the book a unique platform of knowledge.

I would like to give the major credit of this book to the experts from every corner of the world, who took the time to share their expertise with us. Also, I owe the completion of this book to the never-ending support of my family, who supported me throughout the project.

Editor

1

Myocardial Infarction in a 7-Year-Old Girl with Polyarteritis Nodosa

Lina Bayazeed[1,2,3] **Alaa Felimban**[1,2,4] **Abdulsalam Alsaiad**[1,2,4] **Fahd Alsufiani**[1,2,4] **and Jubran Alqanatish**[1,2,3]

[1]*King Saud Bin Abdulaziz University for Health Sciences, Riyadh 14611, Saudi Arabia*
[2]*King Abdullah International Medical Research Center (KAIMRC), Riyadh 14611, Saudi Arabia*
[3]*King Abdullah Specialist Children's Hospital, Riyadh 14611, Saudi Arabia*
[4]*King Abdulaziz Medical City (National Guard Health Affairs), Riyadh 14611, Saudi Arabia*

Correspondence should be addressed to Jubran Alqanatish; qanatishj@ngha.med.sa

Academic Editor: Gregory J. Tsay

Polyarteritis nodosa (PAN) is a rare systemic vasculitis that affects small to medium-sized arteries. It could affect any organ including the heart. However coronary artery involvements are very rare. We describe a young girl who presented following a histopathological diagnosis of PAN with acute chest pain, high serum troponin, and progressive ischemic changes in the electrocardiogram (ECG). Induction of remission of her disease was done with six-moths Cyclophosphamide infusions and pulse corticosteroids. In addition to anticoagulation and dual antithrombotic therapy, the disease remission was maintained with mycophenolate mofetil which helps in the recovery of coronary disease. Our case illustrates the serious cardiac involvement of PAN in a child that responded to intensive management.

1. Introduction

Polyarteritis nodosa (PAN) is a necrotizing vasculitis that affects the wall of small to medium-sized arteries. The clinical spectrum is highly variable where it can be systemic or localized to one organ or system [1]. PAN occurs primarily in middle-aged adults but appears even more rarely in children where both girls and boys are affected equally [2]. It occurs in different forms as cutaneous (the most common form), classic, systemic, or microscopic. Cutaneous PAN is necrotizing vasculitis confined to the skin. It is relatively a benign form that doesn't have deep organ involvement in contrast to systemic PAN which is a potentially life-threatening and involve multiple systems like kidney, heart, lung, gastrointestinal tract, liver, nervous and musculoskeletal systems. Microscopic is localized PAN lesions discovered in surgical specimens, such as the appendix, gallbladder, testes, and other internal organs [3]. Surgical excision is usually curative in this form of PAN [1].

The term classic is used to differentiate idiopathic systemic PAN from a group of patients who have a loss of function mutation of the gene encoding adenosine deaminase 2 (ADA2) [4].

In children's skin, MSK, and GIT are frequently involved while cardiac, brain, and lung are less involved [5, 6]. Cardiac involvement in pediatric PAN is much less compared to adults affected with PAN [7].

We report a pediatric patient diagnosed as a medium-sized vasculitis confirmed based on clinical features, histopathology, and elevated inflammatory markers to have PAN; who presented initially as acute abdominal pain underwent a laparoscopic appendectomy and complicated by acute myocardial infarction (AMI) secondary to Coronary artery vasculitis a few days later.

2. Case Presentation

A previously healthy, 7-year-old girl presented with a history of persistent abdominal pain and vomiting for 4 days. It preceded by upper respiratory tract infection symptoms the week before patient's presentation. She was admitted for the first time in March 2019, as a case of gastritis and to rule out urinary tract infection (UTI). A previous history of intermittent mild abdominal pain since the age of 2 years was reported. Infrequently, associated with vomiting and diarrhea, which occur 1-2 times per year. No history of fever, weight loss, skin rash, respiratory symptoms, headache, or urine changes. Family history was unremarkable for similar presentation, genetic disorders or vasculitis.

Laboratory investigations showed high White cell counts, Erythrocyte Sedimentation Rate, and C-Reactive Protein (WBC 14.6 × 109/L, ESR 70 mm/hr, CRP 179 mg/L). Due to her severe abdominal pain, she underwent an abdominal ultrasound, which was suspicious for appendicitis; the appendix measured 0.65 cm with mild free fluid in the right lower quadrant. The patient was taken to the operating room for laparoscopic appendectomy. Intra-operative the surgeon noticed that the appendix looked non-inflamed so it was sent for histopathological examination. The histopathology report showed; Focal peri-appendicular tissue with 3 medium-sized vessels showing necrotizing vasculitis, there were also few small size vessels with the same finding and no evidence of appendicular inflammation (Figures 1(a) and 1(b)).

The rheumatology team was consulted and the diagnosis of polyarteritis nodosa was made, based on clinical features, laboratory, and histopathology findings. She received three doses of intravenous (I.V) pulse steroid. During hospitalization, an echocardiogram was requested for coronary arteries evaluation and showed normal intra-cardiac anatomy and function with normal coronary arteries' size and branching. No ischemic changes were found in the electrocardiogram. Ophthalmology evaluation showed a normal ocular exam for both eyes. Urinalysis and renal Doppler ultrasound came normal. CT Angiogram of the abdominal vessels (Hepatic, renal, celiac, splenic, mesenteric arteries) showed no findings of vasculitis. Antineutrophil cytoplasmic antibodies (cANCA and pANCA) were negative. Cyclophosphamide was planned to be given in Day Care Treatments Unit (DCTU) 10 days after discharge to allow proper surgical wound healing. The patient was discharged home on prednisolone 2 mg/kg/day divided doses and to be followed in the Rheumatology clinic within a week.

On the 3rd day after discharge, the patient presented to the ER with a complaint of persistent left-sided chest pain, moderate to severe, localized, not radiating. No abdominal pain, fever or other symptoms. Laboratory workup showed a remarkably high Troponin I level of 1682 pg/mL. Initially, ECG and Echocardiogram were normal. The patient was admitted to the Pediatric Intensive Care (PICU) for close monitoring. Nine hours later on the same day, cardiac enzymes kept in trending up (Table 1) and ischemic changes start to appear in the electrocardiogram in form of ST elevation in inferior leads and ST depression in lead I and AVL which is consistent with RCA territory (Figure 2). Urgently repeated echocardiogram showed; impaired left ventricular systolic function involving the septal wall and anterior LV wall; Left anterior descending artery territories (Figure 3(a)). A serial echocardiogram was repeated a few hours later showed multiple echogenic masses at the left ventricular apex (1.5 × 1 cm), LV inferior wall, and in the right ventricle most likely thrombus (Figure 3(b)). The patient's chest pain was progressive and excoriating, that required morphine infusion. Also, she started to have elevated systolic blood pressure, which was controlled by amlodipine and as needed hydralazine. Nitroglycerin and heparin infusion was initiated and she was transferred immediately to the Pediatric Cardiac Intensive Care Unit (PCICU).

The multidisciplinary meeting(MD) was conducted including cardiology, rheumatology, intensive care, and hematology teams, and the patient was taken to the cardiac catheterization lab for a coronary angiogram and possible thrombus removal. Coronary angiography showed no coronary obstruction in both left and right coronary artery systems (Figure 4(a)) but it showed irregularity of the left main coronary artery which indicating vasculitis (Figure 4(b)).

The MD decided to add Aspirin, Clopidogrel, and to give one dose of IVIG 2 g/kg and start intravenous methylprednisolone (2 mg/kg). 2 days later, all cultures came negative and thrombophilia workup was unremarkable. However, the patient was still in critical condition and requiring inotropic and ventilator support so one dose of Infliximab 6 mg/kg/dose was given. ECG at that time is showing ischemic changes in form of ST elevation in inferior leads and ST depression in lead I and AVL (Figure 5(a)).

Follow-up ECG on the 4th day of admission showed no more ischemic changes (Figure 5(b)) and repeated echocardiogram showed improved cardiac function with regression in the size of the left ventricle clot. Further laboratory test results revealed high von willebrand factor >199.5%, negative ANA, normal complements, and immunoglobulins levels. Renal and liver functions remain normal. Whole exome sequencing (WES) was sent to exclude adenosine deaminase 2 deficiency and was negative for CECR1 mutations.

Cyclophosphamide 500 mg/m^2 was initiated as previously planned and the Tropinin I level continues to improve (Table 1). The patient was weaned off inotropes and ventilator over two weeks and was discharged on the third week from hospital in a stable condition with close follow-up.

The patient completed the induction phase of 6 doses of monthly I.V Cyclophosphamide 500 mg/m^2. Then, she was maintained on oral mycophenolate mofetil 600 mg/m^2/day every 12 hrs. Heparin and anti-thrombotic agents were continued. Corticosteroid was weaned off slowly over 10 months with follow up of cardiac enzymes, inflammatory markers, and cardiac function.

Cardiac MRI was done 3 months after discharge which showed mildly dilated LV with normal systolic function 69%. There are LV wall motion abnormalities (hypokinesia), abnormal thinning of the apical septal and lateral wall, and diffuse LV mid-wall scarring involving most of the LV mid &

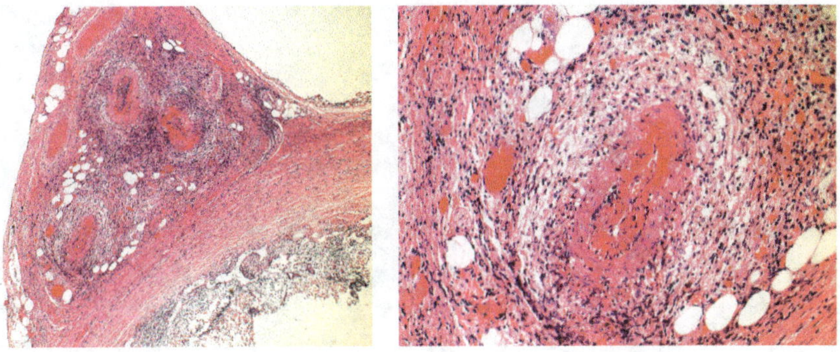

(a) (b)

FIGURE 1: (a) Mesoappendix and part of the appendix. Necrotizing vasculitis in mesoappendix small- to medium-sized arteries is evident. There is no inflammation in the appendix mucosa and muscularis propria. Low magnification. H & E stained slide. (b) Segmental transmural necrotizing inflammation. In the involved artery/arteriole, there is fibrinoid necrosis, neutrophils and eosinophils which associated with lumen narrowing. There are no granulomas. High magnification. H & E stained slide.

TABLE 1: Troponin I trend in the patient over first week of admission.

Exam name	Reference value	1st day of admission	2nd day of admission	3rd day of admission	4th day of admission	5th day of admission
Troponin I	<15.5 pg/mL	1682 then repeated 6019	19835	50.000	42529	29057

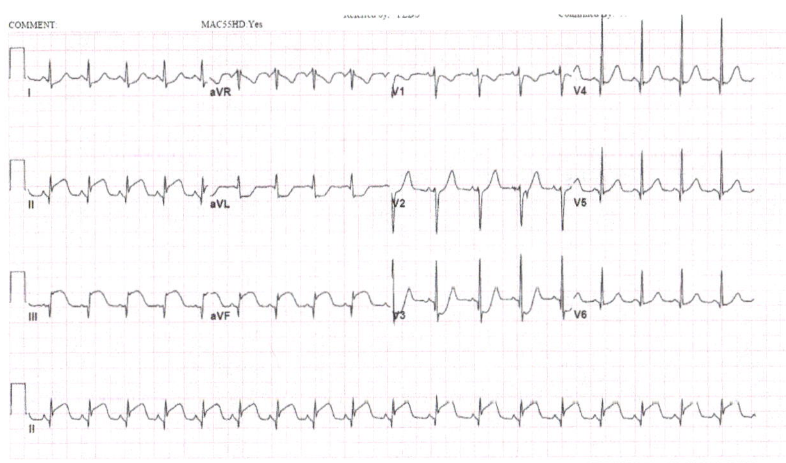

FIGURE 2: Ischemic changes involving right coronary territories.

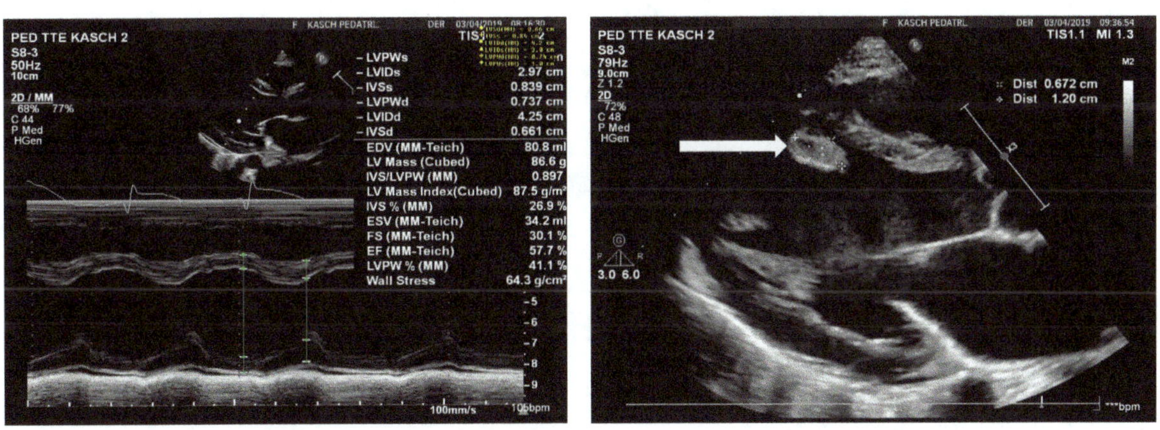

(a) (b)

FIGURE 3: (a) Impaired left ventricular systolic function. (b) Left ventricular thrombus (white arrow).

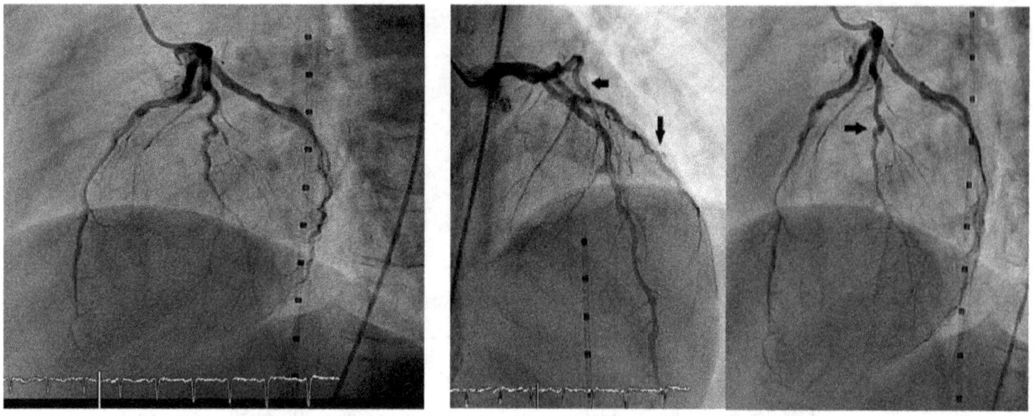

(a) (b)

FIGURE 4: (a) None obstructed coronary arteries. (b) Irregularity of coronary arteries (black arrows).

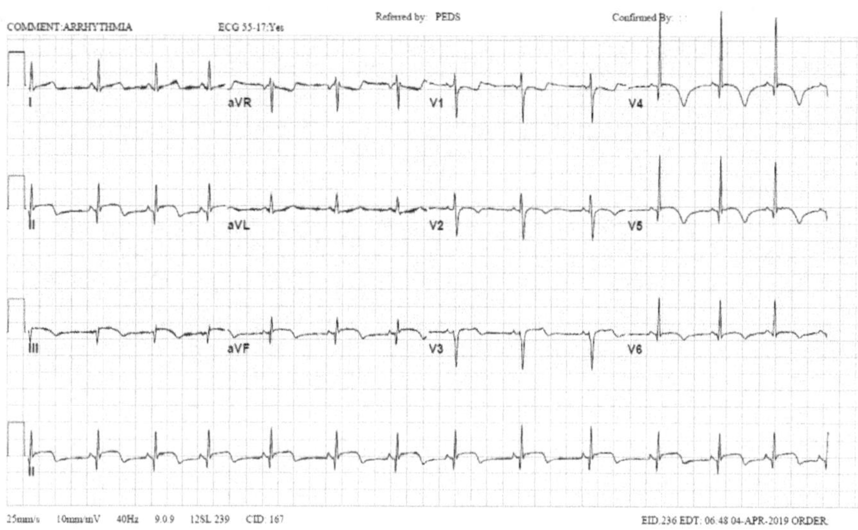

(a)

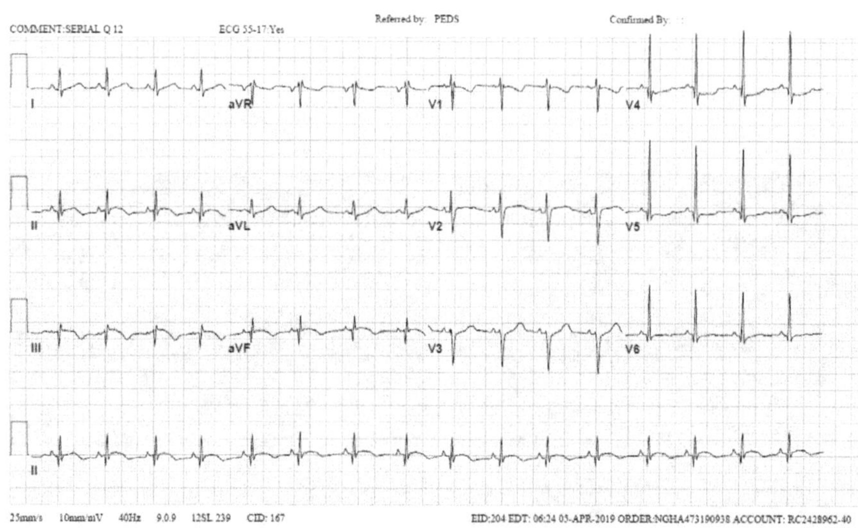

(b)

FIGURE 5: (a) ECG with ischemic changes. (b) Normal ECG on the 4th day after treatment.

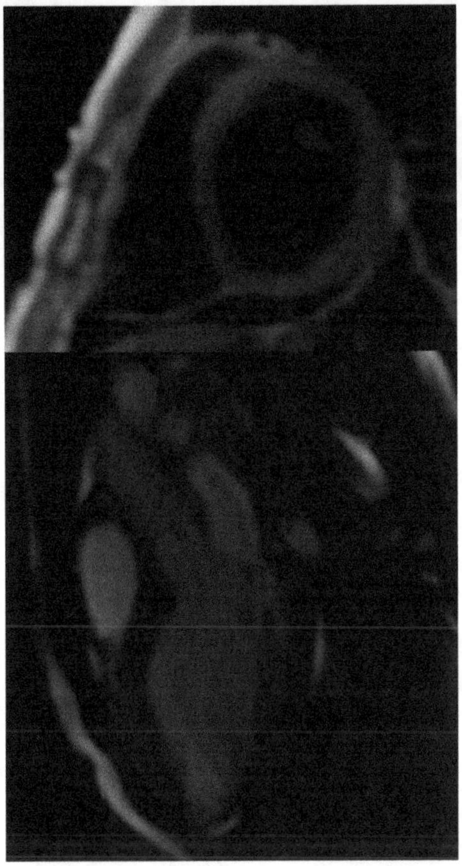

Figure 6: Cardiac MRI showed mildly dilated LV.

apical segments as well as the apical cap with normal coronary arteries (Figure 6).

The patient completed 24 months of follow-up on ASA, Clopidogrel, and mycophenolate mofetil with no signs of inflammation and normal cardiac function.

3. Discussion

In children, Ozen et al. reported gastrointestinal symptoms in 24% of 63 children with PAN [6]. Another study evaluated the cardiac findings of 15 children with childhood PAN [2]. The most common findings were diminished left ventricular systolic function and mild mitral and/or tricuspid valve regurgitation. No cases were reported to have myocardial infarction [2].

In a single center experience over thirty two years, among 69 children diagnosed with PAN, cardiac involvement was present in 3 patients (4%), with 2 of them had valvular heart disease and 1 had pericarditis. Another 3 patients were found to have silent involvement of the coronary arteries during screening echocardiography [5].

In the combined pediatric and adult cohort of polyarteritis nodosa patients reported by Erden et al., gastrointestinal and cardiovascular involvement were more common in adults than children; 31.5% versus 15.5% and 19% versus 4.4% respectively, (P value < 0.001) [5–8]. In a patient with PAN abdominal pain is considered the most common presenting symptom of gastrointestinal involvement [5]. There are multiple cases in the literature reported as PAN presented with acute abdominal pain that mimics appendicitis [9]. However, necrotizing vasculitis of the appendix associated with PAN is uncommon; the largest series in the literature consists of 12 adult cases reported a close relationship between necrotizing arteritis of the appendix and PAN [10]. Similarly, our case presented with acute appendicitis and necrotizing vasculitis.

In clinical and autopsy of five series including 283 adult patients with PAN, congestive heart failure was found to be the most common cardiac involvement (27%), while coronary involvement with myocardial infarction was rare (2%) [11, 12].

Coronary involvement with secondary myocardial infarction in PAN was rarely reported in clinical practice for adults and children, and most of the reported cases were found in postmortem studies [5, 6].

In the largest cohort of 69 children mentioned above, all patients received induction therapy with a combination of corticosteroids and cyclophosphamide, then maintained on either azathioprine or mycophenolate with low-dose corticosteroids. All had achieved remission, with a median of 2 months (range 1–24 months) from diagnosis to remission [5]. The study didn't include specific details about each case; however, it didn't report any relapse, morbidity, or mortality among these cases.

The 5-year survival of patients with PAN without treatment is 13%, while with optimal therapy, it increases to approximately 80% [7]. Early diagnosis and early aggressive treatment are essential and can prevent long-term morbidity and mortality [7].

In the current study, we report a pediatric case of polyarteritis nodosa who presented initially with GI manifestation, treated by 3 doses of pulse methylprednisolone and then complicated after few days by coronary arteritis with secondary myocardial infarction that leads to depressed LV function with small intraventricular thrombus. The patient responded well to systemic steroid, Infliximab, and Cyclophosphamide. In addition to anticoagulation and antithrombotic therapy. Her remission was maintained by mycophenolate mofetil and satisfactory cardiac outcome was achieved on follow up.

Polyarteritis nodosa in pediatric is a rare but serious condition. It is clear that early and aggressive multidisciplinary treatment plan leads to favorable outcome.

References

[1] J. Hernández-Rodríguez, M. A. Alba, S. Prieto-González, and C. C. Maria, "Diagnosis and classification of polyarteritis nodosa," *Journal of Autoimmunity*, vol. 48, pp. 84–89, 2014.

[2] K. M. Beckum, D. J. Kim, D. R. Kelly, P. Weiser, D. A. Lara, and A. Theos, "Polyarteritis nodosa in childhood: recognition of early dermatologic signs may prevent morbidity," *Pediatric Dermatology*, vol. 31, no. 1, pp. e6–e9, 2014.

[3] L. Forbess and S. Bannykh, "Polyarteritis nodosa," *Rheumatic Disease Clinics of North America*, vol. 41, no. 1, pp. 33–46, 2015.

[4] P. Navon Elkan, S. B. Pierce, R. Segel et al., "Mutant adenosine deaminase 2 in a polyarteritis nodosa vasculopathy," *New England Journal of Medicine*, vol. 370, no. 10, pp. 921–931, 2014.
[5] D. Eleftheriou, M. J. Dillon, K. Tullus et al., "Systemic polyarteritis nodosa in the young: a single-center experience over thirty-two years," *Arthritis and Rheumatism*, vol. 65, no. 9, pp. 2476–2485, 2013.
[6] S. Ozen, J. Anton, N. Arisoy et al., "Juvenile polyarteritis: results of a multicenter survey of 110 children," *Journal of Pediatrics*, vol. 145, no. 4, pp. 517–522, 2004.
[7] A. Erden, E. D. Batu, H. E. Sönmez et al., "Comparing polyarteritis nodosa in children and adults: a single center study," *International Journal of Rheumatic Diseases*, vol. 20, no. 8, pp. 1016–1022, 2017.
[8] C. Pagnoux, R. Seror, C. Henegar et al., "Clinical features and outcomes in 348 patients with polyarteritis nodosa: a systematic retrospective study of patients diagnosed between 1963 and 2005 and entered into the French vasculitis study group database," *Arthritis and Rheumatism*, vol. 62, no. 2, pp. 616–626, 2010.
[9] N. Ozçay, K. Arda, T. Sugüneş et al., "Polyarteritis nodosa presenting with necrotising appendicitis and hepatic aneurysm rupture," *Turkish Journal of Gastroenterology: The Official Journal of Turkish Society of Gastroenterology*, vol. 14, no. 1, pp. 68–70, 2003.
[10] T. N. Moyana, "Necrotizing arteritis of the vermiform appendix. a clinicopathologic study of 12 cases," *Archives of Pathology and Laboratory Medicine*, vol. 112, no. 7, pp. 738–741, 1988.
[11] M. Sebastiani, A. Manfredi, and C. Ferri, "Cardiac involvement in systemic vasculitis," *Handbook of Systemic Autoimmune Diseases*, Elsevier, Amsterdam, Netherlands, pp. 335–382, 2017.
[12] R. S. Cassling, J. B. Lortz, D. R. Olson, T. F. Hubbard, and B. M. McManus, "Fatal vasculitis (periarteritis nodosa) of the coronary arteries: angiographic ambiguities and absence of aneurysms at autopsy," *Journal of the American College of Cardiology*, vol. 6, no. 3, pp. 707–714, 1985.

2

Class IV Lupus Nephritis in the Setting of Serologically Quiescent Disease and Normal Urine Sediment in a Patient with Late-Onset Systemic Lupus Erythematosus

Benedicta Nnodum and Lauren Dudley

Berkshire Medical Center, Pittsfield, MA, USA

Correspondence should be addressed to Benedicta Nnodum; bnnodum@bhs1.org

Academic Editor: Mario Salazar-Paramo

Systemic lupus erythematosus (SLE) is a chronic inflammatory autoimmune disease that may affect any organ of the body. Lupus nephritis (LN) is a frequent and serious complication of SLE. We report a case of an 80-year-old woman who was initially diagnosed with late-onset SLE and eventually developed LN in the setting of normal complements, double-stranded DNA, C-reactive protein, erythrocyte sedimentation rate, and urine sediment. She developed abnormal renal function (creatinine of 1.7 mg/dl) and mild proteinuria (1-2+) without hematuria. Renal biopsy showed class IV lupus glomerulonephritis, active and chronic. The patient was started on mycophenolate mofetil which led to improvement of proteinuria and stabilization of creatinine. The suspicion for LN in a patient with late-onset SLE should remain high when there is development of suspicious renal or urinary abnormalities even if laboratory values do not suggest high disease activity and urinary sediment is normal. To our knowledge, this is one of the oldest patients with biopsy-proven LN and late-onset SLE.

1. Introduction

Systemic lupus erythematosus (SLE) is a chronic inflammatory autoimmune disease that may affect many organs of the body such as the skin, joints, kidneys, nervous system, heart, lungs, and the serous membranes [1]. Late-onset SLE refers to a specific group of SLE that begins above 50 years [2] and infrequently causes lupus nephritis (LN). LN significantly increases the morbidity and mortality of SLE patients and requires aggressive immunosuppressive therapy [3]. Prompt diagnosis and treatment are critical for improvement in patient survival, as evidenced by marked improvement in 5-year survival rates from 44% in the 1950s to 95% over the last 50 years [4]. Existing urine and serum biomarkers used to clinically assess patients' disease activity and predict the presence of lupus nephritis include proteinuria, urine sediment activity, creatinine clearance, anti-double-stranded DNA antibodies (anti-dsDNA Abs), complement levels C3 and C4, ESR, and CRP [5]. Nevertheless, the correlation between these markers and LN is imperfect, and their utility in reflecting disease activity and in predicting outcome remains controversial [6]. It is important to note that both C-reactive protein (CRP) and erythrocyte sedimentation rate (ESR) are often elevated in SLE flare. We present a case of a 80-year-old female with late-onset SLE and subsequent class IV lupus nephritis which developed in the setting of normal anti-dsDNA Abs, complement levels C3 and C4, ESR, CRP levels, and an inactive urine sediment.

2. Case Description

An 80-year-old woman with hypertension, chronic obstructive pulmonary disease (COPD), hypothyroidism, hyperlipidemia, congestive heart failure (CHF), and long-standing history of Raynaud's was diagnosed with late-onset SLE 2 years prior to the onset of lupus nephritis. At the time of diagnosis, her disease manifestations included subacute cutaneous lupus erythematosus (SCLE), pancytopenia, Raynaud's with nail-fold capillary changes, sicca symptoms, and photosensitivity. Evaluation for etiology of pancytopenia with bone marrow aspiration/biopsy with flow cytometry and cytogenetic studies, laboratory profile, and CT chest/abdomen/pelvis did not show evidence for primary bone marrow stem cell process or malignant lymphoproliferative disease. Around this time, she developed erythematous plaque lesions with scaling on her upper extremities, and biopsy findings were thought to be consistent with SCLE.

Medications included amlodipine for Raynaud's and Restasis for dry eyes. Family history was notable for a grandson with Crohn's disease but no other autoimmune diseases. Social history was remarkable for secondhand smoke exposure but no active smoking, alcohol, or drug usage.

The pertinent diagnostic tests at the time of SLE diagnosis which were positive include anti-nuclear antibody titer 1 : 1280 finely speckled, elevated rheumatoid factor (RF) of 456 IU/ml (N: 0–20 IU/ml), positive SS-A/Ro > 8.0 and SS-B/La > 8.0 antibodies, anti-beta-2 glycoprotein IgM Ab >100 U/ml, CRP level 3.9 mg/l (N: 0–5 mg/l), and ESR 51 mm/hour (N: 0–20 mm/hour). The serologic tests that were negative include anti-dsDNA Abs, complement C3 level 154 mg/dl (N: 106–194 mg/dl), complement C4 level 38 mg/dl (N: 19–50 mg/dl), cyclic citrullinated peptide IgG, cryoglobulin, serum immunofixation, Scl-70 scleroderma, Smith, RNP, cardiolipin antibodies, and lupus anticoagulant. Urine studies at the time revealed 2 + proteinuria, no hematuria or pyuria, urine protein to creatinine (PC) ratio of 0.2 (N: 0.0–0.1), and creatinine level of 0.93 mg/dl and eGFR >60 ml/min/1.73 m^2.

About 2 years after the diagnosis of late-onset SLE, she was admitted and managed for a CHF exacerbation. During this hospitalization, she developed acute kidney injury (AKI) with creatinine increasing to 1.92 mg/dl during active diuresis. However, the creatinine level never came back to the baseline leaving her with a new baseline of 1.7 mg/dl and eGFR of 28 ml/min/1.73 m^2. The etiology of the AKI was thought to be due to use of diuretics during CHF exacerbation or use of contrast during that hospitalization; however, there was a concern for the development of LN. This prompted repeating urine studies showed 4 + protein on urinalysis, worsening urine PC ratio of 1.9, and 24-hour urine protein of 1170 mg/24 hour (N: 50–150 mg/24 hour). At the time of diagnosis, there was no hematuria, an inactive urine sediment, negative dsDNA, normal ESR and CRP, and normal C3 and C4 levels. There were no symptoms or exam findings consistent with active lupus. Kidney biopsy revealed lupus nephritis, International Society of Nephrology/Renal Pathology Society class IV, activc and chronic with the following findings: mild, focal mesangial hypercellularity, marked thickening of the glomerular capillary wall, segmental duplication of the glomerular baseline membrane in >50% of glomeruli, and a small focal area of interstitial nephritis with a mononuclear infiltrate. There was no necrosis, crescents, vasculitis, or focal segmental glomerulosclerosis (Figure 1). Immunofluorescence showed focal segmental granular staining along the glomerular basement membrane (GBM) for IgG (trace-1+), IgM (4+), IgA (1-2+), Kappa (3-4+), lambda (3-4+), C1q (2-3+), and C3 (1-2+). Electron microscopy showed global glomerular capillary wall thickening, GBM duplication, and subendothelial deposits with no significant podocyte foot effacement (Figure 2).

Upon diagnosis of lupus nephritis, she was started on 60 mg of oral prednisone and mycophenolate mofetil alongside atovaquone for *Pneumocystis jiroveci* pneumonia prophylaxis (sulfa allergic). Repeat urine studies after 4 weeks of being on treatment showed no proteinuria, urine PC ratio of 0.7, and improvement in creatinine to 1.4 mg/dl. She unfortunately died from infection as a complication of therapy despite renal improvement after 2 years of lupus.

3. Discussion

Systemic lupus erythematosus (SLE) is a chronic, inflammatory disease that can affect any organ. It is more prevalent in women than men across all ages. It is of unknown etiology and manifests by the deposition of pathologic autoantibodies and immune complexes into the tissues and cells [1]. Late-onset SLE is a well-described entity seen in older patients above 50 years accounting for 20.4% of SLE diagnoses [2]. They generally have a more benign disease course though with poorer prognosis due to higher frequency of comorbid conditions and higher organ damage in the setting of aging and higher vascular risk factors [7]. Late-onset SLE usually has lower frequency of lupus nephritis (LN) and malar rash but higher frequency of sicca syndrome, pericarditis, and lung involvement as initial manifestations [7, 8]. The atypical presentation with sicca syndrome, pericarditis, and lung involvement often makes it a challenging diagnosis to make in this age group as these symptoms can be attributed to common comorbid conditions seen in elderly patients [9, 10]. This explains the reason time from symptom onset to diagnosis can be 60 months for late-onset SLE compared to 19–24 months for adult-onset SLE [9, 10]. Recent studies that investigated the clinical characteristics between late-onset SLE and adult-onset SLE (18–50 years old) demonstrated that the former has a lower disease activity, decreased renal involvement, and lower cumulative SLE criteria [26, 27]. However, there are varying opinions on the prognosis and mortality as one study showed more favorable result [26] compared to the other [27]. Of note is that the oldest reported age of a patient diagnosed with late-onset SLE and lupus nephritis is 74 years [28]. Our patient was diagnosed with late-onset SLE at 77 years and developed stage IV LN at 79 years.

The presence of lupus nephritis is a major determinant of SLE prognosis [1]. Despite the improvement in the 5- and 10-year survival rates of LN patients, prognosis is unsatisfactory [4]. The manifestations of LN range from asymptomatic urinary findings to nephrotic syndrome and progressive renal impairment. International Society of Nephrology and the Renal Pathology Society (ISN/RPS) classes I and II usually have an indolent course while classes III, IV, and V are often progressive. Class IV LN has been shown to

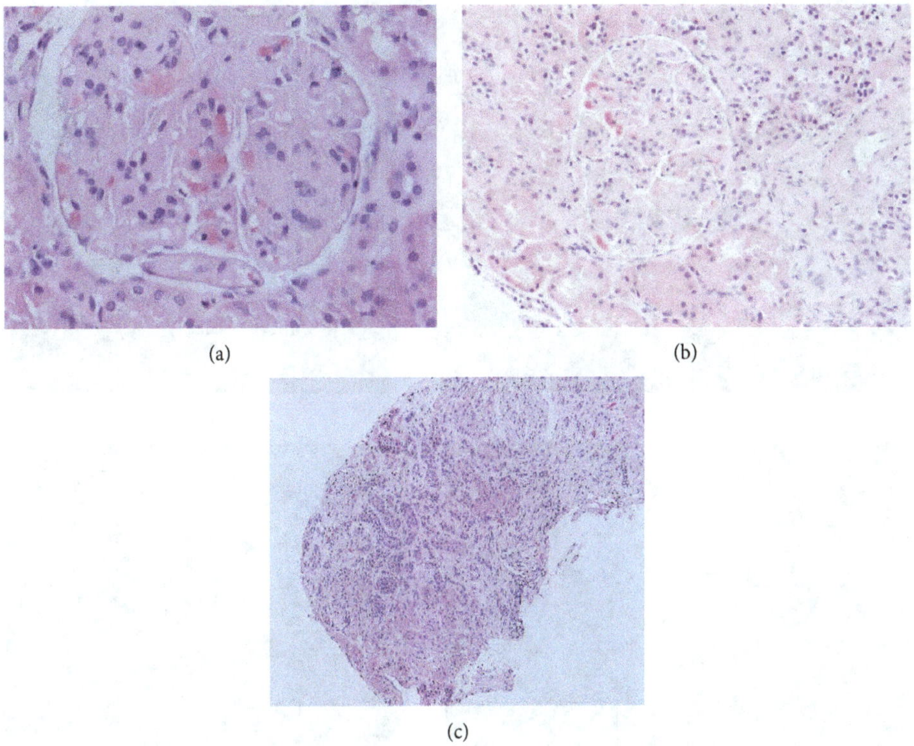

Figure 1: (a) Mild, focal mesangial hypercellularity, lobular architecture, and expanded matrix. The glomerular capillary wall is markedly and uniformly thickened. (b) Arteries are present and have mild arteriosclerosis. (c) Tubular atrophy involving less than 5% of the cortex.

have a 20% 5-year probability of developing end-stage renal disease (ESRD) [11].

Some studies have shown that late-onset SLE patients have increased prevalence of positive RF, hypocomplementemia, anti-Ro/anti-La antibodies [12]. The index patient had elevated RF and anti-Ro/anti-La antibodies. The value of anti-dsDNA Ab is unclear in late-onset SLE as studies have shown mixed results [13]. Sassi et al. and Choi et al. found decreased anti-dsDNA Ab in late-onset SLE [12, 14]. However, an older study on Brazilian patients found slightly higher anti-dsDNA Ab levels in late-onset SLE [15]. Late-onset SLE has a higher incidence of elevated creatinine and decreased creatinine clearance (CrCl) on initial presentation compared to adult-onset SLE. Average CrCl of late-onset SLE was 49.1 ml/min compared to 71.2 ml/min for adult-onset SLE [16]. This is due to a combination of natural loss of renal function with age and increased incidence of hypertension at disease onset [16]. However, nephritis and nephropathy were of lower frequency [10, 12, 14]. Sassi et al. carried out a study on SLE patients that demonstrated nephritis in 26% of late-onset SLE compared to 39.8% of adult-onset SLE [14].

Renal biopsy is an invasive procedure for making a diagnosis of lupus nephritis. Noninvasive biomarkers used to predict the likelihood of lupus nephritis and select appropriate patients for biopsy include urinary protein levels, urinary sediment, complement levels C3 and C4, anti-dsDNA antibodies, and creatinine clearance [3, 5]. The rather insidious onset and fluctuating nature of LN can make early identification difficult [6]. Anti-dsDNA and complement have found to be good markers of disease activity and predictors of outcome in lupus nephritis in some studies [17]. Hsieh et al. carried out a study examining the sensitivity and specificity of these biomarkers which showed the following results: sensitivity and specific for anti-dsDNA was 80–88.6% and 92.3–97.7%, respectively, for decreased C3 level was 64.1 and 88.4%, respectively, and for decreased C4 level was 51.3 and 95.3%, respectively [17]. Anti-dsDNA was found to be the most sensitive and specific biomarker in LN. Although proteinuria measured in 24-hour urine samples or the urine PC ratio is the principal urinary biomarkers for assessing LN, they do not necessarily relate to the histological changes in LN [18]. The presence of acanthocytes or erythrocytes in the urine sediments of patients with proliferative lupus nephritis has been shown to have an 82% positive predictive value (PPV) and 71–85% negative predictive value (NPV), respectively [19]. Interestingly, low total complement hemolytic activity (CH_{50}) and decreased C3 and C4 levels have been found in about 75% of SLE patients with focal nephritis and 90% in patients with diffuse nephritis [20].

Huerta et al. carried out a case series on 4 four adults with renal-limited lupus-like glomerulonephritis, two of them had positive ANA but none had low complement levels or positive anti-dsDNA Abs like our patient. They remained serologically silent with occasional occurrence of low titer of ANA despite follow-up for 8 months to 3.5 years [21]. Our patient is a case of late-onset class IV lupus nephritis occurring in the setting of low disease activity, normal inflammatory markers, complement levels, dsDNA, and urinary sediment.

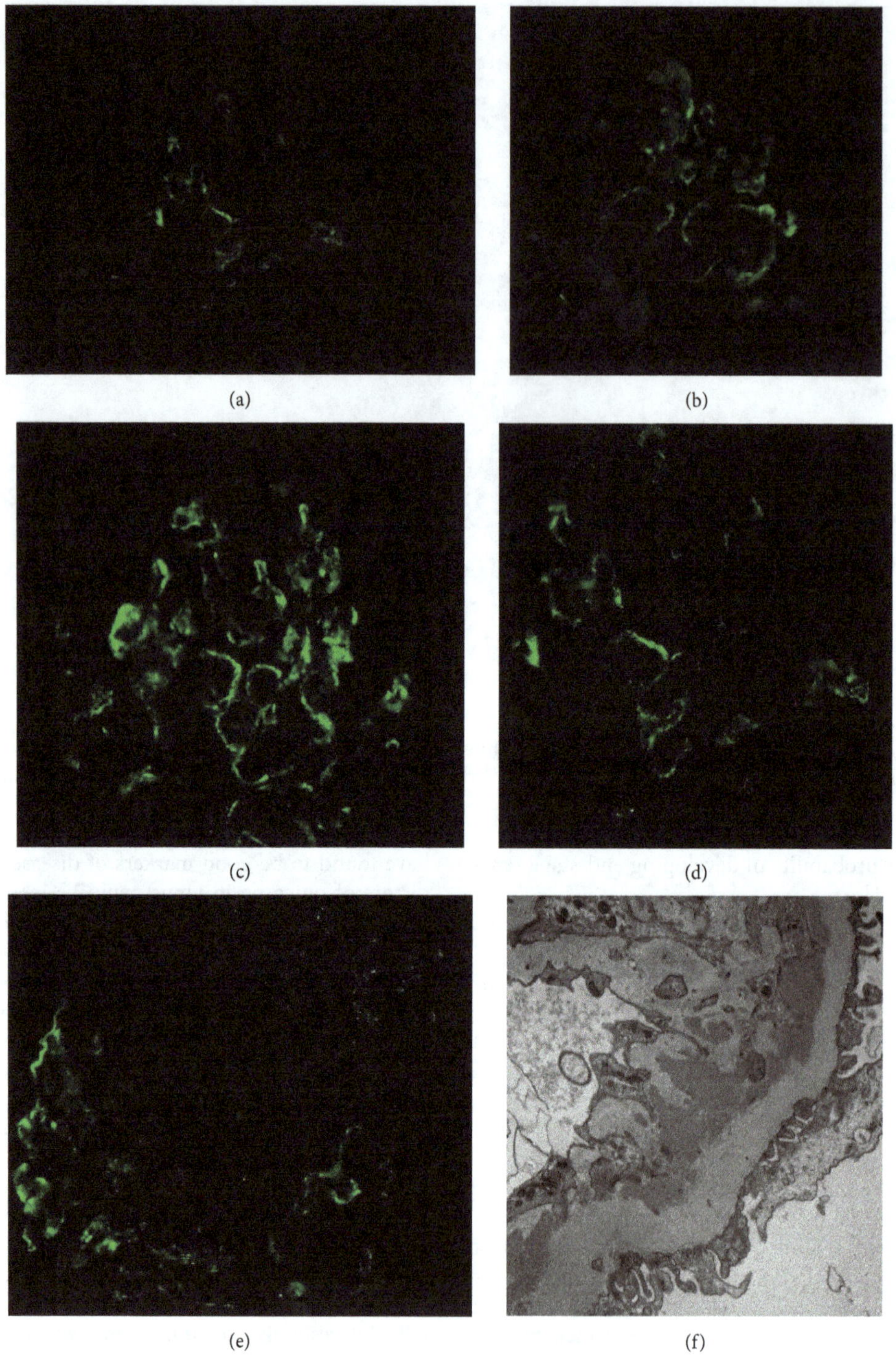

Figure 2: Immunofluorescence pathology slides. Mesangium showing focal moderate granular staining along the (a) GBM IgG (trace to 1+), (b) GBM IgA (1+ to 2+), (c) GBM IgM (4+), (d) GBM C1Q (2+ to 3+), and (e) GBM C3 (1+ to 2+) and (f) electron microscopy slide. No globally sclerotic glomeruli, no significant podocyte foot effacement (about 10%), numerous amorphous electron dense deposits are predominantly subendothelial.

Since currently available biomarkers for lupus nephritis can miss patients such as ours, renal biopsy remains the gold standard for diagnosis and should be performed in patients with SLE who have abnormal renal function or significant proteinuria. There is ongoing research for more sensitive urine biomarkers in LN as urine is easily accessible and directly shows the ongoing pathological state of a kidney through the excretion of immune-related molecules into urine [17].

The recommendation for induction treatment in patients with class IV LN is either oral/intravenous (IV) cyclophosphamide or mycophenolate mofetil (MMF), along with intravenous pulses of high-dose glucocorticoids followed by initiation of oral glucocorticoids [22]. Recent maintenance trials in LN have shown an increased number of patients attaining complete remission and fewer renal flares when MMF is used for at least 3–5 years [23]. Five-year survival rates for late-onset SLE are between 72 and 84% [10, 24], and mortality seen in this group is partly explained by comorbidities at disease onset especially hypertension, altered immune function, and decreased tolerance to immunosuppressive therapy [16, 24, 25]. In summary, majority of patients with class IV lupus nephritis have hematuria, active urine sediments, abnormal complements, positive dsDNA titers, and high measures of disease activity but our patient did not. Late-onset SLE patients are more likely to die from treatment-related complications such as sepsis [10, 24] which is what our patient died from.

4. Conclusion

We reported one of the latest onset cases of lupus nephritis in the literature with class IV lupus nephritis in the setting of serologically quiescent disease and normal urine sediment. Clinical suspicion for lupus nephritis must remain high when a patient with SLE develops proteinuria or abnormal renal function regardless of age or disease activity.

Additional Points

In patients with systemic lupus erythematosus who develop abnormal renal function or proteinuria, there should be a high level of suspicion for lupus nephritis regardless of disease activity or patient's age.

References

[1] A. Salem, A. Meara, and B. H. Rovin, "Update on lupus nephritis," *Clinical Journal of the American Society of Nephrology*, vol. 12, no. 5, pp. 825–835, 2016.

[2] S. Stefanidou, C. Gerodimos, A. Benos et al., "Clinical expression and course in patients with late onset systemic lupus erythematosus," *Hippokratia*, vol. 17, no. 2, pp. 153–156, 2013.

[3] N. Schwartz, B. Goilav, and C. Putterman, "The pathogenesis, diagnosis and treatment of lupus nephritis," *Current Opinion in Rheumatology*, vol. 26, no. 5, pp. 502–509, 2014.

[4] A. Rietveld and J. H. M. Berden, "Renal replacement therapy in lupus nephritis," *Nephrology Dialysis Transplantation*, vol. 23, no. 10, pp. 3056–3060, 2008.

[5] R. Misra and R. Gupta, "Biomarkers in lupus nephritis," *International Journal of Rheumatic Diseases*, vol. 18, no. 2, pp. 219–232, 2015.

[6] N. Schwartz, T. Rubinstein, L. C. Burkly et al., "Urinary TWEAK as a biomarker of lupus nephritis: a multicenter cohort study," *Arthritis Research and Therapy*, vol. 11, no. 5, p. R143, 2009.

[7] A. Tomic-Lucic, R. Petrovic, M. Radak-Perovic et al., "Late-onset systemic lupus erythematosus: clinical features, course, and prognosis," *Clinical Rheumatology*, vol. 32, no. 7, pp. 1053–1058, 2013.

[8] S. Cartella, I. Cavazzana, A. Ceribelli, F. Inverardi, A. Tincani, and F. Franceschini, "Evaluation of mortality, disease activity, treatment, clinical and immunological features of adult and late onset systemicLupus erythematosus," *Autoimmunity*, vol. 46, no. 6, pp. 363–368, 2013.

[9] J. Rovenský and A. Tuchyňová, "Systemic lupus erythematosus in the elderly," *Autoimmunity Reviews*, vol. 7, no. 3, pp. 235–239, 2008.

[10] J. Boddaert, D. L. T. Huong, Z. Amoura, B. Wechsler, P. Godeau, and J.-C. Piette, "Late-onset systemic lupus erythematosus," *Medicine*, vol. 83, no. 6, pp. 348–359, 2004.

[11] L. Ortega, D. Schultz, O. Lenz, V. Pardo, and G. Contreras, "Review: lupus nephritis: pathologic features, epidemiology and a guide to therapeutic decisions," *Lupus*, vol. 19, no. 5, pp. 557–574, 2010.

[12] J. H. Choi, D. J. Park, J. H. Kang et al., "Comparison of clinical and serological differences among juvenile-, adult-, and late-onset systemic lupus erythematosus in Korean patients," *Lupus*, vol. 24, no. 12, pp. 1342–1349, 2015.

[13] S. M. Fu, C. Dai, Z. Zhao, and F. Gaskin, "Anti-dsDNA antibodies are one of the many autoantibodies in systemic lupus erythematosus," *F1000Research*, vol. 4, p. 939, 2015.

[14] R. H. Sassi, J. V. Hendler, G. F. Piccoli et al., "Age of onset influences on clinical and laboratory profile of patients with systemic lupus erythematosus," *Clinical Rheumatology*, vol. 36, no. 1, pp. 89–95, 2016.

[15] L. T. Costallat and A. Coimbra, "Systemic lupus erythematosus: clinical and laboratory aspects related to age at disease onset," *Clinical and Experimental Rheumatology*, vol. 12, no. 6, pp. 603–607, 1994.

[16] A. Mak, C. C. Mok, W. P. Chu, C. H. To, S. N. Wong, and T. C. Au, "Renal damage in systemic lupus erythematosus: a comparative analysis of different age groups," *Lupus*, vol. 16, no. 1, pp. 28–34, 2016.

[17] S. C. Hsieh, C. Y. Tsai, and C. L. Yu, "Potential serum and urine biomakrjers in patients with lupus nephritits and the unsolved problems," *Open Access Rheumatology: Research and Reviews*, vol. 8, pp. 81–91, 2016.

[18] L. Watson and M. W. Beresford, "Urine biomarkers in juvenile-onset SLE nephritis," *Pediatric Nephrology*, vol. 28, no. 3, pp. 363–374, 2012.

[19] M. U. Martinez-Martinez, L. M. Llamazares-Azuara, D. Martinez-Galla et al., "Urinary sediment suggest lupus nephritis histology," *Lupus*, vol. 26, no. 6, pp. 580–587, 2016.

[20] L. Bao, P. N. Cunningham, and R. J. Quigg, "Complement in lupus nephritis: new perspectives," *Kidney Diseases*, vol. 1, no. 2, pp. 91–99, 2015.

[21] A. Huerta, A. S. Bomback, V. Liakopoulos et al., "Renal-limited "lupus-like" nephritis," *Nephrology Dialysis Transplantation*, vol. 27, no. 6, pp. 2337–2342, 2011.

[22] B. H. Hahn, M. A. McMahon, A. Wilkinson et al., "American college of rheumatology guidelines for screening, treatment, and management of lupus nephritis," *Arthritis Care and Research*, vol. 64, no. 6, pp. 797–808, 2012.

[23] F. A. Houssiau, D. D'Cruz, S. Sangle et al., "Azathioprine versus Mycophenolate mofetil for long-term immunosuppression in lupus nephritis: results from the MAINTAIN Nephritis trial," *Annals of the Rheumatic Diseases*, vol. 69, no. 12, pp. 2083–2089, 2010.

[24] M. Padovan, M. Govoni, G. Castellino, N. Rizzo, M. Fotinidi, and F. Trotta, "Late onset systemic lupus erythematosus: no substantial differences using different cut-off ages," *Rheumatology International*, vol. 27, no. 8, pp. 735–741, 2006.

[25] N. Kasitanon, L. S. Magder, and M. Petri, "Predictors of survival in systemic lupus erythematosus," *Medicine*, vol. 85, no. 3, pp. 147–156, 2006.

[26] I. W. Sohn, Y. B. Joo, S. Won, and S. C. Bae, "Late-onset systemic lupus erythematosus: is it "mild lupus"?," *Lupus*, vol. 27, no. 2, pp. 235–242, 2017.
[27] L. J. Catoggio, E. R. Soriano, P. M. Imamura et al., "Late-onset systemic lupus erythematosus in Latin Americans: a distinct subgroup?," *Lupus*, vol. 24, no. 8, pp. 788–795, 2014.
[28] M. Kutky and S. Aloudat, "Late-onset systemic erythematosus with lupus nephritis in a 74-year-old male: a brief case and review," *Canadian Journal of Kidney Health and Disease*, vol. 5, 2018.

3

Successful Treatment of Pulmonary Arterial Hypertension in Systemic Sclerosis with Anticentriole Antibody

Yusho Ishii,[1] Hiroshi Fujii,[1] Koichiro Sugimura,[2] Tsuyoshi Shirai,[1] Yosuke Hoshi,[1] Yoko Fujita,[1] Yuko Shirota,[1] Tomonori Ishii,[3] Hiroaki Shimokawa,[2] and Hideo Harigae[1]

[1]*Department of Hematology and Rheumatology, Tohoku University Graduate School of Medicine, Aoba-ku, Sendai, Japan*
[2]*Department of Cardiovascular Medicine, Tohoku University Graduate School of Medicine, Aoba-ku, Sendai, Japan*
[3]*Clinical Research, Innovation and Education Center, Tohoku University Hospital, Sendai, Miyagi, Japan*

Correspondence should be addressed to Hiroshi Fujii; hfujii@med.tohoku.ac.jp

Academic Editor: Mario Salazar-Paramo

Systemic sclerosis (SSc) is characterized by skin sclerosis and multiple organ damages which may cause mortality and is usually accompanied with several specific autoantibodies, each of which is associated with characteristic complications. Among them, anticentriole antibody is recently reported to be highly associated with SSc-associated pulmonary arterial hypertension (SSc-PAH). In general, several vasodilators are used as therapeutic drugs for SSc-PAH, whereas immunosuppressive therapies are not. Here, we report the case of a 62-year-old female with anticentriole antibody-positive SSc-PAH treated with immunosuppressants and vasodilators. She presented with two-year exertional dyspnea and was diagnosed with PAH and SSc owing to the centriole staining pattern and other symptoms without digital sclerosis. Oral vasodilators were initially administered but were not sufficiently effective on dyspnea. Immunosuppressants such as prednisolone and cyclophosphamide were started. Both of them improved mean pulmonary arterial pressure and 6-minute walk distance, and the anticentriole antibody also disappeared. In this case, SSc-PAH with anticentriole antibody was properly diagnosed and immunosuppressants and vasodilators improved the hemodynamics of PAH with anticentriole antibody and stably maintained it and, in addition, reduced the titer of anticentriole antibody. This indicates that anticentriole antibody might represent a good responsive group to therapies among subgroups of patients with SSc PAH.

1. Introduction

Systemic sclerosis (SSc) is a systemic autoimmune disease and presents with vasculopathy, inflammation, and fibrosis of the skin and internal organs [1, 2]. SSc also presents with heterogeneous organ damages such as pulmonary arterial hypertension (PAH) and interstitial pneumoniae (IP), gastrointestinal dysfunction, cardiac dysfunction, and skin disorder [1, 2]. PAH is one of the serious complications that induce high mortality. Generally, the recommended treatments for SSc-PAH comprise vasodilators, including phosphodiesterase-5 inhibitor (PDE5i), endothelin receptor antagonist, prostacyclin analogs, and soluble guanylate cyclase stimulator [3], which repress the rapid progression of SSc-PAH [4]. Although immunosuppressive therapies are not generally effective for SSc-PAH compared with other connective tissue diseases associated with PAH [2, 5], clinical trials for rituximab, tocilizumab, and dimethyl fumarate for SSc-PAH are underway and are effective in some cases of SSc-PAH [6–9]. Some case reports have indicated that a subpopulation of patients with SSc-PAH is responsive to immunosuppressive therapy [10, 11]; however, it still remains unclear what kind of clinical features or biomarkers are useful to identify SSc-PAH patients on whom immunosuppressive therapies are effective.

Patients with SSc show various types of autoantibodies, and each autoantibody is associated with characteristic clinical phenotypes such as anti-topoisomerase I (diffuse sclerosis, IP, digital ulcer (DU), and severe heart disease), anti-centromere (limited sclerosis, DU, calcinosis, and

PAH), anti-RNA polymerase III (diffuse sclerosis and renal crisis), anti-U3 RNP (diffuse sclerosis, PAH, IP, severe heart disease, myositis, and overlap syndrome), anti-Th/To (limited sclerosis, PAH, and IP), anti-PM-Scl (limited sclerosis and SSc-myositis overlap syndrome), and anti-Ku antibodies (overlap syndrome and myositis) [12–14]. In addition, the anticentriole antibody is recently reported to be highly associated with PAH in patients with SSc [15]. Here, we present the case of a patient with SSc-PAH with anticentriole antibody who was successfully treated with vasodilators and immunosuppressive therapies. The presence of the anticentriole antibody is rare; however, it may be a useful biomarker that affects diagnostic and therapeutic strategies for SSc-PAH.

2. Case Presentation

A 62-year-old female presented with two-year exertional dyspnea. Her dyspnea progressively worsened and severe pitting edema of the lower extremities appeared, so she visited her previous doctor and took an electrocardiography which revealed right heart overload. Blood examination showed that the value of brain natriuretic peptide (BNP) was 537 pg/ml. Echocardiography revealed that the ejection fraction was 78.7%. Tricuspid regurgitation pressure gradient (TRPG) was elevated to 92 mmHg, and the right atrium, right ventricle, and inferior vena cava were enlarged. The cardiac catheter test revealed that the mean pulmonary arterial pressure (mPAP), pulmonary capillary wedge pressure, and pulmonary vascular resistance (PVR) levels were 54 mmHg, 8 mmHg, and 13.7 Wood, respectively. The pulmonary function test revealed the percent vital capacity (%VC), $FEV_{1.0}$%, and percent diffusing capacity of the lung for carbon monoxide (%DLCO) to be 117%, 82%, and 55%, respectively, thus suggesting the involvement of the lungs with impaired diffusion but not with restrictive and obstructive pulmonary disorder. Her chest X-ray and computer tomography did not reveal any pulmonary complications (Figure 1). She was diagnosed with group I PAH according to the Nice classification of PH. Serological analysis revealed antinuclear antibody (ANA) to be negative; however, the centriole pattern of staining was observed with high titers (1 : 640) using indirect immunofluorescence (Figure 2). Then, she was introduced to our hospital. The patient also manifested DUs, nailfold bleeding, telangiectasia (Figure 3), and Raynaud's phenomenon but no skin sclerosis when she visited us. She has never noticed her digital sclerosis. Based on the 2013 classification criteria for SSc by the American College of Rheumatology/European League against Rheumatism, the patient was subsequently diagnosed with SSc [16] (Table 1). She was initially treated with oral vasodilators and diuretics. Beraprost (120 μg/day) and riociguat (1.5 mg/day) as vasodilators were prescribed and azosemide (60 mg/day), spironolactone (25 mg/day), and tolvaptan (3.75 mg/day) as diuretics were also prescribed in order. As edema of the lower limbs worsened immediately after macitentan was started, its use was discontinued. Dyspnea was not completely improved with beraprost and riociguat. Although we considered continuous intravenous infusion of epoprostenol as an additional therapy, the patient refused because of issues concerning aesthetics and quality of life. Therefore, we discussed with cardiologists and

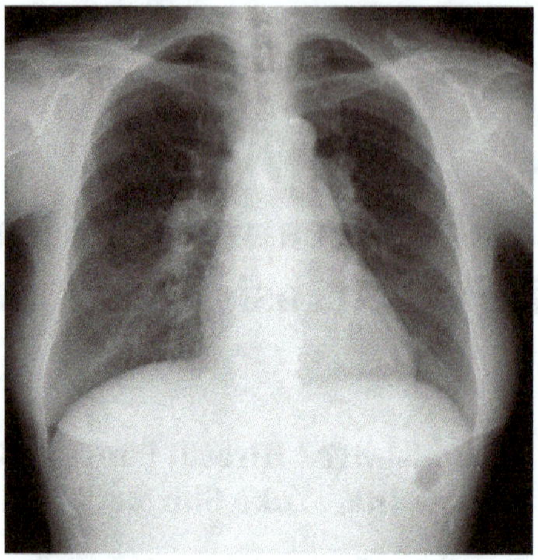

(a)

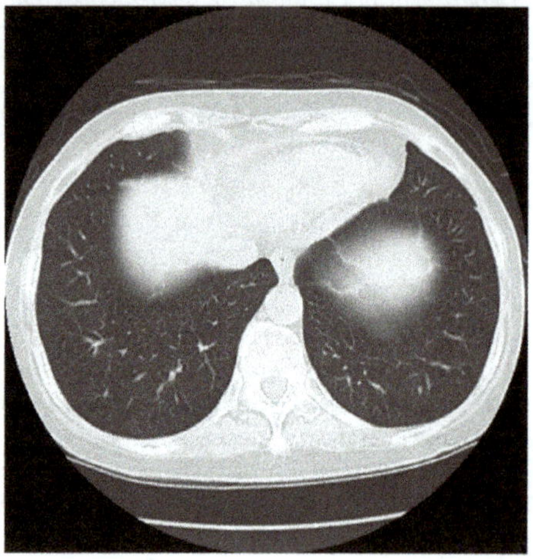

(b)

FIGURE 1: Chest X-ray and computed tomography examination performed.

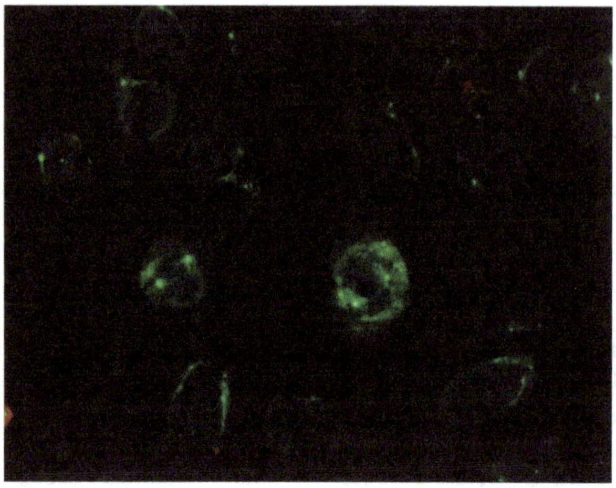

FIGURE 2: Anticentriole antibody in immunofluorescence examination (1 : 640).

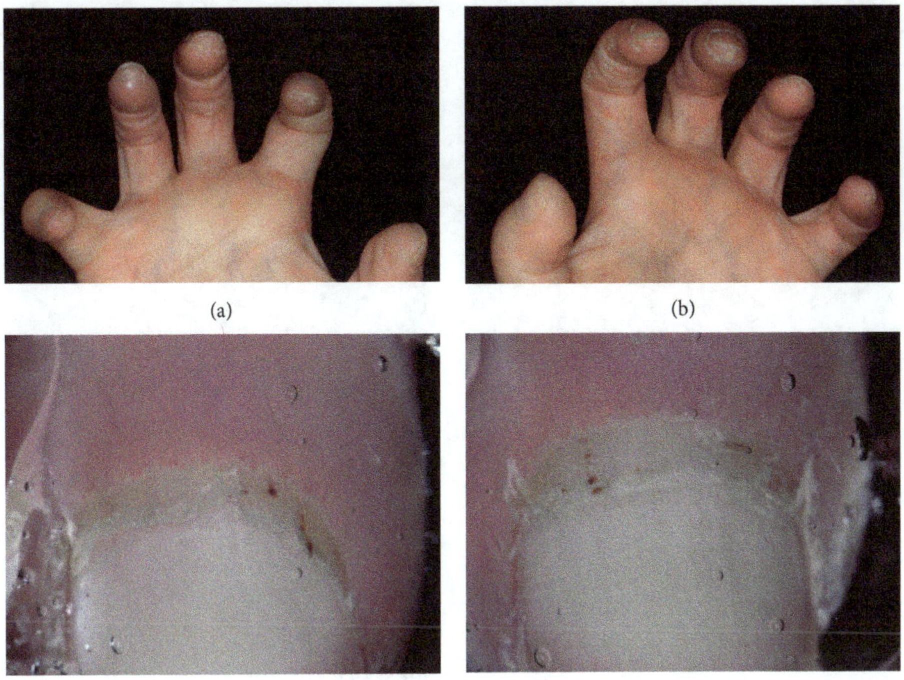

(a) (b) (c) (d)

FIGURE 3: Scar of the digital ulcer found and nailfold bleeding.

suggested the use of immunosuppressive therapy, which might be effective owing to the positivity of the anticentriole antibody, a unique immunological abnormality strongly associated with SSc-PAH. Moderate doses of prednisolone (PSL; 30 mg/day) and intravenous cyclophosphamide (IVCY; 500 mg every four weeks) were initiated. After two months, these immunosuppressive therapies and vasodilators improved mPAP from 47 to 33 mmHg, 6-minute walk distance (6MWD) from 418 to 480 m, and PVR from 8.7 to 6.0 Wood. Interestingly, the anticentriole antibody also disappeared and was not detected 16 months with a slight decrease of immunoglobulin G (IgG) after the treatment. After 10 times IVCY, azathioprine (50 mg/day) was started, and PSL was gradually decreased and maintained at 5 mg/day. To achieve further improvement, a new vasodilator selexipag was added and increased up to 2 mg/day in addition to riociguat (7.5 mg/day) and beraprost (360 mg/day). PAH has been well controlled using these treatments (Figure 4).

3. Discussion

PAH is one of the most severe complications of SSc. Approximately, 10% of all patients with SSc experience PAH [17]. The associated PAHs in SSc, systemic lupus erythematosus (SLE), mixed connective tissue disease (MCTD), and rheumatoid arthritis (RA) are 68%, 19%, 9%, and 5%, respectively [18]. Primary Sjögren syndrome (SS) has a very low prevalence of PAH [19]. SSc-PAH has a worse prognosis compared with other CTD-PAH, partially because the PAH of SLE, MCTD, SS, and RA were improved with the administration of immunosuppressive drugs (cyclophosphamide, prednisolone, azathioprine, and mycophenolate mofetil) [18–23]. Therefore, except for cases of progressive skin and pulmonary fibrosis, we generally do not use immunosuppressive therapies for patients with SSc [24].

Centrosome plays an important role in dividing cells with the mitotic spindle during cell cycle. It is usually located near the nucleus and moves to the bipolar of the cells after its replication during cell division. This means that the centrioles are one of the components of the centrosome located in the cytoplasm. We can detect the anticentriole antibody by the examination of antinuclear antibodies; however, it is not the antinuclear antibody but the anticytoplasmic antibody [25]. Centrosome is composed of centrioles and proteins termed the pericentriolar material (PCM) and is responsible for microtubule nucleation and anchoring [25]. Some centrosomal proteins have autoreactivities such as pericentriolar material 1 (PCM-1), pericentrin, ninein, and Cep250. Antibodies for those proteins were identified from autoimmune disease patients and postinfectious patients [26]. There is high prevalence of centrosome antibodies in SSc among autoimmune diseases [27]. Anticentriole antibody is one of anticentrosome antibodies. Connolly et al. first identified the antibody for centriole in nonimmune rabbit sera in 1978 [28]. Since 1980, several reports have been published regarding the anticentriole antibody. In these reports, the anticentriole antibody was indicated to be related to SSc [29–33]. Recently, Hamaguchi reported that 4 of 5 patients with the anticentriole antibody in SSc develop Raynaud's phenomenon and PAH [15]. Clinically, this autoantibody is not well recognized or elucidated as an SSc-specific antibody. Using previous PubMed reports, we investigated the characteristics of patients with positive

Table 1: Peripheral blood examination inday 20 after treatment.

Blood test (day 20)	
Urinalysis	
Specific gravity	1.021
pH	6
Protein	+
Blood	–
Nitrite	–
WBC	–
Bacteria	–
CBC	
WBC	5,000 mL
Neutrophil	3,000 mL
Eosinophil	0 mL
Basophil	0 mL
Lymphocyte	1,800 mL
Monocyte	200 mL
RBC	4.77×10^6 mL
Hb	13.5 g/dL
MCV	89.5 fl
Plt	212×10^3 mL
Coagulation	
PT	18.7 sec
PT-INR	2.34
APTT	52.9 sec
D-dimer	0.6 mg/mL
Infection	
T-SPOT	(–)
HBs Ab	(–)
HBs Ag	(–)
HCV Ab	(–)
Biochemistry	
T-bil	1.6 mg/dL
D-bil	0.1 mg/dL
ALP	72 U/L
γ – GTP	33 U/L
AST	35 U/L
ALT	34 U/L
LDH	297 U/L
BUN	10 mg/dL
Cre	0.55 mg/dL
UA	4.4 mg/dL
TP	6.4 g/dL
Alb	4 g/dL
Pre-Alb	15 mg/dL
Na	142 mEq/L
K	3.7 mEq/L
Cl	107 mEq/L
Ca	8.4 mg/dL
IP	3.6 mg/dL
TG	101 mg/dL
TC	122 mg/dL
LDL-C	69 mg/dL
CPK	112 U/L
CK-MB	21 U/L
Glucose	98 mg/dL
Hb-A1c (NGSP)	6.2%
CRP	0.07 mg/dL
Hp	≦3.0 mg/dL
Ferritin	69.8 ng/mL
Endocrine	
FT4	1.17 ng/dL
TSH	6.33 mgIU/mL
FT3	2.69 pg/mL
BNP	432.1 pg/mL
Immune system	
IgG	1001 mg/dL
IgA	228 mg/dL
IgM	94 mg/dL
ANA	≦40
C3	90 mg/dL
C4	21.8 mg/dL
CH50	46.9 U/mL
Anti-dsDNA Ab	≦10I U/mL
Anti-RNP Ab	≦5.0 U/mL
Anti-Sm Ab	≦5.0 U/mL
Anti-SS-A/Ro Ab	≦5.0 U/mL
Anti-SS-B/La Ab	≦5.0 U/mL
Anti-Scl 70 Ab	≦5.0 U/mL
Anti-centromere Ab	≦5.0 U/mL
Anti-CL.β2GPI Ab	≦1.3 U/mL
Anti-CALG Ab	≦1.0 U/mL
LAC	≦1.0 U/mL
PR3-ANCA	≦1.0I U/mL
MPO-ANCA	≦1.0 U/mL
RF	≦5.0 U/mL
Anti-CCP Ab	≦0.5 U/mL
Anti-ARS Ab	10 U/mL
Anti-RNA polymerase III Ab	15.2

anticentriole antibody. Although some data were unavailable, we found 16 cases of patients with anticentriole antibody between 1982 and 2015. Based on those reports, 11 of 11 (100%) patients were female. Reynaud phenomenon, DU, and PAH were observed at high rates in 100% (14 of 14), 86% (6 of 7), and 71% (5 of 7) of cases, respectively. The anticentriole antibody was reported to be associated with SSc and 4 of 15 patients (27%) did not show any cutaneous sclerosis (Table 2) [15, 30–32, 34–37]. This ratio of patients without skin sclerosis (27%) was higher than that of all patients with SSc, because only 5%–9% of SSc were classified as SSc sine sclerosis [38–40]. In addition, the anticentriole antibody is not detected as ANA; hence, such patients without clear skin sclerosis may be missed and diagnosed with "idiopathic PAH." When an ANA-negative patient presents with DUs, Raynaud phenomenon, and/or PAH, the original image of immunofluorescence of ANA staining should be reconsidered for the presence of anticentriole antibody.

To the best of our knowledge, this is the first report of an SSc-PAH patient with anticentriole antibody, who was successfully treated. In this case, the hemodynamics of PAH were further improved and stably maintained after the induction of immunosuppressive therapies. The positivity of the anticentriole antibody in SSc is extremely highly associated with PAH among other SSc-associated autoantibodies [15]. Immunosuppressive therapies decreased the titer of the anticentriole antibody. These results indicate that the pathogenesis of SSc-PAH with the anticentriole antibody may be immune-mediated. Thus, the anticentriole antibody could be a useful biomarker to identify a subpopulation of patients with SSc-PAH.

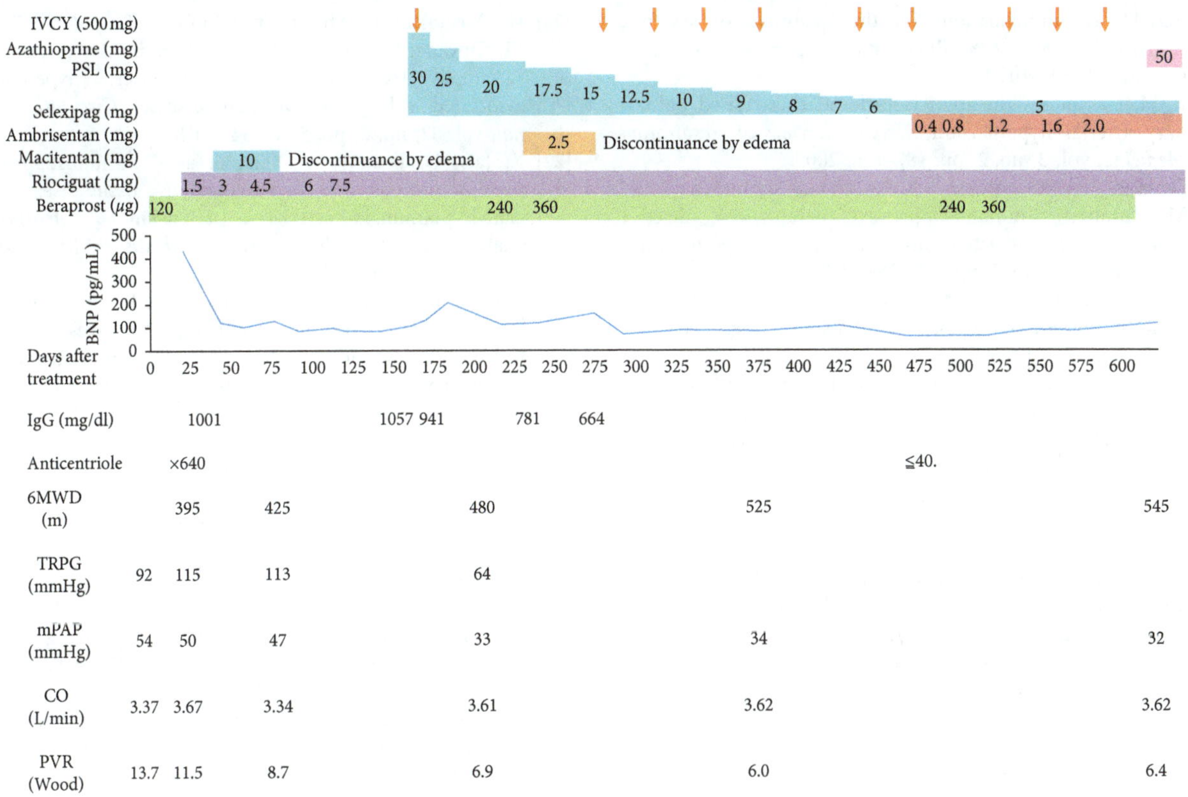

Figure 4: Clinical course.

Table 2: Data about anticentriole antibody positive patients from previous reports Ref [15, 30–32, 34–37].

	The feature of anticentriole antibody positive cases from previous reports			
Total 16 cases n (%)	Positive	Negative	Not described	$P/P+N$ (%)
Sex (female)	11 (69)	0 (0)	5 (31)	100
Raynaud's phenomenon	14 (88)	0 (0)	2 (12)	100
Digital sclerosis	9 (56)	4 (25)	3 (19)	69
Systemic sclerosis	4 (25)	9 (56)	3 (19)	31
Digital ulcer	6 (38)	1 (6)	9 (56)	86
Interstitial pneumonia	4 (25)	6 (38)	6 (38)	40
Reflux esophagitis	5 (31)	6 (38)	5 (31)	45
Telangiectasia	5 (31)	5 (31)	6 (38)	50
Renal crisis	0 (0)	8 (50)	8 (50)	0
Pulmonary hypertension	5 (31)	2 (12)	9 (56)	71

In mitotic phase, centrioles at poles of mitotic spindles were stained like 2 dots.

Anticentriole antibody was detected in 1 : 640 by a commercial examination. The staining disappeared completely after the treatment (no data shown).

Abbreviations

IVCY: Intravenous cyclophosphamide
PSL: Prednisolone
BNP: Brain natriuretic peptide
IgG: Immunoglobulin G
Ab: Antibody
6MWD: 6-minute walk distance
TRPG: Transtricuspid pressure gradient
mPAP: Mean pulmonary arterial pressure
CO: Cardiac output
PVR: Pulmonary vascular resistance.

Acknowledgments

The authors thank the staff of the Department of Hematology and Rheumatology, Tohoku University, for helpful discussion.

References

[1] Y. Allanore, R. Simms, O. Distler et al., "Systemic sclerosis," *Nature Reviews Disease Primers*, vol. 1, p. 15002, 2015.

[2] C. P. Denton and D. Khanna, "Systemic sclerosis," *The Lancet*, vol. 390, no. 10103, pp. 1685–1699, 2017.

[3] O. Kowal-Bielecka, J. Fransen, J. Avouac et al., "Update of

EULAR recommendations for the treatment of systemic sclerosis," *Annals of the Rheumatic Diseases*, vol. 76, no. 8, pp. 1327–1339, 2017.

[4] P. M. Hassoun, "Therapies for scleroderma-related pulmonary arterial hypertension," *Expert Review of Respiratory Medicine*, vol. 3, no. 2, pp. 187–196, 2009.

[5] O. Sanchez, O. Sitbon, X. Jaïs, G. Simonneau, and M. Humbert, "Immunosuppressive therapy in connective tissue diseases-associated pulmonary arterial hypertension," *Chest*, vol. 130, no. 1, pp. 182–189, 2006.

[6] N. F. Chaisson and P. M. Hassoun, "Systemic sclerosis-associated pulmonary arterial hypertension," *Chest*, vol. 144, no. 4, pp. 1346–1356, 2013.

[7] USNLo Medicine, "Rituximab for treatment of systemic sclerosis-associated pulmonary arterial hypertension (SSc-PAH)," 2019, https://ClinicalTrials.gov/show/NCT01086540.

[8] USNLo Medicine, "A therapeutic open label study of tocilizumab in the treatment of pulmonary arterial hypertension (TRANSFORM-UK)," 2018, https://clinicaltrials.gov/show/NCT02676947.

[9] USNLo Medicine, "Dimethyl fumarate (DMF) in systemic sclerosis-associated pulmonary arterial hypertension," 2019, https://ClinicalTrials.gov/show/NCT02981082.

[10] E. Sugawara, M. Kato, T. Sato et al., "Diversity of borderline pulmonary arterial pressure associated with systemic sclerosis: 3 case series," *Modern Rheumatology Case Reports*, vol. 1, no. 1, pp. 9–14, 2017.

[11] Y. Furuya, T. Satoh, and M. Kuwana, "Interleukin-6 as a potential therapeutic target for pulmonary arterial hypertension," *International Journal of Rheumatology*, vol. 2010, Article ID 720305, 8 pages, 2010.

[12] Y. Hamaguchi, "Autoantibody profiles in systemic sclerosis: predictive value for clinical evaluation and prognosis," *The Journal of Dermatology*, vol. 37, no. 1, pp. 42–53, 2010.

[13] R. T. Domsic, "Scleroderma," *Current Opinion in Rheumatology*, vol. 26, no. 6, pp. 646–652, 2014.

[14] C. Liaskos, E. Marou, T. Simopoulou et al., "Disease-related autoantibody profile in patients with systemic sclerosis," *Autoimmunity*, vol. 50, no. 7, pp. 414–421, 2017.

[15] Y. Hamaguchi, T. Matsushita, M. Hasegawa et al., "High incidence of pulmonary arterial hypertension in systemic sclerosis patients with anti-centriole autoantibodies," *Modern Rheumatology*, vol. 25, no. 5, pp. 798–801, 2015.

[16] F. van den Hoogen, D. Khanna, J. Fransen et al., "2013 classification criteria for systemic sclerosis: an American college of rheumatology/European league against rheumatism collaborative initiative," *Annals of the Rheumatic Diseases*, vol. 72, no. 11, pp. 1747–1755, 2013.

[17] R. Condliffe and L. S. Howard, "Connective tissue disease-associated pulmonary arterial hypertension," *F1000Prime Reports*, vol. 7, no. 6, 2015.

[18] L. Chung, J. Liu, L. Parsons et al., "Characterization of connective tissue disease-associated pulmonary arterial hypertension from Reveal," *Chest*, vol. 138, no. 6, pp. 1383–1394, 2010.

[19] D. Launay, E. Hachulla, P.-Y. Hatron, X. Jais, G. Simonneau, and M. Humbert, "Pulmonary arterial hypertension: a rare complication of primary Sjögren syndrome," *Medicine*, vol. 86, no. 5, pp. 299–315, 2007.

[20] J. Zhao, Q. Wang, Y. Liu et al., "Clinical characteristics and survival of pulmonary arterial hypertension associated with three major connective tissue diseases: a cohort study in China," *International Journal of Cardiology*, vol. 236, pp. 432–437, 2017.

[21] H. Yasuoka, Y. Shirai, Y. Tamura, T. Takeuchi, and M. Kuwana, "Predictors of favorable responses to immunosuppressive treatment in pulmonary arterial hypertension associated with connective tissue disease," *Circulation Journal*, vol. 82, no. 2, pp. 546–554, 2018.

[22] X. Jais, D. Launay, A. Yaici et al., "Immunosuppressive therapy in lupus- and mixed connective tissue disease-associated pulmonary arterial hypertension: a retrospective analysis of twenty-three cases," *Arthritis & Rheumatism*, vol. 58, no. 2, pp. 521–531, 2008.

[23] S. Miyamichi-Yamamoto, Y. Fukumoto, K. Sugimura et al., "Intensive immunosuppressive therapy improves pulmonary hemodynamics and long-term prognosis in patients with pulmonary arterial hypertension associated with connective tissue disease," *Circulation Journal*, vol. 75, no. 11, pp. 2688–2674, 2011.

[24] J. Konma, T. Kotani, T. Shoda et al., "Efficacy and safety of combination therapy with prednisolone and oral tacrolimus for progressive interstitial pneumonia with systemic sclerosis: a retrospective study," *Modern Rheumatology*, vol. 28, no. 6, pp. 1009–1015, 2018.

[25] C. L. Rieder, S. Faruki, and A. Khodjakov, "The centrosome in vertebrates: more than a microtubule-organizing center," *Trends in Cell Biology*, vol. 11, no. 10, pp. 413–419, 2001.

[26] G. J. Mack, J. Rees, O. Sandblom, R. Balczon, M. J. Fritzler, and J. B. Rattner, "Autoantibodies to a group of centrosomal proteins in human autoimmune sera reactive with the centrosome," *Arthritis & Rheumatism*, vol. 41, no. 3, pp. 551–558, 1998.

[27] I. Gavanescu, D. Vazquez-Abad, J. McCauley, J.-L. Senecal, and S. Doxsey, "Centrosome proteins: a major class of autoantigens in scleroderma," *Journal of Clinical Immunology*, vol. 19, no. 3, pp. 166–171, 1999.

[28] J. A. Connolly and V. I. Kalnins, "Visualization of centrioles and basal bodies by fluorescent staining with nonimmune rabbit sera," *The Journal of Cell Biology*, vol. 79, no. 2, pp. 526–532, 1978.

[29] S. Brenner, S. Pepper, and S. Berns, "Autoantibodies in human serum selectivity bind to the centriole region in cultured cells," *Journal of Cell Biology*, vol. 87, p. 240, 1980.

[30] T. G. Osborn, N. J. Patel, S. C. Ross, and N. E. Bauer, "Antinuclear antibody staining only centrioles in a patient with scleroderma," *New England Journal of Medicine*, vol. 307, no. 4, pp. 253-254, 1982.

[31] D. L. Tuffanelli, F. McKeon, D. M. Kleinsmith, T. K. Burnham, and M. Kirschner, "Anticentromere and anticentriole antibodies in the scleroderma spectrum," *Archives of Dermatology*, vol. 119, no. 7, pp. 560–566, 1983.

[32] Y. Moroi, I. Murata, A. Takeuchi, N. Kamatani, K. Tanimoto, and R. Yokohari, "Human anticentriole autoantibody in patients with scleroderma and Raynaud's phenomenon," *Clinical Immunology and Immunopathology*, vol. 29, no. 3, pp. 381–390, 1983.

[33] J. B. Rattner, L. Martin, D. M. Waisman, S. A. Johnstone, and M. J. Fritzler, "Autoantibodies to the centrosome (centriole) react with determinants present in the glycolytic enzyme enolase," *Journal of Immunology*, vol. 146, no. 7, pp. 2341–2344, 1991.

[34] D. Tuffanelli, "Persistant anti-kinetochore (centromere) and anti-centriole antibodies in scleroderma and Raynaud's disease," *Clinical Research Journal*, vol. 30, no. 2, p. 612A, 1982.

[35] I. Hayakawa, S. Sato, M. Hasegawa, T. Echigo, and K. Takehara, "A case of scleroderma spectrum disorder with anticentriole antibody and pulmonary hypertension," *Clinical Rheumatology*, vol. 23, no. 3, pp. 266–268, 2004.

[36] S. Sato, M. Fujimoto, H. Ihn, and K. Takehara, "Antibodies to centromere and centriole in scleroderma spectrum disorders," *Dermatology*, vol. 189, no. 1, pp. 23–26, 1994.

[37] T. G. Osborn, J. S. Ryerse, N. E. Bauer, J. M. Urhahn, D. Blair, and T. L. Moore, "Anticentriole antibody in a patient with progressive systemic sclerosis," *Arthritis & Rheumatism*, vol. 29, no. 1, pp. 142–146, 1986.

[38] M. Hinchcliff and J. Varga, "Systemic sclerosis/scleroderma: a treatable multisystem disease," *American Family Physician*, vol. 78, no. 8, pp. 961–968, 2008.

[39] R. G. Marangoni, L. F. Rocha, A. P. T. Del Rio, N. H. Yoshinari, J. F. Marques-Neto, and P. D. Sampaio-Barros, "Systemic sclerosis sine scleroderma: distinct features in a large Brazilian cohort," *Rheumatology*, vol. 52, no. 8, pp. 1520–1524, 2013.

[40] H. Poormoghim, M. Lucas, N. Fertig, and T. A. Medsger Jr., "Systemic sclerosis sine scleroderma: demographic, clinical, and serologic features and survival in forty-eight patients," *Arthritis & Rheumatism*, vol. 43, no. 2, pp. 444–451, 2000.

4

Granulomatosis with Polyangiitis Overlapping with IgG4-Related Disease

Aureliano Pistone and Muhammad Soyfoo

Department of Rheumatology, Cliniques Universitaires de Bruxelles – Hôpital Erasme, Université Libre de Bruxelles (ULB), Bruxelles, Belgium

Correspondence should be addressed to Muhammad Soyfoo; msoyfoo@ulb.ac.be

Academic Editor: James V. Dunne

IgG4-related disease and granulomatosis with polyangiitis share several features as well as the presence of ANCA antibodies and serum IgG4 immunoglobulins. It is often difficult to distinguish between two entities. We hereby report the case of a patient portraying the clinical conundrum with clinical and biological features of the two diseases.

1. Introduction

Granulomatosis with polyangiitis (GPA), previously known as Wegener's granulomatosis is an ANCA-associated vasculitis mainly involving the lungs and kidneys [1, 2]. This disease involves small to medium size blood vessels (more frequently small-sized vessels) with a reported annual incidence of 0.4 to 11.9 cases per million. GPA can affect people from all ethnic origins with predominance for white populations. The male to female ratio is 1 : 1. The cause of GPA is still not known. Although almost every small vessel can be affected by GPA, the upper and lower respiratory system and the kidneys are frequently involved. The disease can present as a continuous spectrum of clinical manifestations ranging from mild to severe organ-threatening conditions jeopardizing the lives of patients. One of the hallmarks of GPA is the presence of the antineutrophil cytoplasmic antibody (ANCA) in nearly 90% of cases, and up to 75% of cases are associated with PR3 (proteinase 3) ANCA [3]. Tailored and adapted targeted therapy is cardinal to decrease the burden of disease while increasing survival [4, 5].

IgG4-related disease (IgG4-RD) is an immune-mediated inflammatory disorder affecting several organs with a wide spectrum of clinical manifestations. The affected organs share several clinical and biological characteristics such as tumor-swelling like of organs, lymphoproliferative infiltration, and a certain extent of fibrosis described as "storiform fibrosis." The pathological hallmark of IgG4-RD is lymphoplasmacytic infiltrates containing IgG4+ plasma cells of the affected tissues [2, 6]. Serum IgG4 levels increased in more than two-thirds of patients. The two main manifestations of this disease are autoimmune pancreatitis and sclerosing sialadenitis, but other organs can be affected. Cholangitis, dacryoadenitis, retro-peritoneal fibrosis, mediastinal fibrosis, tubulointerstitial nephritis, hepatitis interstitial pneumonia, thyroiditis, prostatitis, and gastritis have also been reported [7]. This disease generally responds well to glucocorticoids and immunosuppressants and more specifically in the absence of significant fibrosis [8].

Because of several similar clinical signs and the presence of ANCA antibodies and serum IgG4 immunoglobulins, differentiating IgG4-RD from GPA is not always easy. Furthermore, increased serum concentration of IgG4 has been observed in GPA as well as the presence of infiltration of IgG4 positive cells in tissues in patients with GPA. Currently, the existence of an overlap between the two diseases is not clearly certified [9–12]. We hereby present a case illustrating this situation.

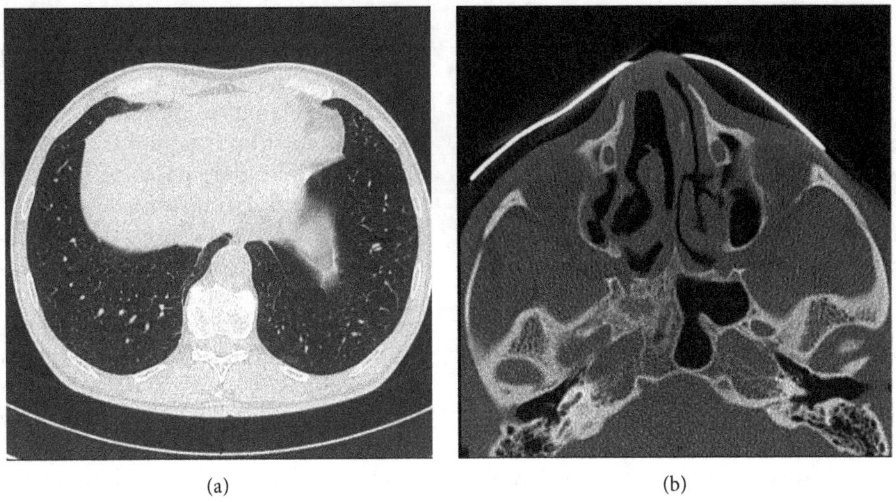

(a) (b)

FIGURE 1: Computed tomography of lungs showing several micronodules (a) and that of sinus showing pansinusitis (b).

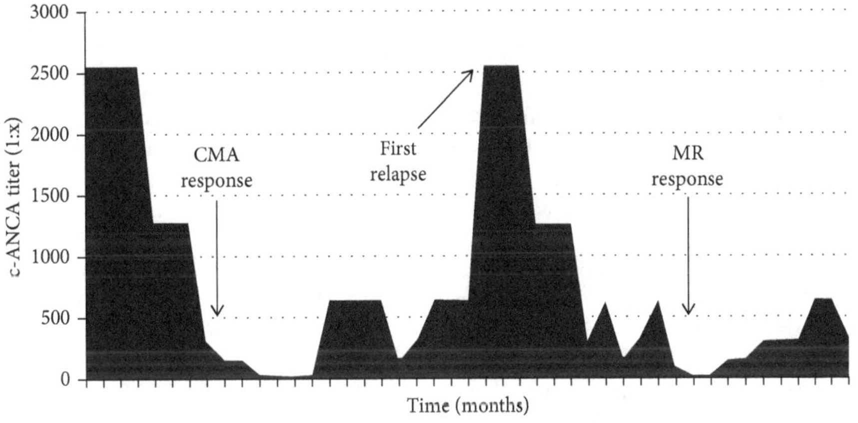

FIGURE 2: Evolution of c-ANCA titers over time. CMA: cyclophosphamide and methylprednisolone-based treatment followed by azathioprine. MR: methylprednisolone and rituximab-based treatment. This figure represents the evolution of c-ANCA titers over time. Peaks correspond to episodes of clinical relapses, and the falls correspond to improvements after treatment.

2. Case Presentation

A 60-year-old patient was admitted to our hospital because of inflammatory syndrome, polyarthralgia, and weight loss. A physical examination showed only pain in the heels and the first metatarsophalangeal joint as well as hypoesthesia of the left foot. The significant biological results showed nonidentified c-ANCA (non-PR3 and non-MPO) with a titer of 1 : 2560 as well as a C-reactive protein of 99 mg/L, and an erythrocyte sedimentation rate of 67 mm/h. The renal function was in the normal range values. The thoracic computed tomography (CT) scan showed several bilateral nonspecific micronodules (Figure 1(a)), and the positron emission tomography computed tomography (PET-CT) scan showed moderately hypermetabolic retroperitoneal and inguinal lymphadenopathy. A sinus CT scan was performed and showed pansinusitis (Figure 1(b)). A biopsy of inguinal adenopathy was performed in favour of reactive inflammatory nodes with no signs of malignancy. The tuberculosis QuantiFERON ELISA test was positive, but the culture and polymerase chain reaction of the biopsied node were negative. The patient later developed arthritis in the ankle confirmed by IRM, and sinus CT confirmed the presence of pansinusitis. The diagnosis of GPA was made on the basis of high c-ANCA titers (non-PR3 and non-MPO), bilateral pulmonary nodules, and pansinusitis, and treatment with cyclophosphamide and methylprednisolone was administered, followed by azathioprine. This treatment was combined with isoniazid for tuberculosis prophylaxis. The patient presented a good clinical evolution with normalisation of the inflammatory syndrome and a significant decrease in c-ANCA (Figure 2). Five years later, the patient's clinical condition deteriorated with asthenia, weight loss, and abdominal pain. There was an increased inflammatory syndrome as well as increased ANCA titers (variation of titers is shown in Figure 2). The PET-CT scan was not in favour of a vasculitis relapse. The node biopsy performed five years ago was retrospectively reviewed for evaluation of IgG4. The histology of the lymph node was described as an inflammatory node with extensive plasmacytosis as depicted with CD138 immunostaining. The infiltrate showed 50 IgG4 positive plasma cells per high-power field. A serum IgG4 assay was performed and very slightly increased at 1.351 g/L ($N < 1.350$). The abdominal CT image did not show retroperitoneal fibrosis despite the presence of bilateral uretero-hydronephrosis without objectified obstacle. A possible diagnosis of IgG4-related disease (IgG4-RD) was then carried out, but GPA diagnosis was not completely excluded. The patient was treated by intravenous methylprednisolone and rituximab with a good clinical and biological evolution. Three years later, he developed another relapse with distal digital ischemia of the foot, multiplex mononeuritis, and external popliteal sciatica deficit, rather in favour of GPA with a BVAS score of 6 (Birmingham Vasculitis Activity Score). Afterwards, the patient was treated only with mycophenolate mofetil (2 g/day) without any relapse.

3. Discussion

GPA and IgG4-RD are today two better known diseases. GPA is an ANCA-associated vasculitis that can be defined by the 1990 ACR criteria and the 2012 Chapel Hill Consensus Conference. Recently, an Iranian team proposed a new algorithm called 2017 ACR/EMA Revised Criteria for Very Early Diagnosis of GPA [13].

IgG4-RD diagnosis can be based on the CDC according to the presence of organ involvement, the presence of IgG4/IgG ratio >40% abd the presence of high power fieds immunostaining for IgG4 more than 10. The diagnosis can be established as either possible, probable or definite [14]. Recently, Wallace et al. proposed the 2019 American College of Rheumatology (ACR)/European League against Rheumatism Classification Criteria for IgG4-Related Disease, which is not yet used in clinical practice [15].

Currently, the existence of an overlap between the two diseases is not clearly certified. Some authors believe that this association is possible and represent as such a particular phenotype. Organ involvement occurring in AAV patients could be related to IgG4-RD rather than to refractory granulomatous lesions, especially in GPA patients [9]. In this latter study, the authors identified some patients depicting clinical and/or histological clues pertaining to both diseases thereby raising the question of a potential overlap syndrome sharing common pathophysiological characteristics. We found only one case report of the patient suffering from GPA, IgG4-RD, and a small cell lung cancer [2].

On the other hand, there is even a case report of GPA mimicking IgG4-RD [16]. It is important to note that GPA biopsy can mimic IgG4-RD portrayed by inflammatory background [17]. It was demonstrated that IgG1 and IgG4 were the predominant subclasses of ANCA in patients with GPA. [18] In 2013, Chang et al. showed that 8/43 GPA patients had IgG4+ biopsy with the IgG4+ cells criteria (average IgG4+ cells greater than 30 per HPF with the ratio of IgG4+/IgG+ cells greater than 40%). However, all patients had histological characteristics of GPA like necrosis, necrotizing granulomas, abscesses, and vasculitis [19].

The association of GPA and IgG4-RD as a potential overlap syndrome with common pathophysiological mechanisms responsible for clinical and biological manifestations is therefore probable. However, both diseases have complex and still yet undeciphered pathological pathways. The link between the pathological role of ANCA and IgG4 in purporting damage in both diseases is still unknown. Certain lines of evidence underscore the role of *T* follicular helper cells that have increased in both diseases [9].

Our patient illustrates the difficulty to differentiate between these two diseases. In fact, the patient presented the characteristics of the two diseases. The presence of c-ANCA with pulmonary micronodules, pansinusitis, multiplex mononeuritis, and a decrease in ANCA with treatment is in favour of GPA. In 2009, the diagnosis was made following the consensus methodology for the classification of ANCA-associated vasculitis despite the presence of nonidentified c-ANCA [20]. Besides, cases of GPA with nonidentified ANCA were described in the literature [21]. However, the lymphadenopathy associated with a high level of IgG4 and node biopsy positive for IgG4 positive plasma cells are compatible with IgG4-RD. But we could not affirm the diagnosis of IgG4-RD if we apply the 2019 ACR criteria [15]. It is therefore difficult to confirm whether the patient has an overlap between GPA and IgG4-RD or GPA mimicking IgG4-RD.

4. Conclusion

This case illustrates well the possible coexistence of characteristics of ANCA vasculitis and IgG4-RD, as well as the difficulty to differentiate between the two diseases and above all, to affirm the presence of an overlap syndrome.

Authors' Contributions

Pistone A was responsible for data collection and writing of the case report. Soyfoo M. S was responsible for editing, revising, and reviewing the case report.

References

[1] Z. X. Yunt, S. K. Frankel, and K. K. Brown, "Diagnosis and management of pulmonary vasculitis," *Therupatic Advances in Respiratory Disease*, vol. 6, no. 6, pp. 375–390, 2012.

[2] K. Abbass and H. Krug, "Granulomatosis with polyangiitis in a patient with biopsy-proven IgG4-related pulmonary disease and coincident small cell lung cancer," *BMJ Case Reports*, vol. 12, no. 3, Article ID e226280, 2019.

[3] J. Savige, D. Davies, R. J. Falk, J. C. Jennette, and A. Wiik, "Antineutrophil cytoplasmic antibodies and associated diseases: a review of the clinical and laboratory features," *Kidney International*, vol. 57, no. 3, pp. 846–862, 2000.

[4] O. Flossmann, A. Berden, K. de Groot et al., "Long-term patient survival in ANCA-associated vasculitis," *Annals of the Rheumatic Diseases*, vol. 70, no. 3, pp. 488–494, 2011.

[5] M. Yates, R. A. Watts, I. M. Bajema et al., "EULAR/ERA-EDTA recommendations for the management of ANCA-associated vasculitis," *Annals of the Rheumatic Diseases*, vol. 75, no. 9, pp. 1583–1594, 2016.

[6] W. Cheuk and J. K. C. Chan, "IgG4-related sclerosing disease:

a critical appraisal of an evolving clinicopathologic entity," *Advances in Anatomic Pathology*, vol. 17, no. 5, pp. 303–332, 2010.

[7] T. Saeki, S. Nishi, N. Imai et al., "Clinicopathological characteristics of patients with IgG4-related tubulointerstitial nephritis," *Kidney International*, vol. 78, no. 10, pp. 1016–1023, 2010.

[8] A. Khosroshahi and J. H. Stone, "Treatment approaches to IgG4-related systemic disease," *Current Opinion in Rheumatology*, vol. 23, no. 1, pp. 67–71, 2011.

[9] F.-X. Danlos, G. M. Rossi, D. Blockmans et al., "Anti-neutrophil cytoplasmic antibody-associated vasculitides and IgG4-related disease: a new overlap syndrome," *Autoimmunity Reviews*, vol. 16, no. 10, pp. 1036–1043, 2017.

[10] E. Della-Torre, M. Lanzillotta, C. Campochiaro et al., "Antineutrophil cytoplasmic antibody positivity in IgG4-related disease: a case report and review of the literature," *Medicine (Baltimore)*, vol. 95, no. 34, Article ID e4633, 2016.

[11] A. Erden, E. C. Bolek, K. G. Yardimci, L. Kilic, S. A. Bilgen, and O. Karadag, "Do ANCA-associated vasculitides and IgG4-related disease really overlap or not?" *International Journal of Rheumatic Diseases*, vol. 22, no. 10, pp. 1926–1932, 2019.

[12] L. Dudley, L. Brown, J. Pettus, C. Black, and N. Orzechowski, "The association of granulomatosis with polyangiitis and IgG4-related disease: a case series," *La Presse Médicale*, vol. 42, no. 4, pp. 706-707, 2013.

[13] I. Salehi Abari, "ACR/EMA revised criteria for too early diagnosis of granulomatosis with polyangiitis (GPA)," *Autoimmune Diseases Therupatic Approaches Open Access*, vol. 33, 2017.

[14] H. Umehara, K. Okazaki, Y. Masaki et al., "Comprehensive diagnostic criteria for IgG4-related disease (IgG4-RD), 2011," *Modern Rheumatology*, vol. 22, no. 1, pp. 21–30, 2012.

[15] Z. S. Wallace, R. P. Naden, S. Chari et al., "The 2019 American College of Rheumatology/European League against rheumatism classification criteria for IgG4-related disease," *Arthritis Rheumatology*, vol. 72, no. 1, pp. 7–19, 2020.

[16] P. Kaushik, J. H. Stone, J. T. Anderson et al., "Medical mirroring: granulomatosis with polyangiitis (formerly Wegener's) mimicking immunoglobulin-G4 related disease," *International Journal of Rheumatic Diseases*, vol. 21, no. 4, pp. 885–889, 2018.

[17] J. Yoo, S. S. Ahn, S. M. Jung, J. J. Song, Y. B. Park, and S. W. Lee, "No overlap between IgG4-related disease and microscopic polyangiitis and granulomatosis with polyangiitis despite elevated serum IgG4 at diagnosis: a retrospective monocentric study," *Clinical Rheumatology*, vol. 38, no. 4, pp. 1147–1154, 2019.

[18] E. Brouwer, J. W. C. Tervaert, G. Horst et al., "Predominance of IgGl and IgG4 subclasses of anti-neutrophil cytoplasmic autoantibodies (ANCA) in patients with Wegener's granulomatosis and clinically related disorders," *Clinical and Experimental Immunology*, vol. 83, no. 3, pp. 379–386, 2008.

[19] S. Y. Chang, K. A. Keogh, J. E. Lewis et al., "IgG4-positive plasma cells in granulomatosis with polyangiitis (Wegener's): a clinicopathologic and immunohistochemical study on 43 granulomatosis with polyangiitis and 20 control cases," *Human Pathology*, vol. 44, no. 11, pp. 2432–2437, 2013.

[20] R. Watts, S. Lane, T. Hanslik et al., "Development and validation of a consensus methodology for the classification of the ANCA-associated vasculitides and polyarteritis nodosa for epidemiological studies," *Annals of the Rheumatic Diseases*, vol. 66, no. 2, pp. 222–227, 2006.

[21] M. Givaudan, F. Vandergheynst, P. Stordeur et al., "Value of non-identified ANCA (non-PR3, non-MPO) in the diagnosis of granulomatosis with polyangiitis (Wegener's granulomatosis)," *Acta Clinica Belgica*, vol. 72, no. 5, pp. 313–317, 2017.

5

Nephrotic Syndrome as an Extramuscular Manifestation of Anti-EJ Antibody-Positive Dermatomyositis: A Case Report and Review of the Literature

Syoko Tsubouchi, Takahiro Mizuuchi, Yusuke Yamamoto, Daiki Fujimori, Kayo Ishii, Mayu Tago, Eri Kato, Hiroaki Mori, Haeru Hayashi, Koichiro Tahara, and Tetsuji Sawada

Department of Rheumatology, Tokyo Medical University Hospital, Shinjuku, Tokyo, Japan

Correspondence should be addressed to Tetsuji Sawada; tsawada@tokyo-med.ac.jp

Academic Editor: Gregory J. Tsay

Renal involvement is underestimated as an extramuscular manifestation of dermatomyositis (DM). Here, we describe a 67-year-old woman with anti-glycyl-transfer ribonucleic acid synthetase (anti-EJ) antibody and anti-ribonucleoprotein antibody-positive DM complicated by systemic sclerosis, who developed nephrotic syndrome concurrently with the exacerbation of DM, as indicated by incremental serum creatine kinase levels, high-intensity lesions on muscle magnetic resonance imaging, and active interstitial pneumonitis on chest computed tomography. Renal biopsy revealed the presence of immune-deposition in the glomerulus by immunofluorescence. To our knowledge, this is the first report describing the coexistence of anti-EJ antibody-positive DM and nephrotic syndrome. More reports of similar cases are warranted to substantiate the association.

1. Introduction

Polymyositis (PM) and dermatomyositis (DM) are two main types of autoimmune inflammatory muscle disease and are clinically characterized by symmetrical weakness and myalgia of proximal muscles with elevated serum levels of muscle enzymes [1]. DM is characterized by distinctive skin manifestations, including Gottron's sign, Gottron's papules, heliotrope rash, and mechanic's hands. Autoimmune abnormalities manifest as the presence of autoantibodies, which can be categorized into myositis-associated and myositis-specific autoantibodies. Anti-aminoacyl-transfer ribonucleic acid (tRNA) synthetase antibodies (anti-ARS Abs) are classified as myositis-specific autoantibodies and are detected in PM and DM patients presenting with myositis, non-erosive polyarthritis, Raynaud's phenomenon, mechanic's hands, and interstitial pneumonitis, designated as anti-synthetase syndrome (ASS) [2]. The characteristics of each anti-ARS Ab vary slightly in terms of incidence and the clinical course of interstitial lung disease, skin rashes, myopathies, and arthritis [3, 4]. Anti-glycyl tRNA synthetase antibodies (anti-EJ Abs) are the second most prevalent anti-ARS Ab in Japan after anti-Jo1 Ab, accounting for approximately a quarter of ASS cases, and are associated with classic DM with a high frequency of interstitial lung disease (ILD) [4].

Renal involvement, which is frequently observed in patients with systemic autoimmune diseases such as systemic lupus erythematosus (SLE), has been considered rare in PM and DM. However, case reports describing the simultaneous occurrence of PM or DM and renal diseases have been reported in the literature [5]. Two main types of renal involvement exist in patients with PM or DM: rhabdomyolysis-induced acute tubular necrosis with deterioration of renal function and chronic glomerulonephritis [6]. In the latter, mesangial proliferative glomerulonephritis is the leading histological type in PM, while membranous nephropathy appears to prevail in DM [6]. Herein, we describe the case of a woman who developed nephrotic syndrome concurrently with the exacerbation of anti-EJ Ab-positive

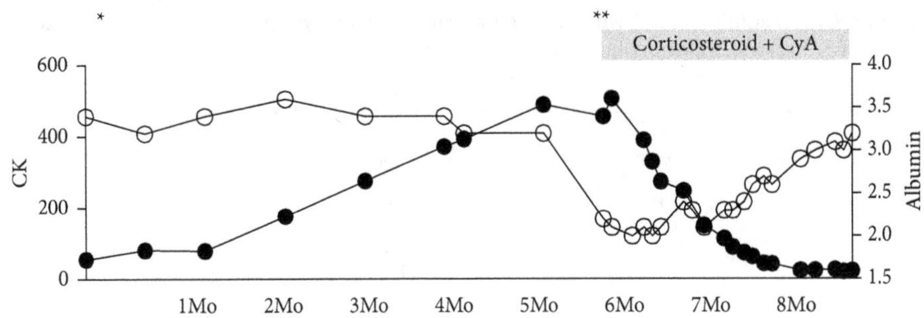

FIGURE 1: Graph showing serum levels of creatine kinase (CK) and albumin (Alb) over time after discharge from first admission to our hospital. The left vertical axis indicates the serum CK levels ((U/L), closed black circles), and the right axis indicates serum albumin (Alb) levels ((mg/dL), open circles). The horizontal line indicates the months (Mo) after discharge from first admission. *indicates the timing of discharge of first admission to our hospital. **indicates readmission to our hospital. CyA: cyclosporine A.

DM with active interstitial pneumonitis. To our knowledge, this is the first description of anti-EJ Ab-positive DM associated with nephrotic syndrome.

2. Case

We describe here the case of a 67-year-old Japanese woman with a 30-year history of DM and a 2-year history of limited cutaneous systemic sclerosis (SSc), who developed nephrotic syndrome that occurred concurrently with the exacerbation of DM.

She developed Raynaud's phenomenon when she was 27 years old. In terms of DM, she developed Gottron's papules, a heliotrope rash, polyarthralgia, and proximal muscle weakness with elevated muscle enzymes at the age of 37. She was diagnosed with DM and treated with corticosteroids. Although the full details of the disease and treatment course were unavailable, she had been treated with a maintenance dose of 10 mg prednisolone daily and 4 mg methotrexate (MTX) weekly, when she developed bilateral hand contracture and subsequent digital ulcers at the age of 66. At this point, the doses of prednisolone and MTX were increased to 15 mg per day and 8 mg per week, respectively, and further increased, 2 months later, to 30 mg per day and 12 mg per week, respectively. Despite the strengthened treatment, the digital ulcers exacerbated, and she was admitted to our hospital, when she was 67 years old (first admission). It was revealed that the case had been complicated by bacterial tenosynovitis refractory to antibiotic treatment, which required amputation of the right middle finger at the base of the proximal phalanx. The digital ulcers were ameliorated by vasodilator treatments, including sympathetic blocks and the administration of calcium antagonists. During the perioperative period, weekly MTX was discontinued, and the dose of prednisolone was reduced over a couple of months to 10 mg per day, when she was discharged from the hospital.

The digital ulcers did not recur during the follow-up period after hospital discharge. However, 3 months after hospital discharge, the patient presented with mechanic's hands and proximal muscle pain and weakness, with elevated serum creatine kinase (CK) levels. The serum CK levels continued to increase over several months (Figure 1), at which point she developed hypoalbuminemia and nephrotic-range proteinuria, and was admitted to our hospital again.

On second admission, the patient measured 149 cm in height and weighed 49.3 kg. Her vital signs were as follows: temperature of 37.5°C, pulse rate of 80 beats per minute, blood pressure of 101/89 mmHg, and oxygen saturation (SpO_2) measured by pulse oximetry of 99% on room air and at rest. The palpebral conjunctiva was not anemic, and the bulbar conjunctiva was not icteric. Cardiac sounds were normal. Fine crackles were heard during late inspiration at the posterior base of both lungs. Abdominal examination revealed no abnormalities. The skin on the ulnar sides of the thumbs and radial sides of the index fingers appeared hyperkeratotic and cracked, compatible with mechanic's hands. No heliotrope rash or Gottron's papules were noted. There was tenderness over her upper arms and thighs bilaterally. Mild pretibial pitting edema was noted in both legs. The laboratory findings are shown in Table 1. Of note, serum levels of muscle-derived enzymes including CK, aspartate aminotransferase, lactate dehydrogenase, myoglobulin, and aldolase were elevated. Muscle magnetic resonance imaging (MRI) revealed the presence of diffuse high signal intensity lesions in the bilateral thigh on T2-weighted and short-tau inversion recovery (STIR) sequences (Figure2). Immunological examination showed positive antinuclear antibodies at a titer of 1 : 320 with speckled patterns and 1 : 40 with cytoplasmic patterns (normal value, <1 : 40). Anti-ARS Ab was positive at an index of 174 (normal value, <5.0 index), and anti-EJ Ab was subsequently demonstrated to be positive by immunoblot analysis. Anti-ribonucleoprotein (RNP) Ab, anti-anti-Sjögren's syndrome A (SSA) Ab, and anti-anti-Sjögren's syndrome B (SS-B) Ab were also positive, but anti-double-stranded deoxyribonucleic acid (dsDNA) Ab, anti-Smith (Sm) Ab, anti-phospholipid Ab, anti-myeloperoxidase (MPO) Ab, and anti-proteinase-3 (PR3) Ab were absent. Electrocardiography showed no abnormalities. Serum Krebs von den Lungen-6 (KL-6) was elevated at 1163 U/mL (normal value, <500 U/mL), and chest computed tomography (CT) showed reticular shadows preferentially at the periphery of the lower lungs bilaterally, indicating the presence of active interstitial pneumonitis. Regarding

TABLE 1: Laboratory values on second admission of a woman with limited cutaneous systemic sclerosis who developed nephrotic syndrome in the setting of recurrence of anti-glycyl-transfer ribonucleic acid synthetase antibody (anti-EJ)-positive dermatomyositis.

Laboratory test	Result	Reference range
CBC		
WBC count (/μL)	10,500	2,700–8,800
Lymphocyte (%)	16.6	19–47
RBC count (/μL)	458	370–540
Hemoglobin (g/dL)	12.6	11.0–17.0
Hematocrit (%)	39.0	34.0–49.0
Platelets ($\times 10^4$/μL)	40.8	14–34
Coagulation		
PT-INR	1.12	
APTT (sec)	33.1	30.0 ± 5.0
Biochemistry		
Total protein (g/dL)	7.0	6.6–8.2
Albumin (g/dL)	2.0	3.9–4.9
AST (U/L)	38	8–38
ALT (U/L)	27	4–44
LDH (U/L)	440	106–211
γGTP (U/L)	9	16–73
Alkaline phosphatase (U/L)	191	104–338
Total bilirubin (mg/dL)	0.50	0.2–1.2
BUN (mg/dL)	17.3	8.0–22.6
Creatinine (mg/dL)	0.56	0.4–0.8
CK (U/L)	1163	43–165
ESR (mm/hour)	19.0	<15
CRP (mg/dL)	2.09	<0.3
KL-6 (U/mL)	1163	<430
SP-A (ng/mL)	124.2	<43.8
SP-D (ng/mL)	202	<110
Urinalysis		
Proteinuria	≥300 mg/dL	(–)
WBC (/HPF)	1–4	<1–4
RBC (/HPF)	1–4	<1–4
Casts (/HPF)	Hyaline casts ≥ 100 Epithelial casts 1–4 Fatty casts 1–4	(–)
Immunological		
IgG (mg/dL)	2,623	870–1,700
IgA (mg/dL)	412	110–410
IgM (mg/dL)	273	35–220
CH50 (U/mL)	47	25–50
C3 (mg/dL)	80	65–135
C4 (mg/dL)	15	13–35
ANA	1 : 320 speckled 1 : 40 cytoplasmic	<1 : 40
Anti-dsDNA IgG Ab (IU/mL)	<10	<12
Anti-SSA Ab	Positive at a titer of 1 : 16	Negative
Anti-SSB Ab	Positive at a titer of 1 : 2	Negative
Anti-RNP Ab	Positive at a titer of 1 : 16	Negative
Anti-Sm Ab	Negative	Negative
Anti-ARS Ab (U/mL)	174.0	<25.0
Anti-EJ Ab	Positive	Negative
LAC	0.83	≤1.16
Ant-cardiolipin Ab (U/mL)	≤8	<10
Anti-β2GPI Ab (U/mL)	≤1.2	<3.5
PR3-ANCA (U/mL)	<1.0	<3.5
MPO-ANCA (U/mL)	<1.0	<3.5

CBC: complete blood count; WBC: white blood cell; RBC: red blood cell; PT-INR: prothrombin time-international normalized ratio; APTT: activated partial thromboplastin time; sec: seconds; AST: aspartate aminotransferase; ALT: alanine aminotransferase; LDH: lactate dehydrogenase; γGTP: γglutamyl transpeptidase; BUN: blood urea nitrogen; CK; creatine kinase; ESR: erythrocyte sedimentation rate; CRP: C-reactive protein; KL-6: krebs von den lungen-6; SP: surfactant protein; HPF: high power field; IgG; immunoglobulin G; IgM; immunoglobulin M; IgA; immunoglobulin A; CH50; 50% hemolytic complement activity; C3: complement 3; C4: complement 4; ANA: antinuclear antibody; dsDNA: double-stranded deoxyribonucleic acid; Ab: antibody; SSA: Sjögren's syndrome-related antigen A; SSB: Sjögren's syndrome type B; RNP: ribonucleoprotein; Sm: Smith; ARS: aminoacyl-transfer ribonucleic acid (tRNA) synthetase; EJ: glycyl-transfer ribonucleic acid synthetase; LAC: lupus anticoagulant; β2GPI: β2-glycoprotein; PR3: proteinase 3; MPO: myeloperoxidase; ANCA: anti-neutrophil cytoplasmic antibody.

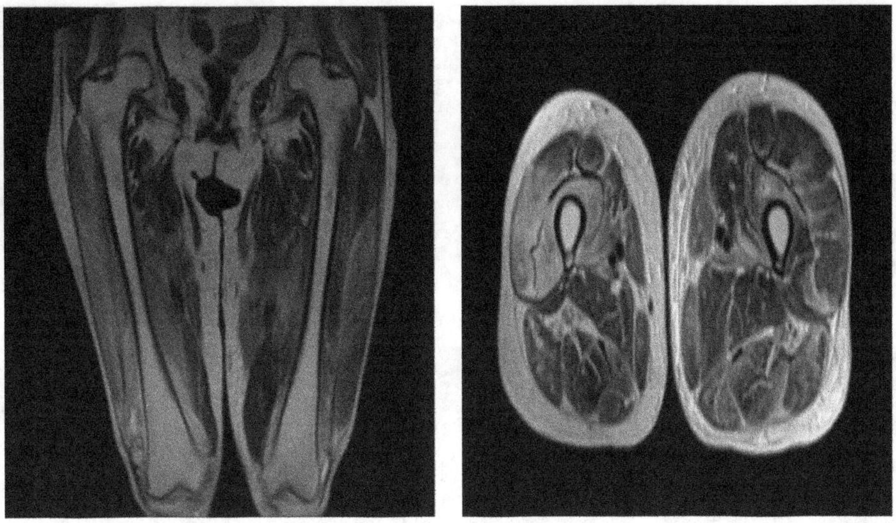

(a) (b)

FIGURE 2: Magnetic resonance imaging (MRI) of bilateral thigh muscles of a woman who developed recurrent anti-glycyl tRNA synthetase (EJ) antibody-positive dermatomyositis concurrently with newly developed nephrotic syndrome shown are sagittal (a) and axial. (b) MRI images demonstrating wide-spread high-intensity lesions on T2-weighted sequences.

musculoskeletal symptoms, she was diagnosed with exacerbation of dermatomyositis complicated by interstitial pneumonitis after reducing immunosuppressive treatments.

As for renal injuries, urinalysis showed 3+ proteinuria, with 1–4 red blood cells per high power field (HPF), 1–4 white blood cells per HPF, >100 hyaline casts per HPF, 1–4 epithelial casts per HPF, and 1–4 fatty casts per HPF, in urinary sediment analysis. The urine protein-to-creatinine ratio was 8.09, and urinary protein excretion was 3.97 g per day. Together with low serum albumin levels (2.0 g/dL) and elevated levels of total cholesterol (295 mg/dL), she was diagnosed with nephrotic syndrome. To determine the underlying renal pathology of nephrotic syndrome, a renal biopsy was performed (Figure 3). Light microscopic examination using hematoxylin-eosin, periodic acid Schiff, Masson's trichrome, and periodic acid methenamine silver staining showed neither thickening nor spike formation of basement membranes. However, the deposition of immunoglobulin G (IgG) (++), IgG1 (+++), IgG2 (+++), IgG3 (−), IgG4 (+++), immunoglobulin A (IgA) (−), immunoglobulin M (IgM) (±), complement 3 (C3) (+++), complement 1q (C1q) (±), and complement 4 (C4) (−) was observed in the glomerulus by immunofluorescence (Figure 3), which suggests the possibility of membranous nephropathy at an early stage, i.e., before the deposition of immune complexes causes apparent basement thickening.

Collectively, the diagnosis of nephrotic syndrome concurrently with exacerbation of anti-EJ Ab-positive DM with interstitial pneumonitis was made. The dose of prednisolone was increased from 10 mg to 40 mg daily, and cyclosporine was initiated at a dose of 100 mg daily, which 2 weeks later was increased to 150 mg daily, together with the anti-platelet drug dipyridamole. This led to normalization of serum CK levels and proteinuria expressed as urine protein-to-creatinine ratio (Figure 4). The dose of prednisolone was gradually decreased thereafter over 6 months to a maintenance dose of 5 mg daily without recurrence.

3. Discussion

In the present study, we describe the case of a woman who presented with nephrotic syndrome concurrent with the recurrence of DM. Renal damage is considered rare as an extramuscular manifestation of PM and DM [1]. However, it has recently been postulated that renal involvement is not as uncommon as previously thought [7]. Yen et al. retrospectively investigated the complications of renal disease in 65 patients with PM or DM over a 10-year period and demonstrated that 14 patients (21.5%) were found to show varying degrees of renal involvement, which were attributed to two disease categories: acute tubular necrosis and chronic glomerulonephritis [8]. Recently, Couvrat-Desvergnes et al. also performed a retrospective study involving 150 patients with inflammatory myopathies, including DM, PM, and ASS [5], with a 4.1-year follow-up period, and demonstrated that renal involvement was present in 35 patients (23.3%) who were categorized into acute kidney injury ($n = 16$) and chronic kidney disease (CKD) ($n = 31$), including those who shifted from AKI to CKD.

Acute kidney injury related to PM or DM can develop during the acute phases of rhabdomyolysis, leading to myoglobinuria, which causes acute tubular necrosis and subsequent renal failure. Patients with PM or DM often have high serum CK levels, usually 10-fold and sometimes up to 50-fold the upper limit of normal values [9, 10]. It was previously considered that rhabdomyolysis leading to acute renal failure was uncommon in PM and DM because the rate and degree of myolysis could be lower than those of myotoxic drug-related necrotizing myopathy [11]. However,

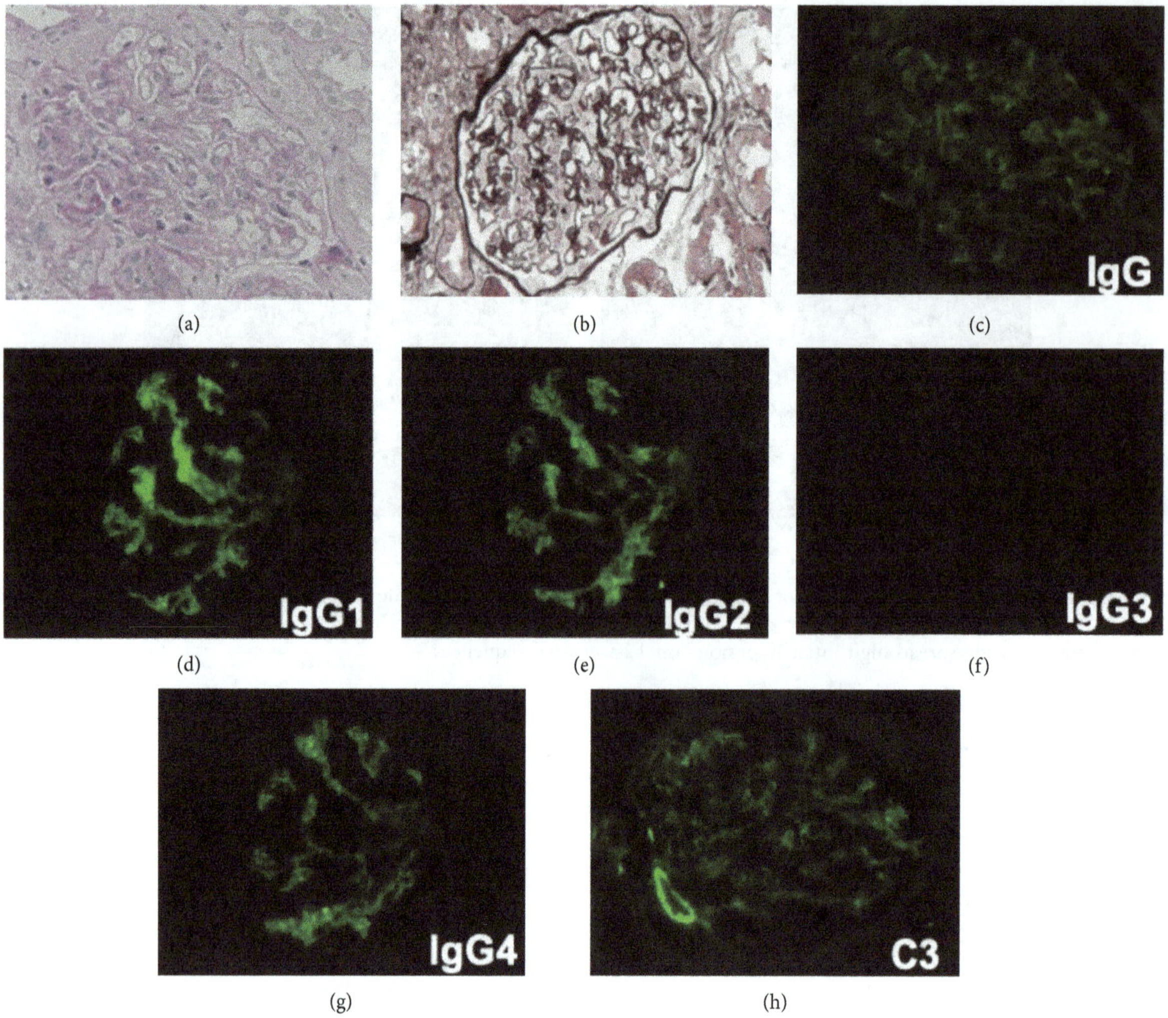

FIGURE 3: Renal biopsy showing deposition of immunoglobulin G (IgG) and complement 3 (C3) in a woman who developed recurrent anti-glycyl tRNA synthetase (EJ) antibody-positive dermatomyositis concurrently with newly developed nephrotic syndrome. (a) Hematoxylin and eosin (HE) stain; (b) periodic acid methenamine silver (PAM) stain; immunofluorescence examination: (c) total IgG; (d) IgG1; (e) IgG2; (f) IgG3; (g) IgG4; (h) C3. Light microscopic examinations using HE and PAM stains show neither thickening nor spike formation of basement membranes. Deposition of IgG, IgG1, IgG2, IgG4, and C3 is noted. Immunoglobulin A (IgA) and immunoglobulin M (IgM) are absent (data not shown).

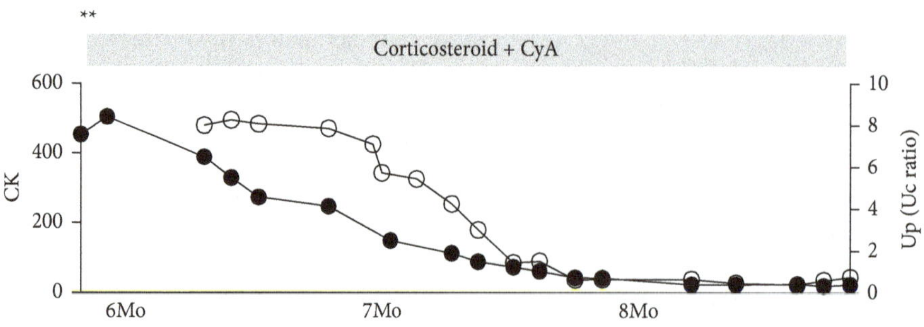

FIGURE 4: Graph showing serum levels of creatine kinase (CK) and urine protein-to-creatinine ratio (Up/Uc ratio) over time after second admission to our hospital. The left vertical axis indicates the serum CK levels ((U/L), closed black circles), and the right axis indicates the degree of proteinuria, expressed as (Up/Uc) ratio (open circles). The horizontal line indicates the months (Mo) after discharge of first admission. Up: urinary protein; Uc: urinary creatinine. **indicates readmission to our hospital. CyA: cyclosporine A.

myoglobinuria-induced acute tubular necrosis caused by PM or DM has been reported in the literature, especially in patients with DM [12–20]. The other type of renal damage related to PM or DM is chronic glomerulonephritis, which is presumed to be immune-mediated, and exhibits a variety of histologic features. From the 65 PM and DM patients reported by Yen et al., a renal biopsy was performed in two DM patients with overt proteinuria and membranous nephropathy was revealed in one and IgA nephropathy in the other [8]. As for the study by Couvrat-Desvergnes et al., they identified 14 patients who had undergone renal biopsy (6 PM, 5 DM, and 3 ASS), which revealed the presence of glomerulonephritis with various pathologic patterns including immune complex-related glomerulonephritis ($n = 4$), membranous nephropathy ($n = 2$), and IgA nephropathy ($n = 2$) [5]. We conducted an additional literature search and retrieved case reports describing the association of PM or DM with a variety of pathological glomerular lesions, including mesangial proliferative glomerulonephritis [21–25], membranous nephropathy [26–31], membranoproliferative glomerulonephritis [32], IgA nephropathy [33–37], diffuse proliferative glomerulonephritis [38], immune complex-type glomerulonephritis [39–42], acute interstitial nephritis [43], lipoid nephrosis and focal glomerulosclerosis [44], focal segmental glomerulosclerosis with evidence of acute tubular injury [45], sclerotic GN with fibrocellular crescent [46], and crescentic glomerulonephritis associated with malignancy [47]. Cases presenting with anti-neutrophil cytoplasmic antibody-associated glomerulonephritis in the context of DM have also been reported [48–50]. As pointed out in previous studies [6, 25], there is a tendency for mesangial proliferative glomerulonephritis to be more frequently observed in PM, while membranous nephropathy is more frequently observed in the context of DM.

The present case was positive for anti-ARS Ab, which was measured using MESACUP anti-ARS tests (MBL, Japan) that detected five anti-ARS Abs (anti-Jo-1, anti-PL-7, anti-PL-12, anti-EJ, and anti-KS Abs). The patient was subsequently found to have anti-EJ Ab using BlueDiver immunoblot kits (D-tek, Belgium) that measured each anti-ARS Ab separately. The frequency of anti-EJ Ab in ASS varies among previous studies, ranging from 1.8% to 23% [4, 51–53]. Thus, Pinal-Fernandez et al. investigated the frequency of anti-ARS Abs based on the Johns Hopkins Myositis Center cohort and demonstrated that anti-Jo1 Ab was most prevalent (73.4%) in ASS, followed by anti-PL12 (13.6%), anti-PL7 (9.5%), anti-EJ (1.8%), and anti-OJ (1.8%) Abs [51]. Based on the AENEAS (American and European Network of anti-synthetase syndrome) collaborative group's cohort database, Cavagna et al. also showed that anti-EJ Ab was the fourth anti-ARS Ab with its frequency of 4.5% (38 out of 828 patients with ASS) [52]. Furthermore, Hamaguchi et al. reported that anti-EJ Ab was detected in 38 out of 166 Japanese patients with ASS (23%) [4]. As for its frequency in China, Zhan et al. demonstrated that anti-EJ Ab was the third most prevalent anti-ARS Ab, preceded by anti-Jo-1 and anti-PL7 Abs in patients with ASS complicated by ILD with its frequency of 21% (23 out of 108 patients) [53].

To our knowledge, this is the first case report describing the association of anti-EJ Ab with nephrotic syndrome. It should be noted here that our patient, who developed nephrotic syndrome concurrently with the recurrence of DM, was positive for anti-RNP Ab and anti-SSB Ab in addition to anti-EJ Ab. Regarding the involvement of anti-SSB Abs, they are immunological markers for Sjögren's syndrome (SS) [54]. Although the renal manifestation of SS is usually type I distal renal tubular acidosis and tubular interstitial nephritis, glomerulonephritis can be found, albeit less frequently [55]. Therefore, the possibility cannot be excluded that nephrotic syndrome developed in relation to SS. However, we consider that the synchronicity of the development of nephrotic syndrome with the exacerbation of DM supports the association with DM in our patient. As for anti-RNP Ab, this can be detected alone in various autoimmune diseases (mixed connective tissue disease (MCTD), rheumatoid arthritis (RA), SS, SSc, and inflammatory myositis) or together with anti-Sm Ab specifically in systemic lupus erythematosus [56]. Although dermatomyositis overlapping with lupus nephritis has been described in the literature [57–59], our patient showed neither anti-Sm Ab, anti-dsDNA IgG Ab, anti-phospholipid Ab, or hypocomplementemia, thereby making the diagnosis of SLE less likely.

In our case, Raynaud's phenomenon and skin changes at the fingertips were so severe that the distal ends of the phalanges were denuded. Since the overlapping features of SSc, SLE, and PM or DM in MCTD are usually mild with favorable outcomes [60], the patient was considered to have SSc rather than MCTD. The simultaneous detection of anti-ARS Ab and anti-RNP Ab is relatively uncommon. Hamaguchi et al. examined the clinical features of 166 adult patients with anti-ARS Abs, including anti-histidyl tRNA synthetase (anti-Jo-1) Ab ($n = 59$), anti-EJ Ab ($n = 38$), anti-threonyl tRNA synthetase (anti-PL-7) Ab ($n = 29$), anti-alanyl tRNA synthetase (anti-PL-12) Ab ($n = 18$), anti-asparaginyl tRNA synthetase (anti-KS) Ab ($n = 13$), anti-isoleucyl tRNA synthetase (anti-OJ) Ab ($n = 8$), anti-PL7/PL12 Ab ($n = 1$), and demonstrated that anti-RNP Ab was detected in only 2 patients, including one with anti-PL7 Ab and another with anti-PL12 Ab [4]. Previous case-based studies described the patients with anti-RNP Ab coexisting anti-Jo1 Ab [61–64]. To our knowledge, this is the first report describing a patient positive with both anti-EJ Ab and anti-RNP Ab who presented with DM and nephrotic syndrome.

The patient in the present case developed nephrotic syndrome at a time when the disease activity of DM had been increasing. The temporal concurrence of nephrotic syndrome and DM suggests that the two diseases share a common pathophysiological process in this patient. Of course, it should be noted that the simultaneous occurrence of nephrotic syndrome and DM could have been a coincidence. Of interest, Fukui et al. previously used immunohistochemical methods to analyze the components of immune complexes deposited in the glomerulus in a patient with DM that was associated with immune complex (IC)-type membranous nephropathy. It was demonstrated that renal tubular epithelial (RTE) antigens were present specifically at the granular IC disposition sites, suggesting that RTE antigens could be autoantigens in this case. Although their findings have not been replicated subsequently, it would be interesting to search for autoantigens in our patients using modern proteomic technologies. It should also be noted here that the present case was positive for anti-RNP Ab, as described elsewhere. Casal-Dominguez et al. have recently demonstrated that anti-RNP Ab was related to glomerulonephritis in patients with inflammatory myositis [64], in which the clinical phenotypes of 21 patients with anti-RNP Ab-positive myositis were compared to those of 178 patients with DM, 135 patients with immune-mediated necrotizing myopathy, and 132 patients with ASS. They demonstrated that arthritis (60%), DM-specific skin features (60%), and interstitial lung disease (45%) were the most common extramuscular clinical features of anti-RNP Ab-positive myositis. Notably, glomerulonephritis and pericarditis were less common but uniquely found during the disease course in 25% and 40% of patients with anti-RNP Ab-positive myositis, respectively. Further accumulation of cases with anti-EJ Ab-positive dermatomyositis complicated by nephrotic syndrome in the presence or absence of anti-RNP Ab is warranted.

A limitation of this case report is that we did not perform electromyography or muscle biopsy for the evaluation of inflammatory myositis. However, the patient presented with symmetrical proximal muscle weakness and pain, increased serum CK levels, and muscle signal on MRI, together with rashes typical of DM. Furthermore, she was positive for anti-EJ Ab specific for DM [65]. Collectively, we diagnosed her with overlap of dermatomyositis and SSc rather than MCTD. Another limitation was that we did not measure anti-M-type phospholipase A2 receptor antibody, which has been demonstrated to be associated with primary membranous nephropathy [66–68].

In conclusion, we have described a woman with limited cutaneous SSc who developed nephrotic syndrome in the setting of the recurrence of anti-EJ Ab-positive DM. The association of membranous nephropathy with anti-Jo1 Ab-positive DM has been described in the literature. However, to the best of our knowledge, the association of nephrotic syndrome with anti-EJ Ab-positive DM is described for the first time in the present case report. We believe that this report is a valuable addition to the literature since the renal manifestations of PM and DM remain to be firmly established. Further studies investigating patients with DM complicated by nephrotic syndrome according to category of different patterns of autoantibodies, such as myositis-specific and myositis-related Abs, are warranted to better understand the renal manifestations of DM.

Authors' Contributions

ST and TS were the lead investigators of the study, including preparation of the manuscript. All authors participated in management of the case, interpretation of the data, critically reviewed the manuscript, and approved the final version of the article for publication.

Acknowledgments

This case study was supported by Tokyo Medical University Hospital.

References

[1] D. Ascherman, R. Aggarwal, and C. Oddis, "Classification, epidemiology, and clinical features of inflammatory muscle disease," in *Rheumatology*, M. Hochberg, E. Gravallese, A. Silman, J. Smolen, M. Weinblatt, and M. Weisman, Eds., Elsevier, Amsterdam, Netherlands, 2019.

[2] J. L. Marco and B. F. Collins, "Clinical manifestations and treatment of antisynthetase syndrome," *Best Practice & Research Clinical Rheumatology*, vol. 34, no. 4, Article ID 101503, 2020.

[3] A. L. Mammen, Y. Allenbach, W. Stenzel et al., "239th ENMC international workshop: classification of dermatomyositis, Amsterdam, Netherlands," *Neuromuscular Disorders*, vol. 30, no. 1, pp. 70–92, 2020.

[4] Y. Hamaguchi, M. Fujimoto, T. Matsushita et al., "Common and distinct clinical features in adult patients with anti-aminoacyl-tRNA synthetase antibodies: heterogeneity within the syndrome," *PLoS One*, vol. 8, no. 4, Article ID e60442, 2013.

[5] G. Couvrat-Desvergnes, A. Masseau, O. Benveniste et al., "The spectrum of renal involvement in patients with inflammatory myopathies," *Medicine (Baltimore)*, vol. 93, no. 1, pp. 33–41, 2014.

[6] A. Kronbichler and G. Mayer, "Renal involvement in autoimmune connective tissue diseases," *BMC Medicine*, vol. 11, no. 1, p. 95, 2013.

[7] D. Cucchiari and C. Angelini, "Renal involvement in idiopathic inflammatory myopathies," *Clinical Reviews in Allergy and Immunology*, vol. 52, no. 1, pp. 99–107, 2017.

[8] T. H. Yen, P. C. Lai, C. C. Chen, S. Hsueh, and J. Y. Huang, "Renal involvement in patients with polymyositis and dermatomyositis," *International Journal of Clinical Practice*, vol. 59, no. 2, pp. 188–193, 2004.

[9] M. C. Dalakas, "Inflammatory muscle diseases," *New England Journal of Medicine*, vol. 372, no. 18, pp. 1734–1747, 2015.

[10] J. Jones and R. Wortmann, "Idiopathic inflammatory myopathies-a review," *Clinical Rheumatology*, vol. 34, no. 5, pp. 839–844, 2015.

[11] L. G. Rider and F. W. Miller, "Laboratory evaluation of the inflammatory myopathies," *Clinical and Diagnostic Laboratory Immunology*, vol. 2, no. 1, pp. 1-9, 1995.

[12] E. Kessler, I. Weinberger, and J. B. Rosenfeld, "Myoglobinuric acute renal failure in a case of dermatomyositis," *Israel Journal of Medical Sciences*, vol. 8, no. 7, pp. 978–983, 1972.

[13] P. C. Singhal, M. R. Narayanan-Nampoory, R. K. Visweswaran, R. L. Mehta, V. Gupta, and K. S. Chugh, "Myoglobinuric renal failure associated with dermatomyositis," *Journal of the Association of Physicians of India*, vol. 33, no. 10, pp. 672-673, 1985.

[14] S. K. Park, K. H. Cho, and S. K. Kang, "Acute renal failure associated with dermatomyositis and colon cancer," *Nephron*, vol. 55, no. 2, pp. 225-226, 1990.

[15] D. V. Caccamo, C. Y. Keene, J. Durham, and D. Peven, "Fulminant rhabdomyolysis in a patient with dermatomyositis," *Neurology*, vol. 43, no. 4, pp. 844-845, 1993.

[16] A. I. Lazar, "Acute myositis complicated by myoglobinuric acute renal failure," *Journal of the Association of Physicians of India*, vol. 42, no. 6, pp. 507-508, 1994.

[17] M. R. Rose, J. T. Kissel, L. S. Bickley, and R. C. Griggs, "Sustained myoglobinuria: the presenting manifestation of dermatomyositis," *Neurology*, vol. 47, no. 1, pp. 119–123, 1996.

[18] D. Joshi, N. Kumar, and A. Rai, "Dermatomyositis presenting with rhabdomyolysis and acute renal failure; an uncommon manifestation," *Annals of Indian Academy of Neurology*, vol. 12, no. 1, pp. 45–47, 2009.

[19] M. M. Sabha, H. T. Simo, R. M. Shadid, and N. I. Altorok, "Successful treatment of antisynthetase syndrome presenting as rhabdomyolysis with rituximab," *Rheumatology International*, vol. 38, no. 6, pp. 1125–1130, 2018.

[20] M. Hamadeh, S. Boustany, and J. Fares, "Acute kidney injury following dermatomyositis," *Clinical Medicine and Research*, vol. 17, no. 3-4, pp. 102–104, 2019.

[21] R. F. Dyck, A. Katz, D. A. Gordon et al., "Glomerulonephritis associated with polymyositis," *Journal of Rheumatology*, vol. 6, no. 3, pp. 336–344, 1979.

[22] N. A. Frost, E. F. Morand, C. L. Hall, P. J. Maddison, and A. K. Bhalla, "Idiopathic polymyositis complicated by arthritis and mesangial proliferative glomerulonephritis: case report and review of the literature," *Rheumatology*, vol. 32, no. 10, pp. 929–931, 1993.

[23] P. Picco, M. Gattomo, G. C. Barbano, A. Trivelli, V. Pistoia, and A. Buoncompagni, "Mesangial glomerulonephritis and transient SLE manifestations in an adolescent with dermatomyositis," *Lupus*, vol. 6, no. 1, pp. 72-73, 1997.

[24] O. F. Valenzuela, I. W. Reiser, and J. G. Porush, "Idiopathic polymyositis and glomerulonephritis," *Journal of Nephrology*, vol. 14, no. 2, pp. 120–124, 2001.

[25] Y. Takizawa, H. Kanda, K. Sato et al., "Polymyositis associated with focal mesangial proliferative glomerulonephritis with depositions of immune complexes," *Clinical Rheumatology*, vol. 26, no. 5, pp. 792–796, 2007.

[26] I. Hara, N. Kurata, K. Hyozu, and H. Tamao, "A case of polymyositis complicated with membranous nephritis," *Nihon Naika Gakkai Zasshi*, vol. 80, no. 1, pp. 108-109, 1991.

[27] H. Makino, K. Hirata, M. Matsuda, T. Amano, and Z. Ota, "Membranous nephropathy developing during the course of dermatomyositis," *Journal of Rheumatology*, vol. 21, no. 7, pp. 1377-1378, 1994.

[28] J. D. Rose, "Membranous glomerulonephritis, dermatomyositis, and bronchial carcinoma," *BMJ*, vol. 2, no. 6191, p. 641, 1979.

[29] A. Soylu, S. Kavukçu, M. Türkmen, and S. Saroğlu, "Dermatomyositis with membranous nephropathy," *Turkish Journal of Pediatrics*, vol. 43, no. 2, pp. 143–145, 2001.

[30] Y. Akashi, M. Inoh, N. Gamo et al., "Dermatomyositis associated with membranous nephropathy in a 43-year-old female," *American Journal of Nephrology*, vol. 22, no. 4, pp. 385–388, 2002.

[31] M. Hanaoka, H. Tsutsumi, T. Sano et al., "A case of membranous nephropathy associated with polymyositis," *Kitasato Medicine*, vol. 29, no. 6, pp. 385–390, 1999.

[32] M. B. Owlia, R. Hemayati, S. Taghipour Zahir, and M. Moeini Nodeh, "Dermatomyositis sine myositis with membranoproliferative glomerulonephritis," *Case Reports in Rheumatology*, vol. 2012, Article ID 751683, 3 pages, 2012.

[33] A. H. Vilppula and R. A. T. Aine, "Polymyositis associated with several immunological disorders," *Clinical Rheumatology*, vol. 3, no. 4, pp. 533–539, 1984.

[34] T. H. Yen, J. Y. Huang, and C. Y. Chen, "Unexpected IgA nephropathy during the treatment of a young woman with idiopathic dermatomyositis: case report and review of the literature," *Journal of Nephrology*, vol. 16, no. 1, pp. 148–153, 2003.

[35] M. Civilibal, N. Selcuk Duru, A. Ozagari, K. Durali, and M. Elevli, "Immunoglobulin A nephropathy associated with juvenile dermatomyositis," *Pediatric Nephrology*, vol. 24, no. 10, pp. 2073–2075, 2009.

[36] T. B. M. Barros, F. H. C. Souza, D. M. A. C. Malheiros, M. Levy-Neto, and S. K. Shinjo, "IgA nephropathy and polymyositis: a rare association," *Revista Brasileira de Reumatologia*, vol. 54, no. 3, pp. 231–233, 2014.

[37] M. R. Mantoo, S. K. Tripathy, R. H. Phulware, N. K. Bagri, P. Hari, and A. Barwad, "Juvenile dermatomyositis with IgA nephropathy: case-based review," *Rheumatology International*, vol. 39, no. 3, pp. 577–581, 2019.

[38] Q. Xie, Y. Liu, G. Liu, N. Yang, and G. Yin, "Diffuse proliferative glomerulonephritis associated with dermatomyositis with nephrotic syndrome," *Rheumatology International*, vol. 30, no. 6, pp. 821–825, 2010.

[39] T. Moriyama, Y. Uruta, H. Yamaguchi et al., "A case of immune-complex type glomerulonephritis associated with dermatomyositis," *Nihon Naika Gakkai Zasshi*, vol. 78, no. 7, pp. 994-995, 1989.

[40] H. Fukui, T. Kimura, K. Nakabayashi, and T. Nagasawa, "Dermatomyositis associated with immune-complex type nephritis induced by tubular epithelial antigen," *Nihon Jinzo Gakkai Shi*, vol. 18, no. 8, pp. 523–533, 1976.

[41] H. Kaneoka, Y. Sasatomi, K. Miyagi et al., "A rare case of dermatomyositis associated with immune-complex type glomerulonephritis, idiopathic thrombopenic purpura, pulmonary fibrosis and lung cancer," *Clinical & Experimental Rheumatology*, vol. 21, no. 6, pp. 801-802, 2003.

[42] K. Kamata, Y. Kobayashi, H. Shigematsu, and T. Saito, "Childhood type polymyositis and rapidly progressive glomerulonephritis," *Pathology International*, vol. 32, no. 5, pp. 801–806, 1982.

[43] J. Das, P. George, B. Pawar, and N. Calton, "Acute interstitial nephritis in association with polymyositis," *Journal of Postgraduate Medicine*, vol. 54, no. 2, pp. 170-171, 2008.

[44] H. Moutsopoulos and K. H. Fye, "Letter: lipoid nephrosis and focal glomerulosclerosis in a patient with polymyositis," *The Lancet*, vol. 305, no. 7914, p. 1039, 1975.

[45] A. Nickavar and M. Mehr Azma, "Nephrotic syndrome and juvenile dermatomyositis," *Rheumatology International*, vol. 32, no. 9, pp. 2933–2935, 2012.

[46] M. Tsunemi, E. Ishimura, K. Tsumura et al., "A case of crescentic glomerulonephritis associated with polymyositis," *Nephron*, vol. 64, no. 3, pp. 488-489, 1993.

[47] K. C. Chiu, T. C. Tsai, W. T. Lin, W. J. Lee, C. C. Su, and C. Y. Chen, "Paraneoplastic polymyositis associated with crescentic glomerulonephritis," *Renal Failure*, vol. 30, no. 9, pp. 939–942, 2008.

[48] H. Kawai, W. Kitagawa, N. Suzuki et al., "Myeloperoxidase-antineutrophil cytoplasmic antibody-related crescentic glomerulonephritis after treatment for clinically amyopathic dermatomyositis: a coincidental combination or not?" *Clinical and Experimental Nephrology*, vol. 15, no. 4, pp. 577–581, 2011.

[49] C. Yuste, M. Rapalai, B. A. Pritchard et al., "Overlap between dermatomyositis and ANCA vasculitides," *Clinical Kidney Journal*, vol. 7, no. 1, pp. 59–61, 2014.

[50] P. K. Panda, T. M. Suri, R. Sood, A. S. Bhalla, M. C. Sharma, and P. Ranjan, "Overlap syndrome: juvenile dermatomyositis

and perinuclear antineutrophil cytoplasmic autoantibody vasculitis, a case report and review of literature," *International Journal of Rheumatic Diseases*, vol. 20, no. 12, pp. 2219–2224, 2017.

[51] I. Pinal-Fernandez, M. Casal-Dominguez, J. A. Huapaya et al., "A longitudinal cohort study of the anti-synthetase syndrome: increased severity of interstitial lung disease in black patients and patients with anti-PL7 and anti-PL12 autoantibodies," *Rheumatology*, vol. 56, no. 6, pp. 999–1007, 2017.

[52] L. Cavagna, E. Trallero-Araguás, F. Meloni et al., "Influence of antisynthetase antibodies specificities on antisynthetase syndrome clinical spectrum time course," *Journal of Clinical Medicine*, vol. 8, no. 11, Article ID E2013, 2019.

[53] X. Zhan, W. Yan, Y. Wang et al., "Clinical features of anti-synthetase syndrome associated interstitial lung disease: a retrospective cohort in China," *BMC Pulmonary Medicine*, vol. 21, no. 1, p. 57, 2021.

[54] E. Feist and G. Burmester, "Laboratory tests in rheumatic disorders," in *Rheumatology*, M. Hochberg, E. Gravallese, A. Silman, J. Smolen, M. Weinblatt, and M. Weisman, Eds., Elsevier, Amsterdam, Netherlands, 2019.

[55] A. Goules, D. Geetha, L. J. Arend, and A. N. Baer, "Renal involvement in primary Sjögren's syndrome: natural history and treatment outcome," *Clinical & Experimental Rheumatology*, vol. 7, no. 3, pp. 123–132, 2019.

[56] F. Quismorio and A. Quismorio, "Clinical application of serologic tests, serum protein abnormalities, and other clinical laboratory tests in systemic lupus erythematosus," in *Dubois' Lupus Erythematosus and Related Syndromes*, D. Wallace and B. Hahn, Eds., pp. 579–597, Elsevier, Amsterdam, Netherlands, 2019.

[57] G. Ristic, Z. Paunić, D. Vojvodić, M. Petronijević, B. Glisić, and D. Stefanović, "Systemic lupus erythematosus and dermatomyositis--case report," *Srpski Arhiv Za Celokupno Lekarstvo*, vol. 133, pp. 137–140, 2005.

[58] I. Nakaya, Y. Iwata, Y. Sugiyama, T. Abe, and G. Nomura, "Dermatomyositis relapse complicated with gastric carcinoma and lupus nephritis five years after the initial diagnosis of dermatomyositis," *Internal Medicine*, vol. 41, no. 6, pp. 502-503, 2002.

[59] N. Bitencourt, E. B. Solow, T. Wright, and B. L. Bermas, "Inflammatory myositis in systemic lupus erythematosus," *Lupus*, vol. 29, no. 7, pp. 776–781, 2020.

[60] S. Reiseter, R. Gunnarsson, J. Corander et al., "Disease evolution in mixed connective tissue disease: results from a long-term nationwide prospective cohort study," *Arthritis Research and Therapy*, vol. 19, no. 1, p. 284, 2017.

[61] I. Lundberg, I. Nennesmo, and E. Hedfors, "A clinical, serological, and histopathological study of myositis patients with and without anti-RNP antibodies," *Seminars in Arthritis and Rheumatism*, vol. 22, no. 2, pp. 127–138, 1992.

[62] R. Brouwer, G. J. Hengstman, W. Vree Egberts et al., "Autoantibody profiles in the sera of European patients with myositis," *Annals of the Rheumatic Diseases*, vol. 60, no. 2, pp. 116–123, 2001.

[63] E. Feist, M. L. Schneider, M. Brychcy, T. Dörner, G. R. Burmester, and F. Hiepe, "A unique autoantibody pattern of positive anti-Jo-1, anti-U1RNP, and anti-proteasome antibodies in autoimmune myositis as a diagnostic challenge," *Annals of the Rheumatic Diseases*, vol. 62, no. 4, pp. 370-371, 2003.

[64] M. Casal-Dominguez, I. Pinal-Fernandez, A. M. Corse et al., "Muscular and extramuscular features of myositis patients with anti-U1-RNP autoantibodies," *Neurology*, vol. 92, no. 13, pp. e1416–e1426, 2019.

[65] F. M. Alenzi, "Myositis specific autoantibodies: a clinical perspective," *Open Access Rheumatology Research and Reviews*, vol. 12, pp. 9–14, 2020.

[66] S. Akiyama, M. Akiyama, E. Imai, T. Ozaki, S. Matsuo, and S. Maruyama, "Prevalence of anti-phospholipase A2 receptor antibodies in Japanese patients with membranous nephropathy," *Clinical and Experimental Nephrology*, vol. 19, no. 4, pp. 653–660, 2015.

[67] N. Hayashi, S. Akiyama, H. Okuyama et al., "Clinicopathological characteristics of M-type phospholipase A2 receptor (PLA2R)-related membranous nephropathy in Japanese," *Clinical and Experimental Nephrology*, vol. 19, no. 5, pp. 797–803, 2015.

[68] Y. Katsumata, Y. Okamoto, T. Moriyama et al., "Clinical usefulness of anti-M-type phospholipase-A-receptor antibodies in patients with membranous nephropathy and the comparison of three quantification methods," *Immunological Medicine*, vol. 43, no. 1, pp. 47–56, 2020.

Pyoderma Gangrenosum as a Presenting Feature of Undifferentiated Spondyloarthropathy with Erosive Inflammatory Arthritis

Jaspreet Kaler,[1] Sandra Sheffield,[2] Myint Thway,[1] Karishma Ramsubeik,[1] and Gurjit Kaeley[1]

[1]*Department of Rheumatology, University of Florida Health, 653 W 8th Street, Jacksonville, 32209 Florida, USA*
[2]*Department of Medicine, University of Florida Health, 653 W 8th Street, Jacksonville, 32209 Florida, USA*

Correspondence should be addressed to Jaspreet Kaler; jessiekaler01@gmail.com

Academic Editor: Jamal Mikdashi

Pyoderma gangrenosum is a rare inflammatory condition with varying clinical presentations and severity. It is commonly seen in association with an underlying condition, most common of which is inflammatory bowel disease. We report a case of a 26-year-old male who came to the emergency department with increasing lower extremity ulcers, intermittent hematochezia, and pain in the small joints of his hands. After excluding a broad list of differentials for lower extremity ulcers, the diagnosis of pyoderma gangrenosum was made. He was also found to have erosive changes at multiple proximal interphalangeal joints and jug-like syndesmophytes at T12 and L1 on CT scan. Although there was evidence of a spondyloarthropathy, there was no evidence of inflammatory bowel disease on colonoscopy, psoriasis, or sexually transmitted infections. After multiple failed trials of medications including azathioprine and sulfasalazine, 4 weeks of Adalimumab resulted in rapid healing of pyoderma gangrenosum lesions and improvement in his synovitis. Coupled together, this suggests a diagnosis of pyoderma gangrenosum associated with undifferentiated spondyloarthropathy and erosive inflammatory arthritis. This case is suggestive of spondyloarthropathy going underdiagnosed and untreated in other patients with pyoderma gangrenosum as lower extremity ulcerations can be the primary complaint for seeking treatment. Although rare, axial spondyloarthropathy associated with pyoderma gangrenosum should be kept as an associated differential diagnosis when faced with pyoderma gangrenosum.

1. Introduction

Pyoderma gangrenosum is a rare inflammatory condition with varying clinical presentations and severity. Typically, it presents as a papule or pustule that rapidly evolves to an ulcerative lesion with irregular, erythematous to violaceous edges. Pathergy is a characteristic feature of pyoderma gangrenosum as lesions often occur at sites of trauma. It has an estimated annual incidence of 3–10 cases per million people [1]. It can affect people of any age, but incidence peaks between the ages of 20 and 50 years old and affects men and females equally [2]. Although pyoderma gangrenosum can be found independently, it is more commonly found in association with an underlying disease. In fact, up to 75% of pyoderma gangrenosum cases are associated with inflammatory bowel diseases, inflammatory arthritis, or hematological disorders [2]. Of the accompanying disorders, inflammatory bowel diseases, such as Crohn's disease and ulcerative colitis, are the associated disease in 65% of cases [2]. We present a case of pyoderma gangrenosum as a presenting feature of undifferentiated spondyloarthropathy, with erosive inflammatory arthritis, without any evidence of inflammatory bowel disease.

2. Case Report

A 26-year-old Hispanic male with no significant past medical history came to the emergency department complaining of multiple wounds that gradually developed over the past 3 years. He reported a wound at the vertex of his scalp, posterior aspect of his neck, and on bilateral lower extremities. He reported the wounds initially started as small pimples, with progression in size and pain severity. The patient also reported serosanguineous drainage from his wounds, hematochezia, and pain in the small joints of his hands bilaterally, 9/10 in severity, associated with swelling and stiffness. The patient reported that his scalp lesions started 3 years prior to this admission and remained the same size since then. The lesions over his lower extremities started within 3 months of this admission and progressed so rapidly that it prompted him to go to the emergency department and seek help. He reported that his joint pain started approximately the same time as his scalp lesions and has progressively gotten worse over the past 3 years. He denied diarrhea, back pain, uveitis, iritis, sexually transmitted infections, abdominal pain, fever, or night sweats.

Physical exam was significant for a morbidly obese male in mild distress due to pain. Triage vitals were significant for mild tachycardia of 103 but otherwise were unremarkable. He had multiple wounds with serosanguineous drainage: ulcer at the vertex of the scalp measured $7\,cm \times 3\,cm$, posterior neck ulceration $5\,cm \times 2\,cm$, and multiple ulcers, of varying stages, circumferentially on bilateral lower extremities (Figure 1). Furthermore, there was tenderness and synovitis at the right 2nd and 4th proximal interphalangeal (PIP) joints and the left 5th PIP joint. There was associated fusiform swelling of the second and fourth right digits, suggestive of dactylitis.

Initial admission labs revealed leukocytosis of $12.0 \times 10^3\,\mu L$ (reference range $4.5–11.0 \times 10^3$) with 74% neutrophils, hemoglobin of 12.4 g/dL (reference range 13.0–17.0), ESR of 43 mm/hr (reference range 0–20), and CRP 54 mg/L (reference 0.0–5 mg/L). X-ray of bilateral hands revealed marginal erosions at the right second and fourth PIP joints and left 5th PIP joint (Figure 2). In view of the severity of the wounds in association with synovitis, infectious workup and rheumatological workup were initiated while he was empirically started on vancomycin and ceftriaxone.

Rheumatoid factor (RF), anticyclic citrullinated peptide (CCP), antinuclear antibodies (ANA), anti-Ro/SSA, anti-La/SSB, anti-RNP, complements levels, double-stranded DNA, anti-smith antibodies, anti-neutrophil cytoplasmic antibodies, HLA-B27, HIV, hepatitis B, hepatitis C, Quantiferon, and blood cultures were all negative. Punch biopsy of the left lower extremity edge revealed mixed dermal infiltrate with neutrophils and vasculitis. The tissue culture was positive for *Pseudomonas aeruginosa*. In lieu of the positive culture, he was subsequently treated for ecthyma gangrenosum with a cumulative six-week course of piperacillin/tazobactam and ciprofloxacin. Despite treatment for 6 weeks, his ulcerations did not improve. His hospital course was complicated by hematochezia, for which CT enterography and colonoscopy were completed. The colonoscopy revealed internal hemorrhoids, and small bowel biopsies were negative for findings suggestive of inflammatory bowel disease. CT enterography revealed jug-like syndesmophytes at T12 and L1 with sclerosis at the sacroiliac joints (Figure 3). The gastroenterology team planned on completing a repeat colonoscopy as an outpatient as pyoderma gangrenosum can precede inflammatory bowel disease. Ultrasound of bilateral hands revealed extensive enthesitis and erosions. Right second and fourth proximal interphalangeal (PIP) joints revealed a markedly thickened extensor tendon insertion with a mild effusion. Medial and lateral aspect of these joints revealed thickened collateral ligaments with underlying erosions and periostitis. The fifth left PIP had a similarly thickened extensor tendon insertion with periostitis and erosions medially and laterally.

As there was no improvement of the ulcerative lesions with antibiotics, and in conjunction with syndesmophytes, enthesitis, and dactylitis, we started treatment for undifferentiated spondyloarthropathy associated with pyoderma gangrenosum. The patient was initially started on solumedrol 120 mg intravenously for 3 days followed by tapering doses of prednisone in combination with sulfasalazine. There was poor response after 6 weeks; thus, prednisone was discontinued and azathioprine was added to sulfasalazine. Azathioprine 100 mg daily and sulfasalazine 1000 mg twice daily were continued for 8 weeks with minimal response. In fact, the lower extremities ulcerations coalesced and increased in circumference. Due to lack of response to corticosteroids, sulfasalazine and azathioprine, he was subsequently started on adalimumab 40 mg subcutaneously every 14 days. Within four weeks, there was significant improvement (Figure 4). Unfortunately, we do not have pictures of complete healing as the patient moved out of state and subsequently did not follow-up. Written consent was obtained from the patient to publish his case and case-related imaging.

3. Discussion

Pyoderma gangrenosum can have many different clinical presentations with varying degrees of severity. Clinically, it can present as classic or ulcerative subtype, bullous, pustular, vegetative, drug-induced, postsurgical, or peristomal types [2]. Our patient had clinical manifestations compatible with classic or ulcerative pyoderma gangrenosum with two distinct phases. The ulcerative phase in this patient consisted of an initial pustule that rapidly progressed to a necrotic center with erythematous, irregular, and undermined edges, associated with severe pain. The healing stage consisted of projections of epithelium extending into the center of the ulcer, termed Gulliver's sign [2]. Gulliver's sign can be seen in Figures 4(c) and 4(d). While lower extremity involvement in pyoderma gangrenosum is common, head and neck involvement is quite rare [3]. Our patient had both lower extremity, head, and neck involvement. In fact, Ashchyan et al. completed a retrospective cohort study and found that lower extremity involvement can be found in 62% of patients, as opposed to head or neck involvement which occurs in 5% of pyoderma gangrenosum cases [3]. Despite this fact, multiple case reports have been published where head and neck involvement was the only presenting clinical feature of pyoderma gangrenosum [4–10]. In fact, Yco et al. reported a

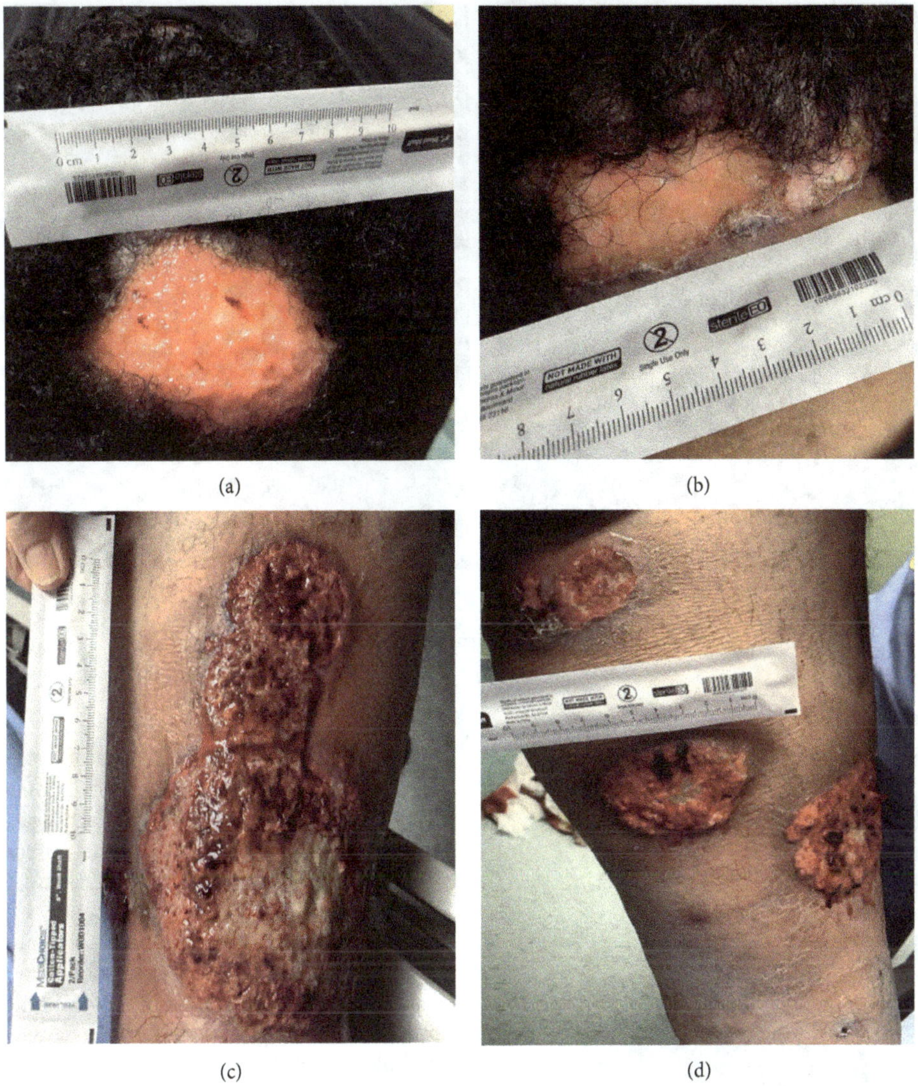

Figure 1: Ulcerations on initial presentation. (a) Vertex of the scalp. (b) Base of the posterior neck. (c) Right lower extremity. (d) Left lower extremity.

case similar to our patient with neck, lower extremity, and oral pyoderma gangrenosum in a patient with a background history of inflammatory bowel disease [10].

The exact pathophysiology of pyoderma gangrenosum is poorly understood but is believed to be a combination of genetics, irregular activation of inflammasomes, and both innate and adaptive immune systems [11]. There is a variety of disorders associated with pyoderma gangrenosum, and review of literature revealed that the most commonly associated condition is inflammatory bowel disease [2, 3, 10]. Other associated conditions with pyoderma gangrenosum include rheumatoid arthritis, seronegative arthritis, psoriatic arthritis, ankylosing spondylitis, solid organ malignancies, myelodysplasia, monoclonal gammopathy, polycythemia vera, hidradenitis suppurativa, PAPA syndrome (pyogenic arthritis, pyoderma gangrenosum, and acne syndrome), PASH syndrome (pyogenic sterile arthritis, pyoderma gangrenosum, and acne syndrome), and PA-PASH syndrome (pyogenic arthritis, pyoderma gangrenosum, acne and suppurative hidradenitis syndrome) [2]. Other case reports with suggested associations with pyoderma gangrenosum include sarcoidosis [12, 13], Sjogren's syndrome [14], systemic lupus erythematosus [15–18], Behcet's disease [19], thyroid disease [15, 20], autoimmune hepatitis [7, 21], takayasu arteritis [21], HIV [22], and cryoglobulinemia [14, 23]. Ashchyan et al. completed a cohort study of patients with pyoderma gangrenosum to determine frequency of associated conditions [3]. Specific to spondyloarthropathies, inflammatory bowel disease was associated with pyoderma gangrenosum in 41% of patients, ankylosing spondylitis in 0.6%, and psoriatic arthritis in 2.2% of patients in their cohort [3]. Unique to our case is that the patient did not have any associated inflammatory bowel disease, as colonoscopy biopsies revealed normal mucosa, and instead he had features of undifferentiated spondyloarthropathy with syndesmophytes, dactylitis, and erosive inflammatory arthritis. The incidental discovery of syndesmophytes on a CT scan did not establish a diagnosis of spondyloarthropathy in our

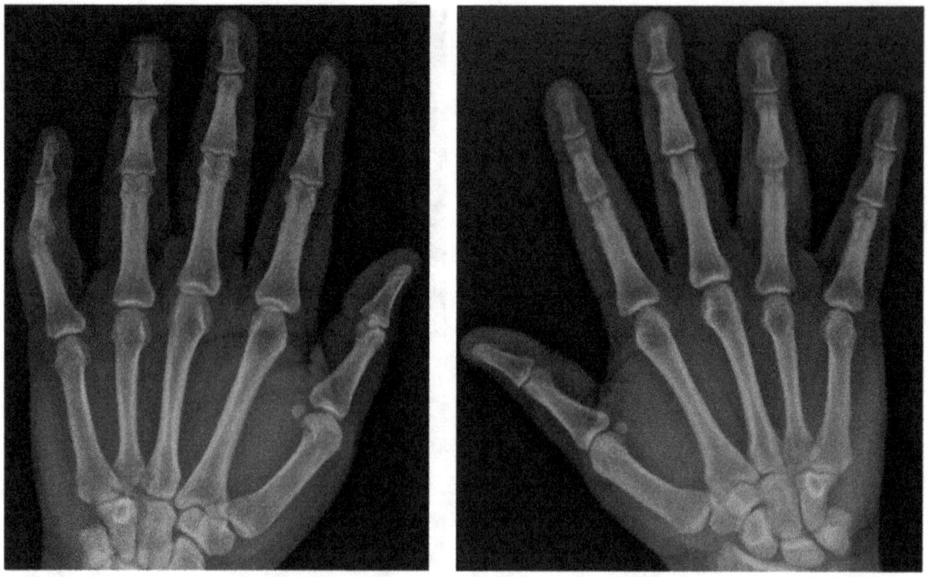

(a) (b)

FIGURE 2: (a) X-ray of the left hand with erosive changes at the 5th PIP joint. (b) X-ray of the right hand with erosive changes at the 2nd and 4th PIP joints.

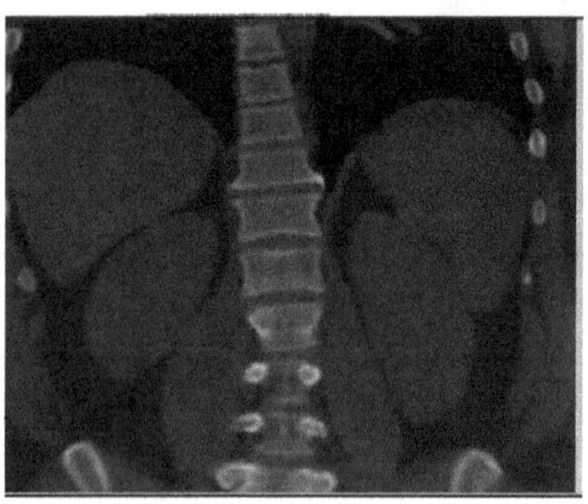

FIGURE 3: CT enterography revealing jug-like syndesmophytes at T12 and L1, suggestive of spondyloarthropathy.

patient; however, on ultrasound examination, there was evidence of enthesitis and periostitis at regions where our patient had severe pain and marginal erosions on X-ray. Evidence of enthesitis is a characteristic feature of spondyloarthropathy and thus helped establish a diagnosis of undifferentiated spondyloarthropathy. Inflammatory arthritis has been associated with pyoderma gangrenosum in 20 to 37 percent of cases based on different cohort studies [3, 15]. Ashchyan et al. completed a retrospective cohort study and found that a diagnosis of arthritis preceded pyoderma gangrenosum in 20% of patients [3]. Of these cases, 41% had rheumatoid arthritis, 11% had psoriatic arthritis, 3% had ankylosing spondylitis, and 45% had an unspecified inflammatory arthritis [3].

The diagnosis of pyoderma gangrenosum is challenging, as it is ultimately a diagnosis of exclusion. Su et al. have proposed diagnostic criteria for pyoderma gangrenosum and require two major and two out of four minor criteria to establish the diagnosis [24]. Major criteria include rapid progression of painful, necrolytic, cutaneous ulcer with an irregular violaceous border and exclusion of other causes of cutaneous ulceration [24]. Minor criteria include history suggestive of pathergy or clinical findings of cribriform scarring, systemic diseases associated with pyoderma gangrenosum, compatible histopathological findings, and response to treatment [24]. Our patient met both of the two major criteria, and all four of the minor criteria were proposed as diagnostic criteria by Su et al. [24]. Histopathologic findings included in these diagnostic criteria consist of sterile dermal neutrophilia with or without mixed inflammation and with or without lymphocytic vasculitis [24]. Pyoderma gangrenosum can be associated with pathergy in one-third of patients [25]. Pathergy refers to an overwhelming skin injury with minor skin trauma [25]. Our patient denied any history of trauma or surgery prior to the development of his ulcers, and thus his clinical features were not suggestive of pathergy.

Treatment of these cutaneous ulcerations is based upon the severity and the associated medical conditions. Although a direct association between severity of an associated condition and pyoderma gangrenosum has not been established, it is important that medications ideally be used that are beneficial for both conditions. Limited disease can be managed with wound care, topical, and intralesional therapy, whereas aggressive disease requires systemic immunomodulatory agents. However, no gold standard treatment exists as there are limited randomized controlled trials [25]. Topical agents can be used for ulcerations that are less than 2 cm [2], including corticosteroids, tacrolimus, sodium cromoglycate, dapsone, nicotine, and 5-aminosalicylic acid [25]. Systemic corticosteroids are first line for severe disease as either oral prednisone (0.5–1 mg/kg/day) or pulse

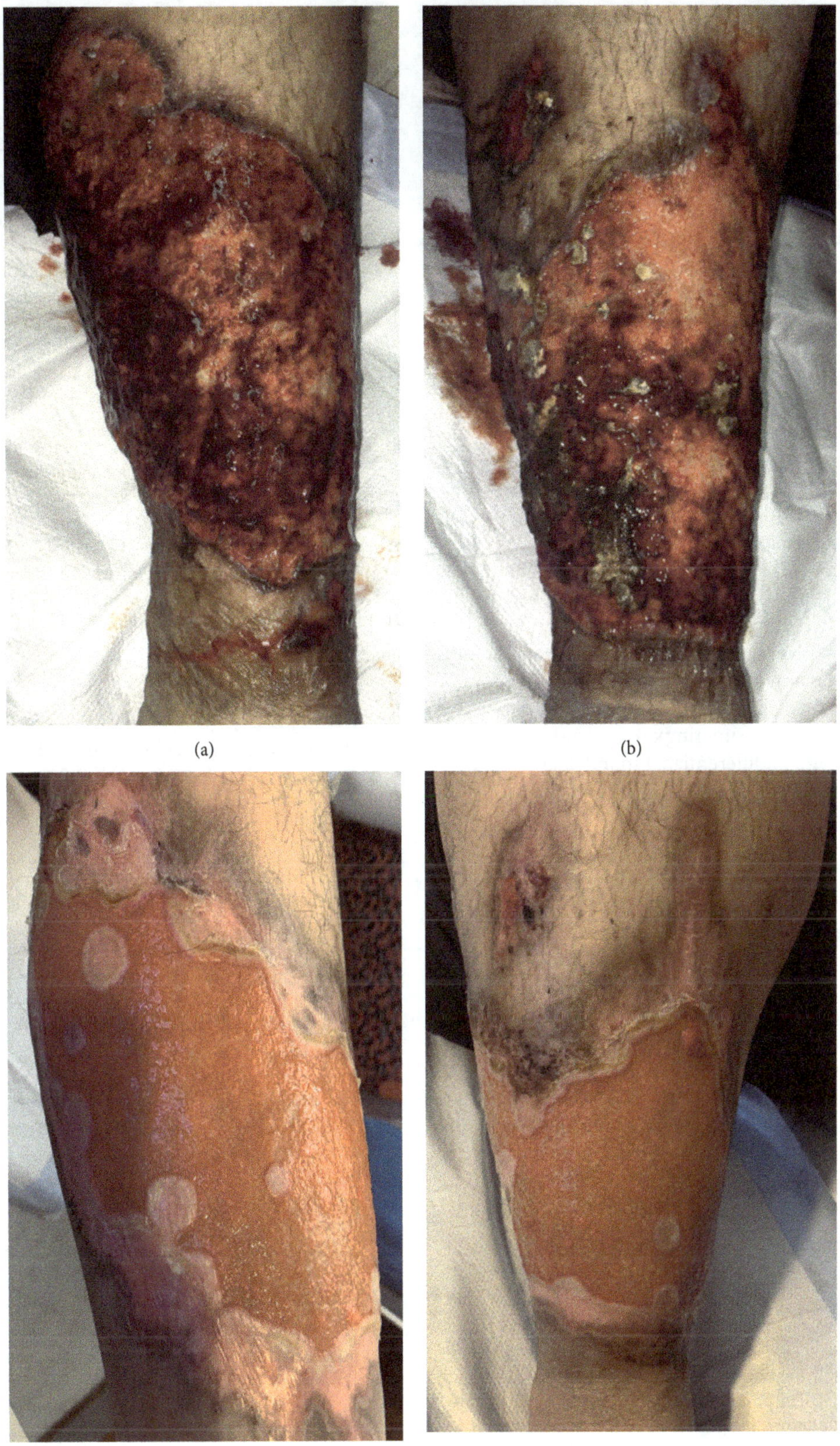

FIGURE 4: (a, b) Bilateral lower extremities prior to adalimumab initiation. (c, d) Bilateral lower extremities 4 weeks after Adalimumab treatment.

intravenous methylprednisone 1000 mg/day [25]. Other systemic agents that can be added with steroid-sparing benefits include cyclosporine, tacrolimus, thalidomide, colchicine, dapsone, sulfasalazine, azathioprine, methotrexate, mycophenolate, cyclophosphamide, chlorambucil, minocycline, IVIG, anti-TNFs, anti-interleukin-1, anti-interleukin-12, and anti-interleukin-23 agents [25]. Our patient was given corticosteroids and then transitioned to sulfasalazine and azathioprine but did not respond. Subsequently, adalimumab was started and the patient had a drastic response within 4 weeks (Figure 4).

Initially, sulfasalazine was started for our patient's pyoderma gangrenosum as there was suspicion for an associated inflammatory bowel disease, and colonoscopy had not been completed at this point. Subsequently after minimal response, azathioprine was added as a mild immunosuppressant because our patient was considered high risk for infection with his large, open wounds. However, he did not respond. Finally, adalimumab was started instead of other longer-acting biologics such as infliximab. We preferred adalimumab as it is dosed every two weeks and thus has a shorter half-life, in case the medication had to be discontinued in the future due to an infection. Our indication for an anti-TNF agent was our patient's refractory pyoderma gangrenosum and enthesitis seen on ultrasound examination. The final diagnosis for our patient was pyoderma gangrenosum with superimposed pseudomonas infection associated with undifferentiated spondyloarthropathy.

4. Conclusion

Traditionally, pyoderma gangrenosum is commonly associated with inflammatory bowel disease, but this was not the case in our patient. He initially sought out treatment for ulcerations from pyoderma gangrenosum and then was subsequently found to have erosive inflammatory arthritis and undifferentiated axial spondyloarthropathy. This is suggestive of spondyloarthritis possibly going underdiagnosed and subsequently untreated in other patients with pyoderma gangrenosum. Thus, even though axial spondyloarthropathy may be rarely associated with pyoderma gangrenosum, it should be kept as an associated differential diagnosis when faced with pyoderma gangrenosum.

References

[1] E. Ruocco, S. Sangiuliano, A. G. Gravina, A. Miranda, and G. Nicoletti, "Pyoderma gangrenosum: an updated review," *Journal of the European Academy of Dermatology and Venereology*, vol. 23, no. 9, pp. 1008–1017, 2009.

[2] I. Ahronowitz, J. Harp, and K. Shinkai, "Etiology and management of pyoderma gangrenosum," *American Journal of Clinical Dermatology*, vol. 13, no. 3, pp. 191–211, 2012.

[3] H. J. Ashchyan, D. C. Butler, C. A. Nelson et al., "The association of age with clinical presentation and comorbidities of pyoderma gangrenosum," *JAMA Dermatology*, vol. 154, no. 4, pp. 409–413, 2018.

[4] R. E. Kleinfelder, N. Hin, S. Cubelli, A. Snyder, F. Kerdel, and B. Glick, "Multiple facial lesions of recalcitrant pyoderma gangrenosum successfully treated with adalimumab," *The Journal of Clinical and Aesthetic Dermatology*, vol. 12, no. 12, pp. 28–32, 2019.

[5] H. S. Chae, S. M. Han, H. N. Lee, H. J. Jeon, and Y. J. Seo, "Pyoderma gangrenosum of the preauricular area with ulcerative colitis: a case report and review," *Journal of Audiology and Otology*, vol. 22, no. 4, pp. 248–252, 2018.

[6] C. Bissonnette, A. Kauzman, and G. N. Mainville, "Oral pyoderma gangrenosum: diagnosis, treatment and challenges: a systematic review," *Head and Neck Pathology*, vol. 11, no. 4, pp. 427–441, 2017.

[7] B. McConnell, M. S. Said, and V. R. Ramakrishnan, "Nasal septal perforation associated with pyoderma gangrenosum," *Allergy & Rhinology*, vol. 6, no. 2, 2015.

[8] D. H. Kim, J.-H. Oh, J. J. Lee, and H. J. Kim, "A case of pyoderma gangrenosum on the nasal dorsum," *Archives of Otolaryngology-Head & Neck Surgery*, vol. 136, no. 2, pp. 193–196, 2010.

[9] C. Wittekindt, J.-C. Lüers, J.-P. Klussmann, and K.-B. Hüttenbrink, "Pyoderma gangrenosum in the head and neck," *Archives of Otolaryngology-Head & Neck Surgery*, vol. 133, no. 1, pp. 83–85, 2007.

[10] M. S. Yco, G. R. Warnock, J. C. Cruickshank, and J. R. Burnett, "Pyoderma gangrenosum involving the head and neck," *The Laryngoscope*, vol. 98, no. 7, pp. 765–768, 1988.

[11] S. F. Braswell, T. C. Kostopoulos, and A. G. Ortega-Loayza, "Pathophysiology of pyoderma gangrenosum (PG): an updated review," *Journal of the American Academy of Dermatology*, vol. 73, no. 4, pp. 691–698, 2015.

[12] F. C. Powell, A. L. Schroeter, W. D. Su, and H. O. Perry, "Pyoderma gangrenosum and sarcoidosis," *Archives of Dermatology*, vol. 120, no. 7, pp. 959-960, 1984.

[13] P. A. Eaton and J. P. Callen, "Mycophenolate mofetil as therapy for pyoderma gangrenosum," *Archives of Dermatology*, vol. 145, no. 7, pp. 781–785, 2009.

[14] R. B. Mlika, I. Riahi, S. Fenniche et al., "Pyoderma gangrenosum: a report of 21 cases," *International Journal of Dermatology*, vol. 41, no. 2, pp. 65–68, 2002.

[15] F. C. Powell, A. L. Schroeter, W. P. Su, and H. O. Perry, "Pyoderma gangrenosum: a review of 86 patients," *QJM: An International Journal of Medicine*, vol. 55, no. 2, pp. 173–186, 1985.

[16] A. K. Kole and A. Ghosh, "Cutaneous manifestations of systemic lupus erythematosus in a tertiary referral center," *Indian Journal of Dermatology*, vol. 54, no. 2, p. 132, 2009.

[17] D. O. Hasselmann, G. Bens, W. Tilgen, and J. Reichrath, "Pyoderma gangrenosum: clinical presentation and outcome in 18 cases and review of the literature," *JDDG*, vol. 5, no. 7, pp. 560–564, 2007.

[18] S. P. Masatlıoğlu, F. Göktay, A. T. Mansur, A. D. Akkaya, and P. Güneş, "Systemic lupus erythematosus presenting as pyoderma gangrenosum in two cases," *Rheumatology International*, vol. 29, no. 7, pp. 837–840, 2009.

[19] H. F. S. Fonseka, S. M. B. Ekanayake, and M. Dissanayake, "Two percent topical phenytoin sodium solution in treating pyoderma gangrenosum: a cohort study," *International Wound Journal*, vol. 7, no. 6, pp. 519–523, 2010.

[20] C. Livideanu, D. Lipsker, C. Paul, J. Juillard, and B. Schubert, "Pyoderma gangrenosum as initial manifestation of Graves' disease," *Clinical and Experimental Dermatology*, vol. 31, no. 5, pp. 659–661, 2006.

[21] J. P. H. Byrne, M. Hewitt, and R. Summerly, "Pyoderma gangrenosum associated with active chronic hepatitis," *Archives of Dermatology*, vol. 112, no. 9, pp. 1297–1301, 1976.

[22] A. S. Paller, E. E. Sahn, P. D. Garen, R. L. Dobson, and E. G. Chadwick, "Pyoderma gangrenosum in pediatric ac-

quired immunodeficiency syndrome," *The Journal of Pediatrics*, vol. 117, no. 1, pp. 63–66, 1990.

[23] P. Driesch, "Pyoderma gangrenosum: a report of 44 cases with follow-up," *British Journal of Dermatology*, vol. 137, no. 6, pp. 1000–1005, 1997.

[24] W. P. D. Su, M. D. P. Davis, R. H. Weenig, F. C. Powell, and H. O. Perry, "Pyoderma gangrenosum: clinicopathologic correlation and proposed diagnostic criteria," *International Journal of Dermatology*, vol. 43, no. 11, pp. 790–800, 2004.

[25] A. Alavi, L. E. French, M. D. Davis, A. Brassard, and R. S. Kirsner, "Pyoderma gangrenosum: an update on pathophysiology, diagnosis and treatment," *American Journal of Clinical Dermatology*, vol. 18, no. 3, pp. 355–372, 2017.

7

Microscopic Polyangiitis with Pulmonary Fibrosis: An Often-Recognized Manifestation of the Disease

Liam M. Clifford,[1] **Jamma Li**,[2,3,4] **Christopher J. Renaud**,[5] **and Suran L. Fernando**[2,3,4]

[1]*Department of General Medicine, Gosford Hospital, Gosford, NSW, Australia*
[2]*Department of Clinical Immunology and Allergy, Royal North Shore Hospital, Sydney, NSW, Australia*
[3]*Immunorheumatology Laboratory, New South Wales Health Pathology, Royal North Shore Hospital, Sydney, NSW, Australia*
[4]*University of Sydney, Sydney, NSW, Australia*
[5]*Department of Anatomical Pathology, Royal North Shore Hospital, Sydney, NSW, Australia*

Correspondence should be addressed to Liam M. Clifford; liamclifford@live.co.uk

Academic Editor: Gregory J. Tsay

Background. Microscopic polyangiitis (MPA) can manifest with atypical features such as pulmonary fibrosis and chronic obstructive pulmonary disease (COPD), which are atypical and unusual features of small vessel vasculitis. *Case Presentation.* This paper presents two patients with microscopic polyangiitis and respiratory symptoms attributable to atypical pulmonary manifestations. Pulmonary fibrosis was present in both cases, with COPD also present in one patient. Management involved methylprednisone, prednisone, and cyclophosphamide. The second patient also received azathioprine. Both patients responded well to immunosuppressive treatment; however, pulmonary fibrosis and COPD were refractory to immunosuppression. *Conclusion.* Pulmonary manifestations including pulmonary fibrosis, emphysema, and bronchiectasis are observed in MPA. Evaluation of MPA in unexplained cases should be performed to avoid delays in diagnosis and management. Patients who present with MPA with pulmonary manifestations may respond to treatment, but their pulmonary features demonstrate a refractory nature to such management.

1. Background

Microscopic polyangiitis (MPA) as defined by the Chapel Hill Consensus Conference criteria 2012 is a pauci-immune necrotizing systemic small vessel vasculitis usually associated with the presence anti-neutrophil cytoplasmic antibodies (ANCA) and anti-myeloperoxidase (MPO) antibodies [1]. Other pauci-immune vasculitides include granulomatosis with polyangiitis (GPA) and eosinophilic granulomatosis with polyangiitis (EGPA). In contrast to these other entities, MPA does not involve granulomatous inflammation. The European Medicines Agency (EMA) algorithm [2] established the criteria for MPA by firstly excluding EGPA by either the American College of Rheumatology (ACR) criteria (4 of 6 criteria comprising asthma, >10% eosinophils on the differential leukocyte count, mononeuropathy (including multiplex) or polyneuropathy, migratory or transient pulmonary opacities detected radiographically, paranasal sinus abnormality, and biopsy containing a blood vessel showing the accumulation of eosinophils in extravascular areas) [3] or the Lanham criteria (presence of asthma, peak eosinophilia $>1.5\times10^9$/L, and systemic vasculitis in ≥2 extrapulmonary sites) [4]. Then, secondly excluding GPA by the CHCC definition (necrotizing granulomatous inflammation usually involving the upper and lower respiratory tract and necrotizing vasculitis affecting predominantly small to medium vessels) and the ACR criteria (presence of 2 of 4 criteria comprising nasal or oral inflammation, abnormal chest radiograph showing nodules, fixed infiltrates, or cavities, abnormal urinary sediment, granulomatous inflammation on biopsy of an artery or perivascular area, or positive ANCA in the absence of a biopsy). These algorithms do not reliably differentiate between GPA and MPA in all patients;

the defining pathological difference between GPA and MPA is the presence of granulomatous changes on biopsy which may be missed due to the sampling error; there is overlap in the clinical features and in the ANCA serologies between GPA and MPA, and some patients present initially with manifestations consistent with MPA and subsequently develop features consistent with GPA. The ability to establish a diagnosis is important given the higher rate of relapse with PR3-ANCA vasculitis [5], and the different manifestations associated with each of the vasculitides such as subglottic stenosis in GPA [6] and interstitial lung disease (ILD) in MPA [7] may require different monitoring and therapies. The Diagnostic and Classification of the Systemic Vasculitides (DCVAS) study has proposed a scoring system for MPA with pauci-immune glomerulonephritis scoring +3, p-ANCA or anti-MPO antibody positive +6, fibrosis or interstitial lung disease (ILD) on chest imaging +3, bloody nasal discharge/ulcers/crusting/congestion or blockage/septal defect/perforation −3, c-ANCA or anti-PR3 antibody −1, and eosinophil count $>1\times10^9$/L −4 with a total score of ≥6 needed for classification with a sensitivity 87% and specificity 96% [8].

Despite the difficulties in classification, pulmonary disease is an important manifestation of MPA in addition to constitutional symptoms, glomerulonephritis, peripheral neuropathy, and skin rash. A retrospective chart review of 115 patients in a Western Spain multicentre survey revealed the presence of lung infiltrates in 28% of 74 individuals with MPO-ANCA disease and 16% of 51 individuals with MPA as classified by EMA [9].

Some forms of interstitial lung disease in MPA include pulmonary fibrosis with or without emphysema and are considered atypical manifestations and are usually resistant to conventional therapy for ANCA-associated vasculitis (AAV) [7, 10].

We describe two cases of MPA with pulmonary fibrosis, one with accompanying emphysema to illustrate the pertinent clinical, laboratory, and histological features and the response to treatment.

2. Case Presentation

2.1. Case One. A 64-year-old female presented with significant weight loss over several months (20 kg), a chronic dry cough, exertional dyspnoea, paraesthesiae in her feet and a left foot drop, erythematous maculopapular rash affecting her feet, and peripheral oedema. Her past medical history included hypertension, a previous occipital infarct, pulmonary fibrosis, falls, hypothyroidism, osteoarthritis, and osteopenia and was a previous smoker. There was no history of haemoptysis. Her CXR showed diffuse bronchiectasis in the left lung and the right perihilar region. A high-resolution CT scan demonstrated marked loss of the left lung volume, reduction in hemithorax size, left-sided honey combing, inter- and intralobular septal thickening, traction bronchiectasis, and mediastinal shift to the left in keeping with compensatory right lung hypertrophy. The right lung field also showed fibrotic changes with peripheral nodules affecting predominantly the left upper lobes but also evident in the right middle and lower lobes and diffuse interlobular and intralobular septal thickening with traction bronchiectasis more prominent in the left than right lung. HRCT findings were consistent with usual interstitial pneumonia (UIP) according to the American Thoracic Society (ATS) and the European Respiratory Society (ERS) guidelines (Figure 1).

MRI and angiography of the brain demonstrated punctuate foci of an elevated diffusion signal within the left basal ganglia and the splenium of the corpus callosum as well as the deep temporal and frontal white matter, suggesting a vasculitic process. Additionally, an MRI spine showed loss of normal high signal intensity within the L4/L5 and L5/S1 intervertebral disc spaces, consistent with a degenerative process without nerve root or cord encroachment. Cerebrospinal fluid (CSF) analysis showed normal levels of protein and glucose, an absence of white cells, no culture growth, and no oligoclonal bands. Subsequent nerve conduction studies revealed a severe length-dependent sensorimotor axonal neuropathy, while a sural nerve biopsy demonstrated fibrinoid necrosis and a lymphocytic infiltrate but no evidence of granulomas (Figure 2). Initial respiratory function tests revealed severe restrictive disease with a forced expiratory volume in one second (FEV1)/forced vital capacity (FVC) ratio of 1.15. Her FEV1 was 39.6%, FVC was 37.9%, total lung capacity (TLC) was 45.2%, and diffuse lung capacity for binding carbon monoxide (DLCO) of 40.9% was predicted, respectively. A transthoracic echocardiogram (TTE) showed normal systolic function, no significant valvular disease, and an ejection fraction (EF) of 65%. The subsequent transoesophageal echocardiogram revealed no mural thrombus or signs of pulmonary hypertension. A skin biopsy of the rash demonstrated deep perivascular lymphocytic inflammation with no deposition of immunoglobulins or complement on direct immunofluorescence.

Laboratory investigations revealed a C-reactive protein (CRP) level of 250 mg/L (<5), erythrocyte sedimentation rate (ESR) 84 mm/hr (<15), and perinuclear-ANCA (p-ANCA) (titre 80) with elevated anti-myeloperoxidase (MPO) antibodies of 20 U/mL (<6). Her full blood count (FBC) including the eosinophil count (0.2×10^9/L) was normal. The renal function and urine albumin-creatinine ratio were normal. A diagnosis of microscopic polyangiitis was established with the atypical pulmonary manifestation of pulmonary fibrosis/UIP.

The patient was commenced on intravenous (IV) pulse methylprednisolone 750 mg daily for three days followed by a tapering course of oral prednisone commenced at 1 mg/kg daily. She underwent seven cycles of IV cyclophosphamide over six months before switching to a maintenance therapy of azathioprine 150 mg daily. Prednisone was completely weaned after twelve months. Her maintenance treatment was complicated by an episode of atypical community-acquired pneumonia. She responded to a course of IV ceftriaxone and azithromycin followed by oral amoxicillin/clavulanic acid. Subsequently, the azathioprine was reduced to 100 mg daily. After four years of azathioprine therapy, she remained in remission with near-complete resolution of her left foot drop. A recent anti-MPO antibody level was 10 U/ml. Nerve conduction studies demonstrated resolution of the axonal sensorimotor neuropathy. Her progress CT scans of the chest revealed no change in her pulmonary fibrosis

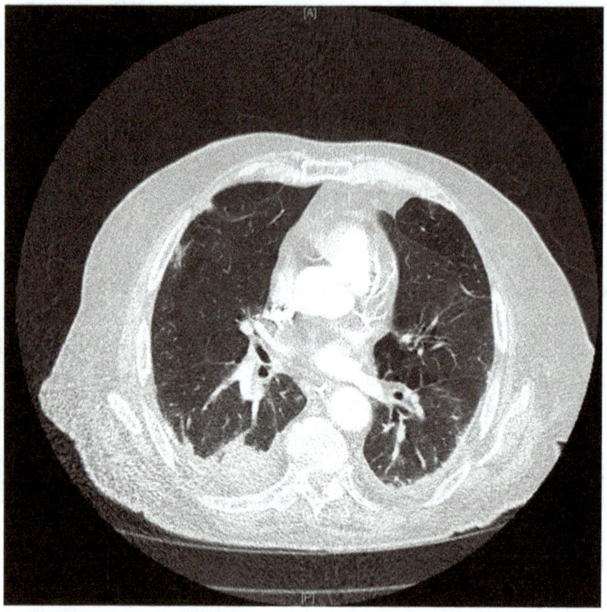

Figure 1: An axial CT chest image of patient 1 demonstrating longstanding bilateral fibrosis and nodular opacities with honey combing and traction bronchiectasis affecting the left lung.

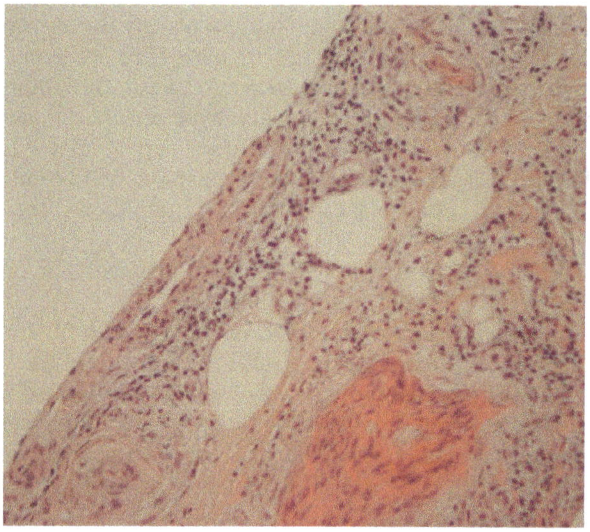

Figure 2: A sural nerve biopsy showing subcutaneous vessels with leukocytoclasis, fibrinoid necrosis, and a perivascular lymphocytic infiltrate (H&E).

and bronchiectasis. Progress respiratory function tests revealed a persistent restrictive pattern with an FEV1/FVC of 91.1 but with an improvement in the FEV1 of 53.6% and FVC of 46.3% predicted, respectively. This appeared consistent with the resolution of her pulmonary nodules. The TLC and DLCO were unchanged. Her progress TTE was normal, in particular there has been no changes suggestive of pulmonary hypertension. Her azathioprine will be slowly weaned over the next year.

2.2. Case Two. A 69-year-old male presented with a six-month history of dyspnoea, anorexia, weight loss (40 kg), and a glove-and-stocking paraesthesia. His past medical history included chronic obstructive pulmonary disease (COPD), ischaemic heart disease, hyperlipidaemia, hypertension, hyperthyroidism, a thyroid nodule, a previous pulmonary embolus, L4/L5 laminectomy, and iron-deficiency anaemia. The patient was an ex-smoker and had previous significant environmental exposure to asbestos. Prior to admission, his colonoscopy was normal whilst a CXR and CT pulmonary angiogram (CTPA) revealed several small (up to 8 mm) spiculated lesions in the right upper lobe, bilateral calcified pleural plaques, bilateral subpleural fibrosis, bilateral subpleural emphysematous change, and a small region of honey combing in the right lower lobe base laterally (Figure 3(a)). HRCT findings were consistent with UIP (ATS/ERS guidelines) and in combination with bronchiectasis, a finding of combined IPF and emphysema (CPFE) was noted. A core biopsy of the right lung lesion demonstrated a mixed inflammatory infiltrate with no evidence of malignancy or asbestos bodies, but cytology revealed giant cells. A CT chest six months later revealed resolution of the spiculated lesions of the right upper lobe, but increase in subpleural fibrosis parenchyma was noted in the previous scan (Figure 3(b)). Respiratory function tests at this time revealed a FEV1/FVC ratio of 1.04, indicating severe restrictive lung disease. A TTE showed normal systolic function, no significant valvular disease, and an EF of 55%. There were no changes suggestive of pulmonary hypertension. The biopsy of the left lung pleura demonstrated macronodular collections of plasma cells, lymphocytes, and histiocytes with histiocytic multinucleated giant cells and foci of young fibrous nodules. No necrotizing granulomas were evident. There were changes of emphysema with plentiful intra-alveolar pigmented histiocytes (Figure 4). Direct immunofluorescence stains were negative for immunoglobulins and complement.

Laboratory investigations revealed a positive p-ANCA (titre 160) and MPO antibodies 90 U/mL (<6). He had normal levels of anti-proteinase 3 antibodies at 2 IU/mL (<6). The remainder of his autoimmune serology: antinuclear, extractable antigen nuclear, antidouble-stranded DNA, anticitrullinated peptide antibodies, and rheumatoid factor and his complement levels (C3, C4) was normal. His CRP level was 58 mg/L (<5) and ESR was 106 mm/hr (<15). FBC showed anaemia with a haemoglobin level of 114 g/L (135–160) and ferritin of 1512 ng/mL (30–300). His eosinophils were normal (0.4×10^9/L).

His CT of the sinuses showed pansinusitis characterised by mucosal thickening without adjacent bone erosion. There was also suspected renal involvement due to 90% dysmorphic red cells in the context of normal renal function with a protein-creatinine ratio of 19 mg/mmol (<30) and a normal renal tract ultrasound.

A diagnosis of AAV was established based on pulmonary giant cell inflammation, dysmorphic haematuria, peripheral neuropathy, and constitutional symptoms in the absence of malignancy. The atypical feature of CPFE was noted on presentation.

Initial management was IV pulse methylprednisone 1 g daily for three days followed by a five-month tapering course of oral prednisone commenced at 1 mg/kg. IV cyclophosphamide was initiated (15 mg/kg every four weeks for six months). Following the completion of the prednisone, he was commenced on azathioprine 150 mg daily.

He responded well to treatment with resolution of his constitutional symptoms and peripheral neuropathy. A repeat

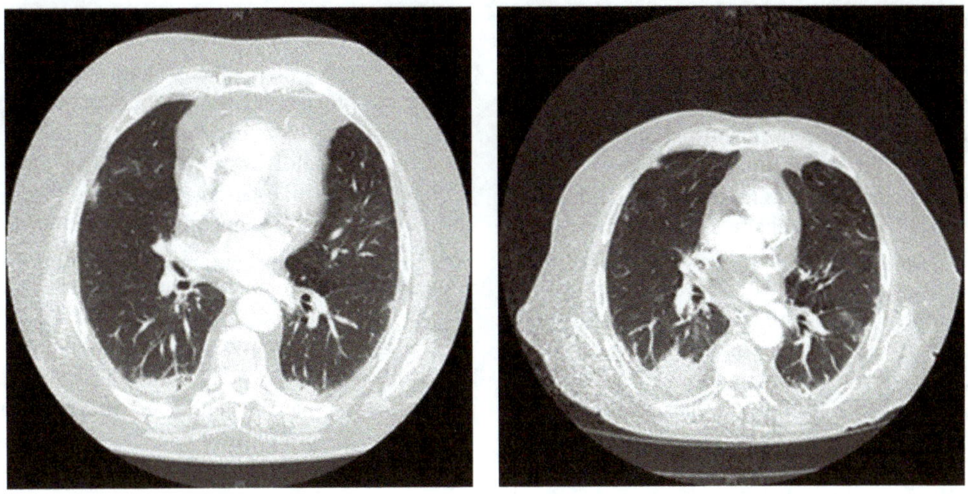

(a) (b)

FIGURE 3: (a) CT pulmonary angiogram of patient 2 reveals bilateral calcified pleural plaques, subpleural fibrosis, paraseptal emphysematous change, and a small region of honey combing in the right lower lobe base laterally. (b) CT chest six months later revealing interval increase in the size of the consolidation, resolution of the right upper lobe spiculated lesions, and stable pulmonary fibrosis.

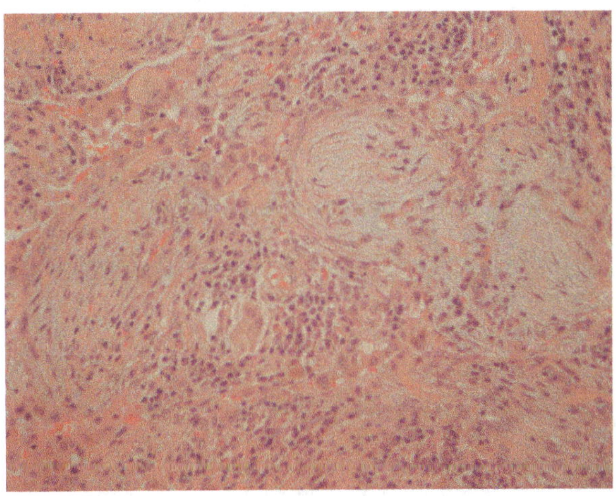

FIGURE 4: Left lung biopsy of patient two showed subpleural proliferative fibroblastic foci and a nodular infiltrate of plasma cells, histiocytes, and multinucleated giant cells.

CT chest performed following cyclophosphamide therapy and three months of azathioprine therapy revealed resolution of parenchymal airspace opacities but stable pleural plaques. He had a normal repeat TTE. There was normalisation of CRP, anti-MPO antibody, haemoglobin, and ferritin levels.

3. Discussion

Our two cases demonstrated the clinical, laboratory, and histological features of MPA with accompanying atypical pulmonary disease.

Diffuse alveolar haemorrhage secondary to pulmonary capillaritis is the most frequently described respiratory manifestation of MPA [11]. However, PF is becoming increasingly appreciated as a manifestation of the disease. A Greek study showed 39% of 33 patients with MPA followed for a median period of 13 months had PF with only one of these patients developing this feature after presentation [7]. A retrospective review over 15 years of an Argentinian cohort with MPA revealed 9 of 28 (32%) patients had PF. Five of these patients had clinical symptoms related to their fibrosis prior to the development of their manifestations of vasculitis by up to 108 months [12]. In a retrospective study of 61 consecutive Japanese patients with an initial diagnosis of IPF, MPO-ANCA was positive in 3 patients (5%) and MPO-ANCA positive conversion occurred in 6 patients (10%), of whom 2 developed manifestations of MPA [13]. In a Japanese retrospective study of 31 patients with pulmonary fibrosis and MPO-ANCA, the histopathological features were analyzed in 15 patients with 13 patients demonstrating interstitial fibrosis extending from the alveolar walls to the proximal interstitial tissues and interlobular septa. Honeycomb lesions were detected in 12 cases. Evidence of vasculitis was found in 8 cases [14], but this finding was not evident in another Japanese study consisting of 9 patients [13].

The pathogenesis of IPF is yet to be fully elucidated, but a number of possibilities exist. Recurrent alveolar haemorrhage including subclinical alveolar bleeding due to pulmonary capillaritis could result in pulmonary fibrosis [15]. MPO-ANCA may play a direct role in the pathogenesis of pulmonary fibrosis. Oxidative stress through the production of hypochlorous acid from the interaction of MPO with anti-MPO antibodies may trigger the fibrosis. IPF may induce ANCA during the chronic inflammation process as a result of neutrophil destruction accounting for the extent of IPF seen at presentation of MPA [7]. There is speculation that tobacco smoke exposure may be involved in the pathogenesis of PF by activating and stimulating MPO expression on epithelial cells. A Japanese retrospective study of 9 patients with PF and MPO-ANCA were all smokers [13]. Exposure to tobacco leads to macrophage activation and neutrophil recruitment, with consequent elastin and collagen breakdown, and subsequent accelerated matrix destruction and emphysema [16]. A Japanese study multicentre longitudinal retrospective CT imaging study comprising 150 hospital patients with MPA revealed 7% of patients had PF and 4% had CPFE [17]. Although 34% of this cohort had a history of smoking, it is unclear whether this to the PF and CPFE patients. However, Cottin et al. showed that combined PF and emphysema (CPFE) occurs independently of smoking in connective tissue diseases such as rheumatoid arthritis and systemic sclerosis [18]. CPFE, characteried by dyspnoea, upper-lobe emphysema, lower-lobe fibrosis, and abnormalities of gas exchange, is complicated by pulmonary hypertension, acute lung injury, and lung cancer and associated with high mortality rates (median survival rates 2.1 to 8.5 years) [19]. One-year survival rate for those with pulmonary hypertension confirmed by right heart catheterization is 60% [20]. IPF without coexistent emphysema confers a worse prognosis. In a Japanese retrospective study of 31 patients with pulmonary fibrosis and MPO-ANCA, the 5-year survival rate of 50% was comparable to those with idiopathic pulmonary fibrosis and worse than patients with MPO-ANCA-negative pulmonary fibrosis with collagen vascular diseases [14]. The causes of death include progressive respiratory failure and its complications (pulmonary haemorrhage, and pneumonia) as well as lung cancer. PF increases the risk of lung malignancy, mainly non-small-cell lung cancer, by 7–20% [21].

Current EULAR/ERA-EDTA recommendations for the induction of remission in organ-threatening AAV involve high-dose corticosteroids and IV cyclophosphamide or rituximab for three to six months [22]. Once remission is induced, azathioprine, methotrexate, or rituximab is continued for a minimum of 2 years. The recent findings of the RITAZAREM randomized control study involved 170 patients with AAV who experienced a relapse and then achieved remission during 4 months of induction therapy with rituximab and corticosteroids, and rituximab demonstrated that maintenance with rituximab 1 g every 4 months was superior in the prevention of relapse than azathioprine 2 mg/kg daily (13 vs. 38%) [23]. Specific therapy for AAV patients with PF is not well established, and further studies are required. A French retrospective multicentre study including 49 patients with AAV and PF demonstrated that the 3-year survival rate in patients initially treated with cyclophosphamide or rituximab combined with corticosteroids was superior to patients treated with corticosteroids alone (94% vs. 64%, $P = 0.03$) [24]. It remains to be determined whether pirfenidone, an antifibrotic agent that inhibits transforming growth factor-beta-stimulated collagen synthesis, extracellular matrix deposition, and fibroblast proliferation, or nintedanib, a receptor blocker for multiple tyrosine kinases that mediate elaboration of fibrogenic growth factors, will be efficacious in these patients. These agents appear to slow disease progression [25, 26] and decrease mortality rates [27, 28] in patients with IPF.

This report comprises two patients, but we aim to alert clinicians to the atypical pulmonary features of MPA that are chronic, resistant to conventional immunosuppression, and are associated with a poor prognosis due to progressive respiratory insufficiency and associated complications such as pulmonary haemorrhage, pneumonia, and lung cancer. Further studies are required to elucidate optimal treatment for patients with AAV and their treatment resistant-pulmonary manifestations.

4. Conclusion

MPA presents with a systemic and nonspecific symptom and can mimic other vasculitides. Laboratory tests including ANCA are useful for evaluating suspected vasculitis. It is important that a confirmatory tissue diagnosis of AAV is established. Pulmonary manifestations including fibrosis, CPFE, and bronchiectasis are frequently associated with MPA, but the underlying mechanisms require further elucidation. Recognition of these manifestations as a feature of the patient's vasculitis may avoid a delay in the diagnosis and implementation of appropriate therapy. Such manifestations are treatment-resistant to conventional immunosuppression for AAV, and further studies are required to determine other treatment modalities to reverse these changes in symptomatic patients.

Abbreviations

AAV: ANCA-associated vasculitides
ANCA: Anti-neutrophil cytoplasmic antibodies
COPD: Chronic obstructive pulmonary disease
CPFE: Combined pulmonary fibrosis and emphysema
CRP: C-reactive protein
CT: Computed tomography
CXR: Chest X-ray
DLCO: Diffusion capacity for carbon monoxide
EF: Ejection fraction
EGPA: Eosinophilic granulomatosis with polyangiitis
ESR: Erythrocyte sedimentation rate
FBC: Full blood count
FEV1: Functional expiratory volume in 1 second
FVC: Functional vital capacity
GPA: Granulomatosis with polyangiitis
IV: Intravenous
MPA: Microscopic polyangiitis
MPO: Myeloperoxidase
MRI: Magnetic resonance imaging
p-ANCA: Perinuclear anti-neutrophil cytoplasmic antibodies
TLC: Total lung capacity
TTE: Transthoracic echocardiogram.

Authors' Contributions

LMC and SLF developed the concept. JL assisted with case analyses. CJR analyzed the pathology and assisted with interpretation of findings. All four authors edited and approved the final manuscript.

Acknowledgments

The authors would like to acknowledge the Immunology laboratory staff at New South Wales Health Pathology for the performance of autoimmune serology. The authors also thank Dr. Sriram Mahadev, respiratory physician at Royal North Shore Hospital and Dr. Christina Liang, neurologist at Royal North Shore Hospital for their involvement in the investigation and management of one of the patients.

References

[1] J. C. Jennette, R. J. Falk, P. A. Bacon et al., "2012 revised international chapel hill consensus conference nomenclature of vasculitides," *Arthritis & Rheumatism*, vol. 65, no. 1, pp. 1–11, 2013.

[2] R. Watts, S. Lane, T. Hanslik et al., "Development and validation of a consensus methodology for the classification of the ANCA-associated vasculitides and polyarteritis nodosa for epidemiological studies," *Annals of the Rheumatic Diseases*, vol. 66, no. 2, pp. 222–227, 2006.

[3] A. T. Masi, G. G. Hunder, J. T. Lie et al., "The American college of rheumatology 1990 criteria for the classification of Churg-Strauss syndrome (allergic granulomatosis and angiitis)," *Arthritis & Rheumatism*, vol. 33, no. 8, pp. 1094–1100, 2010.

[4] J. G. Lanham, K. B. Elkon, C. D. Pusey, and G. R. Hughes, "Systemic vasculitis with asthma and eosinophilia," *Medicine*, vol. 63, no. 2, pp. 65–81, 1984.

[5] S. L. Hogan, R. J. Falk, H. Chin et al., "Predictors of relapse and treatment resistance in antineutrophil cytoplasmic antibody-associated small-vessel vasculitis," *Annals of Internal Medicine*, vol. 143, no. 9, pp. 621–631, 2005.

[6] C. A. Langford, M. C. Sneller, C. W. Hallahan et al., "Clinical features and therapeutic management of subglottic stenosis in patients with Wegener's granulomatosis," *Arthritis & Rheumatism*, vol. 39, no. 10, pp. 1754–1760, 1996.

[7] G. E. Tzelepis, M. Kokosi, A. Tzioufas et al., "Prevalence and outcome of pulmonary fibrosis in microscopic polyangiitis," *European Respiratory Journal*, vol. 36, no. 1, pp. 116–121, 2010.

[8] J. C. Robson, P. C. Grayson, C. Ponte et al., "OP0021 draft classification criteria for the anca associated vasculitides," *Annals of the Rheumatic Diseases*, vol. 77, no. 2, 2018.

[9] L. Corral-Gudino, E. González-Vázquez, I. Calero-Paniagua et al., "The complexity of classifying ANCA-associated small-vessel vasculitis in actual clinical practice: data from a multicenter retrospective survey," *Rheumatology International*, vol. 64, no. 4, pp. 1–9, 2019.

[10] H. Lin and S. Jiang, "Combined pulmonary fibrosis and emphysema (CPFE): an entity different from emphysema or pulmonary fibrosis alone," *Journal of Thoracic Disease*, vol. 7, no. 4, pp. 767–779, 2015.

[11] L. Guillevin, B. Durand-Gasselin, R. Cevallos et al., "Microscopic polyangiitis: clinical and laboratory findings in eighty-five patients," *Arthritis & Rheumatism*, vol. 42, no. 3, pp. 421–430, 1999.

[12] M. Fernandez Casares, A. Gonzalez, M. Fielli, F. Caputo, Y. Bottinelli, and M. Zamboni, "Microscopic polyangiitis associated with pulmonary fibrosis," *Clinical Rheumatology*, vol. 34, no. 7, pp. 1273–1277, 2015.

[13] M. Ando, E. Miyazaki, T. Ishii et al., "Incidence of myeloperoxidase anti-neutrophil cytoplasmic antibody positivity and microscopic polyangitis in the course of idiopathic pulmonary fibrosis," *Respiratory Medicine*, vol. 107, no. 4, pp. 608–615, 2013.

[14] S. Homma, H. Matsushita, and K. Nakata, "Pulmonary fibrosis in myeloperoxidase antineutrophil cytoplasmic antibody-associated vasculitides," *Respirology*, vol. 9, no. 2, pp. 190–196, 2004.

[15] A. Schnabel, M. Reuter, E. Csernok, C. Richter, and W. L. Gross, "Subclinical alveolar bleeding in pulmonary vasculitides: correlation with indices of disease activity," *European Respiratory Journal*, vol. 14, no. 1, pp. 118–124, 1999.

[16] A. Churg, K. Zay, S. Shay et al., "Acute cigarette smoke-induced connective tissue breakdown requires both neutrophils and macrophage metalloelastase in mice," *American Journal of Respiratory Cell and Molecular Biology*, vol. 27, no. 3, pp. 368–374, 2002.

[17] M. Yamagata, K. Ikeda, K. Tsushima et al., "Prevalence and responsiveness to treatment of lung abnormalities on chest computed tomography in patients with microscopic polyangiitis: a multicenter, longitudinal, retrospective study of one hundred fifty consecutive hospital-based Japanese patients," *Arthritis & Rheumatology*, vol. 68, no. 3, pp. 713–723, 2016.

[18] V. Cottin, H. Nunes, L. Mouthon et al., "Combined pulmonary fibrosis and emphysema syndrome in connective tissue disease," *Arthritis & Rheumatism*, vol. 63, no. 1, pp. 295–304, 2011.

[19] M. D. Jankowich and S. I. S. Rounds, "Combined pulmonary fibrosis and emphysema syndrome," *Chest*, vol. 141, no. 1, pp. 222–231, 2012.

[20] V. Cottin, J. Le Pavec, G. Prevot et al., "Pulmonary hypertension in patients with combined pulmonary fibrosis and emphysema syndrome," *European Respiratory Journal*, vol. 35, no. 1, pp. 105–111, 2010.

[21] B. Ballester, J. Milara, and J. Cortijo, "Idiopathic pulmonary fibrosis and lung cancer: mechanisms and molecular targets," *International Journal of Molecular Sciences*, vol. 20, no. 3, p. 593, 2019.

[22] M. Yates, R. A. Watts, I. M. Bajema et al., "EULAR/ERA-EDTA recommendations for the management of ANCA-associated vasculitis," *Annals of the Rheumatic Diseases*, vol. 75, no. 9, pp. 1583–1594, 2016.

[23] R. Smith, D. Jayne, and P. Merkel, "A randomized, controlled trial of rituximab versus azathioprine after induction of remission with rituximab for patients with ANCA-associated vasculitis and relapsing disease [abstract]," *Arthritis & Rheumatology*, vol. 71, no. 10, 2019.

[24] C. Comarmond, B. Crestani, A. Tazi et al., "Pulmonary fibrosis in antineutrophil cytoplasmic antibodies (ANCA)-associated vasculitis," *Medicine*, vol. 93, no. 24, pp. 340–349, 2014.

[25] G. Raghu, B. Rochwerg, Y. Zhang et al., "An official ATS/ERS/JRS/ALAT clinical practice guideline: treatment of idiopathic pulmonary fibrosis: an update of the 2011 clinical practice guideline," *American Journal of Respiratory and Critical Care Medicine*, vol. 192, no. 2, pp. e3–e19, 2015.

[26] W. G. Carlos, M. E. Strek, T. S. Wang et al., "Treatment of idiopathic pulmonary fibrosis," *Annals of the American Thoracic Society*, vol. 13, no. 1, pp. 115–117, 2016.

[27] W. J. Canestaro, S. H. Forrester, G. Raghu, L. Ho, and B. E. Devine, "Drug treatment of idiopathic pulmonary fibrosis," *Chest*, vol. 149, no. 3, pp. 756–766, 2016.

[28] S. D. Nathan, C. Albera, W. Z. Bradford et al., "Effect of pirfenidone on mortality: pooled analyses and meta-analyses of clinical trials in idiopathic pulmonary fibrosis," *The Lancet Respiratory Medicine*, vol. 5, no. 1, pp. 33–41, 2017.

A Case of Severe Seronegative Inflammatory Arthritis due to Nivolumab and Review of the Literature

Bicky Thapa,[1] **Asad Ali**,[2] **Raunak Nair**,[1] **Rishik Vashisht**,[3] **and Cassandra Calabrese**[4]

[1]*Department of Internal Medicine, Cleveland Clinic Fairview Hospital, Cleveland, Ohio, USA*
[2]*Neurological Institute, Taussig Center Institute, Cleveland Clinic Foundation, Cleveland, Ohio, USA*
[3]*Respiratory Institute, Cleveland Clinic Foundation, Cleveland, Ohio, USA*
[4]*Department of Rheumatic & Immunologic Disease, Cleveland Clinic Foundation, Cleveland, Ohio, USA*

Correspondence should be addressed to Cassandra Calabrese; calabrc@ccf.org

Academic Editor: Suleyman Serdar Koca

Immune-checkpoint inhibitors (ICIs) have revolutionized the treatment of cancer, yet therapy is often hampered by immune-related adverse events (irAEs) which range from mild to severe life-threatening events. Musculoskeletal (MSK) irAEs leading to discontinuation of ICIs are uncommon but increasingly recognized. We report a challenging case of severe immune-related seronegative inflammatory arthritis due to nivolumab in a patient with stage IV metastatic adenocarcinoma.

1. Introduction

Immune-checkpoint inhibitors (ICIs) have increasingly demonstrated promising outcomes which have led to accelerated approval in many advanced malignancies such as metastatic melanoma, metastatic non-small cell lung cancer, urothelial carcinoma, mismatch repair-deficient solid tumors, head and neck squamous cancers, renal cell carcinoma, and Merkel cell carcinoma [1].

Activated or primed cytotoxic CD8+ T cells along with CD4+ helper T cells identify the antigen present on tumor cells which produces interferon and cytotoxin leading to an antitumor activity [2, 3]. Many tumor cells express program cell death ligand 1 (PD-L1). ICIs target ligand expressed on the surface of T cells [4]. Nivolumab, anti-PD-1 human monoclonal antibody, binds to PD-L1, thereby preventing binding of a ligand to T-cell surface receptor program death 1 (PD-1), subsequently leading to the continued activation of an immune response against tumor cells [4]. Additionally, this mechanism will result in an unrestricted immune response which can lead to immune-related adverse effects (irAEs) affecting various organ systems in the body [5]. The immunologic basis of musculoskeletal irAEs has not been completely elucidated.

We report a rare and challenging case of new-onset seronegative inflammatory arthritis complicated by baker cyst rupture during the course of treatment with nivolumab in a patient with stage IV adenocarcinoma.

2. Case Report

A 65-year-old previously healthy male presented with an episode of seizure associated with garbled speech, weakness, and abnormal sensation which on further workup revealed a left frontal brain mass with an unknown etiology which was managed with stereotactic radiosurgery. Whole-body computed tomography (CT) scan showed enlarged lymph nodes in the left supraclavicular area, right hilum, and right aortocaval region. Biopsy of the left supraclavicular lymph node demonstrated poorly differentiated adenocarcinoma with unknown primary; the immune phenotype was not specific and was consistent with metastasis from virtually any visceral organ including lung (pulmonary adenocarcinomas TTF-1 negative 20%). The patient also had elevated CA 19-9, which made it difficult to delineate the primary malignancy site (lung vs. gastrointestinal).

He received six cycles of gemcitabine and carboplatin as first-line therapy; however, restaging scans revealed an increase in lymphadenopathy along with elevated CA 19-9. The patient also received other chemotherapeutic agents (2nd line) but continued to have the progression of the disease. Because of the failure of two lines of chemotherapies, the third line of therapy with nivolumab (3 mg/kg/dose every two weeks) was initiated. The patient reported new onset of mild neuropathy of the hands and feet along with occasional bilateral knee joint pain after two cycles of nivolumab. The joint pain improved on its own; however, the patient continued to have persistent neuropathy. At the time, the differential diagnosis for this patient's neuropathy includes chemotherapy-induced (especially carboplatin), paraneoplastic syndrome, thiamine/B12 deficiency, or nivolumab induced.

The follow-up restaging scan revealed a partial response of the tumor burden after eight cycles of nivolumab. During the course of treatment with nivolumab (after the 10th cycle), the patient also reported fatigue and mild pruritus of hand, which responded to antihistamines.

Subsequently, after the 11th cycle of nivolumab, the clinical course was complicated by joint pain involving knees, elbows, and great toes associated with joint stiffness, swelling, and muscle weakness. Physical examination was significant for left leg swelling along with calf tenderness, and muscle strength was noted to be 5/5 in bilateral knee and ankle joints. Routine blood workup including the liver function test and creatine phosphokinase (CPK) was within the normal range. Ultrasound (US) of the left lower extremity demonstrated a Baker's cyst measuring $3.7 \times 0.9 \times 1.1$ cm (Figure 1(a)) which increased to $8.0 \times 6.5 \times 2.3$ cm (Figure 1(b)) on repeat US four days later. Follow-up US after two weeks revealed cyst rupture with hematoma (Figure 1(c)). At this point, the patient was experiencing severe left knee pain that affected his mobility and quality of life. The patient was also evaluated by orthopedics for the left knee pain and calf swelling, as well as elbow pain and swelling. X-rays revealed unremarkable left knee joint and findings consistent with osteoarthritis of the left elbow (Figure 2).

Based on clinical evaluation and worsening symptoms, the patient was started on prednisone 20 mg twice daily for severe immune-related arthritis with improvement in symptoms. However, on a tapering dose of steroids, the patient had worsening arthritis and neuropathy as well.

The patient reported improvement in arthritis symptoms with an initial dose of prednisone (20 mg twice daily dose) but had an intermittent flare-up of arthritis with a change in weather and exertion.

Rheumatology was consulted and started on weekly oral methotrexate 10 mg (MTX) along with prednisone 10 mg daily. The RAPID-3 score (routine assessment of patient index data 3) [6] was 4.4 on the initial evaluation, indicating low disease severity. Laboratory evaluation revealed a positive antinuclear antibody (ANA) with the titer of 1 : 160 (Table 1); the remainder of autoimmune serology was negative (Table 1).

The patient's joint symptoms were well controlled on MTX and prednisone; however, arthritis worsened upon tapering of prednisone, so MTX dose was increased from 10 to 20 mg weekly. After six months of treatment, his RAPID-3 score was 3.9, prednisone was ultimately tapered off, and hydroxychloroquine and sulfasalazine were added. Five months later, his RAPID-3 was 1.3, and he was off DMARDs and did not experience recurrence of rheumatic irAE.

Although the patient's tumor responded to nivolumab (Figure 3), it was stopped after 12 cycles due to MSK irAE. Unfortunately, the patient had severe inflammatory arthritis which worsened the quality of life due to nivolumab; the shared decision was made not to reintroduce nivolumab (Figure 4).

In summary, our patient had initial irAEs in the form of grade 1 neuropathy and grade 1 inflammatory arthritis which resolved on its own; but subsequently, during the treatment course with anti-PD1, the patient developed fatigue and grade 1 pruritus which improved with an antihistamine. Eventually, our patient had grade 2 inflammatory arthritis based on the recommendations from the society for the immunotherapy of cancer toxicity management working group [7], which was managed with glucocorticoids, DMARDs, and discontinuation of ICI.

3. Discussion

A better understanding of irAEs is crucial to ensure the safety and quality of care for cancer patients. The spectrum of irAEs is quite diverse, and while they have been described in essentially every organ system, the most common irAEs are dermatologic, gastrointestinal, and endocrine toxicities such as hypothyroidism and hypophysitis [5, 8, 9]. Less common but life-threatening toxicities include myocarditis, amongst others [10–12].

Arthralgia and myalgia are the most frequent musculoskeletal (MSK) irAEs and have been reported up to 40% in clinical trials [13–15]. However, severe immune-mediated arthritis is rare and has been described in the literature in the form of case reports and case series [13, 14, 16–21].

MSK irAEs have been manifested in varied clinical forms such as arthralgia, myalgia, myositis, fasciitis, tenosynovitis, mild to severe arthritis, psoriatic arthritis, and polymyalgia rheumatica (PMR) (Table 2). Early recognition of rheumatological irAEs and management by rheumatologists play a crucial role in improving outcomes in patients receiving ICI and the continuation of ICI for the treatment of underlying malignancy [15].

As per the literature review, MSK irAEs have heterogeneous phenotypical presentation, mostly symmetrical polyarthritis associated with synovitis. Clinical manifestation varies from large joint oligoarthritic to polyarthritis involving small joints, sometimes accompanied by reactive symptoms such as conjunctivitis and urethritis [13]. Furthermore, some of the most recent case series also reported myositis and fasciitis due to ICI, broadening the clinical presentations of MSK irAEs [33, 34].

While popliteal (Baker's) cyst has not been specifically described in the literature as being a manifestation of rheumatic irAEs, it is well known that rates of popliteal cysts are higher in the patients with inflammatory arthritis, including rheumatoid arthritis [35].

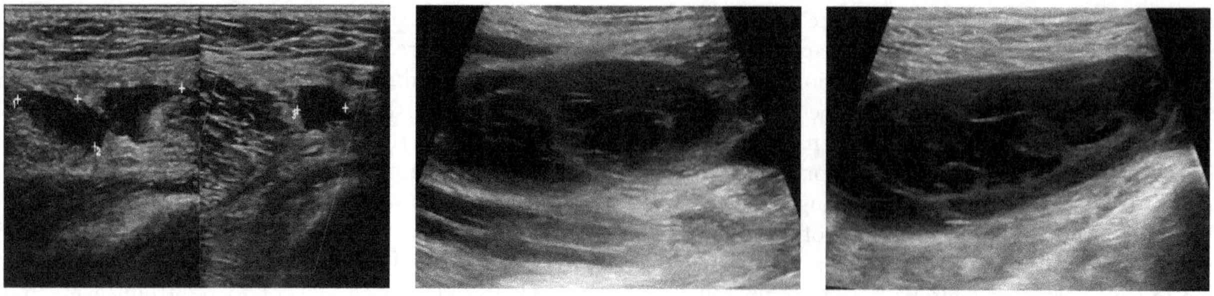

(a) (b) (c)

FIGURE 1: Ultrasound (US) of the left lower extremity: (a) Baker's cyst. (b) Follow-up US showing the increased size of baker's cyst. (c) Image depicting ruptured Baker's cyst.

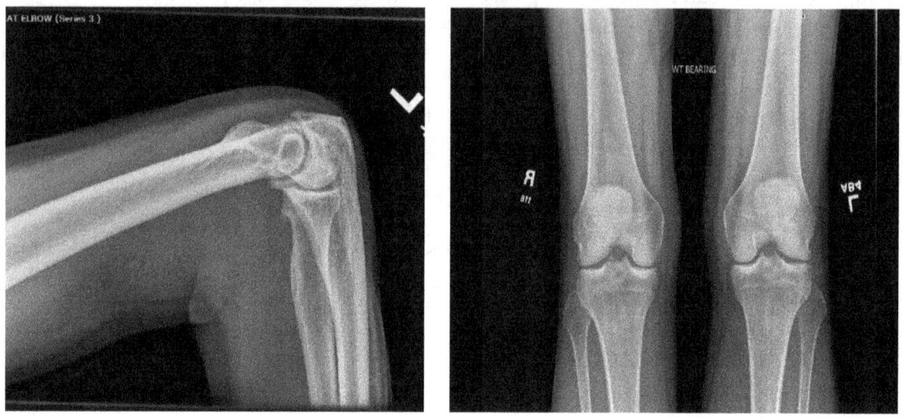

(a) (b)

FIGURE 2: X-ray of the left elbow joint and bilateral knee joints. (a) Moderate osteophytosis at the humeroulnar articulation and involving the radial head with mild joint space narrowing and no joint effusion. (b) Anterior-posterior weight-bearing view; no acute fracture/dislocation, and joint spaces grossly preserved.

TABLE 1: Immunologic workup.

Immunology/serology	Reference range	Result
ANA	Negative	Positive
ANA titer	Negative	1 : 160
ANA pattern	Unknown	Nucleolar
DNA antibody	<30 IU/mL	22
RNP antibody	<1.0	<0.2
Ribosomal RNP	<1.0	<0.2
SSB antibody	<1.0	<0.2
Sm antibody	<1.0	<0.2
SSA antibody	<1.0	<0.2
Scleroderma Ab, IgG	<1.0	<0.2
Jo 1 antibody	<1.0	<0.2
Chromatin antibody	<1.0	<0.2
Centromere Ab	<1.0	<0.2
Rheumatoid factor	<16 IU/mL	<10
CCP antibody, IgG	<20 units	<15

ANA: antinuclear antibody; DNA: deoxyribonucleic acid; RNP: ribonucleoprotein; SSB: anti-Sjögren's syndrome type B; SSA: anti-Sjögren's syndrome type B; Ab: antibody; CCP: cyclic citrullinated peptide; IU: international unit.

Rheumatic auto-antibodies such as rheumatoid factor (RF) and anti-CCP antibody are generally negative [33, 34]; however, there are case series and case reports of seropositive rheumatoid arthritis [26, 27, 30, 32, 33]. Our patient had a low-positive ANA, which was unlikely to be of any clinical significance, as this is a nonspecific test, and his clinical picture was not consistent with an autoimmune connective tissue disease such as systemic lupus erythematosus and the more specific auto-antibodies were negative. To date, there has been no association found between positive ANA and the development of rheumatic irAEs.

It has been observed from most of the case series and case reports, MSK irAEs are more prevalent in the patient population treated with an anti-PD1 single agent than in combination with anti-CTLA-4; only two patient has been found to have inflammatory arthritis after single-agent anti-CTLA-4 [31, 32]. There are rare irAE reports of psoriatic arthritis which responded well to either steroid alone or in combination with synthetic DMARDs [22, 23, 27, 32].

Patients also demonstrated a variable clinical course with unpredictable onset and difference in response to different therapeutic agents such as nonsteroidal anti-inflammatory drugs (NSAIDs), steroid, intraarticular steroid, synthetic, or biologic DMARDs. Most of the patients had a good response with a low to moderate dose of steroid alone, and DMARDs were used to taper off the steroid for better control of the symptoms [25–29, 31, 33, 34]. Moreover, refractory MSK

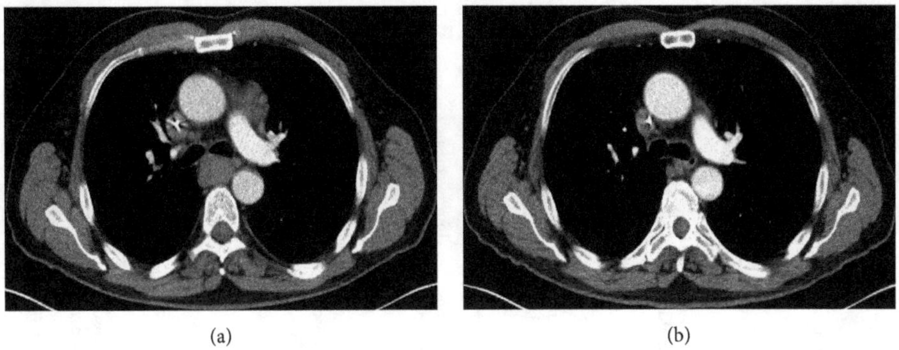

Figure 3: Computed tomography (CT) scan of the chest with contrast before and after nivolumab. (a) CT chest before initiation of nivolumab; an axial image depicting significant mediastinal and right hilar lymphadenopathy. (b) CT chest after 12 cycles of nivolumab; no hilar or mediastinal lymphadenopathy identified.

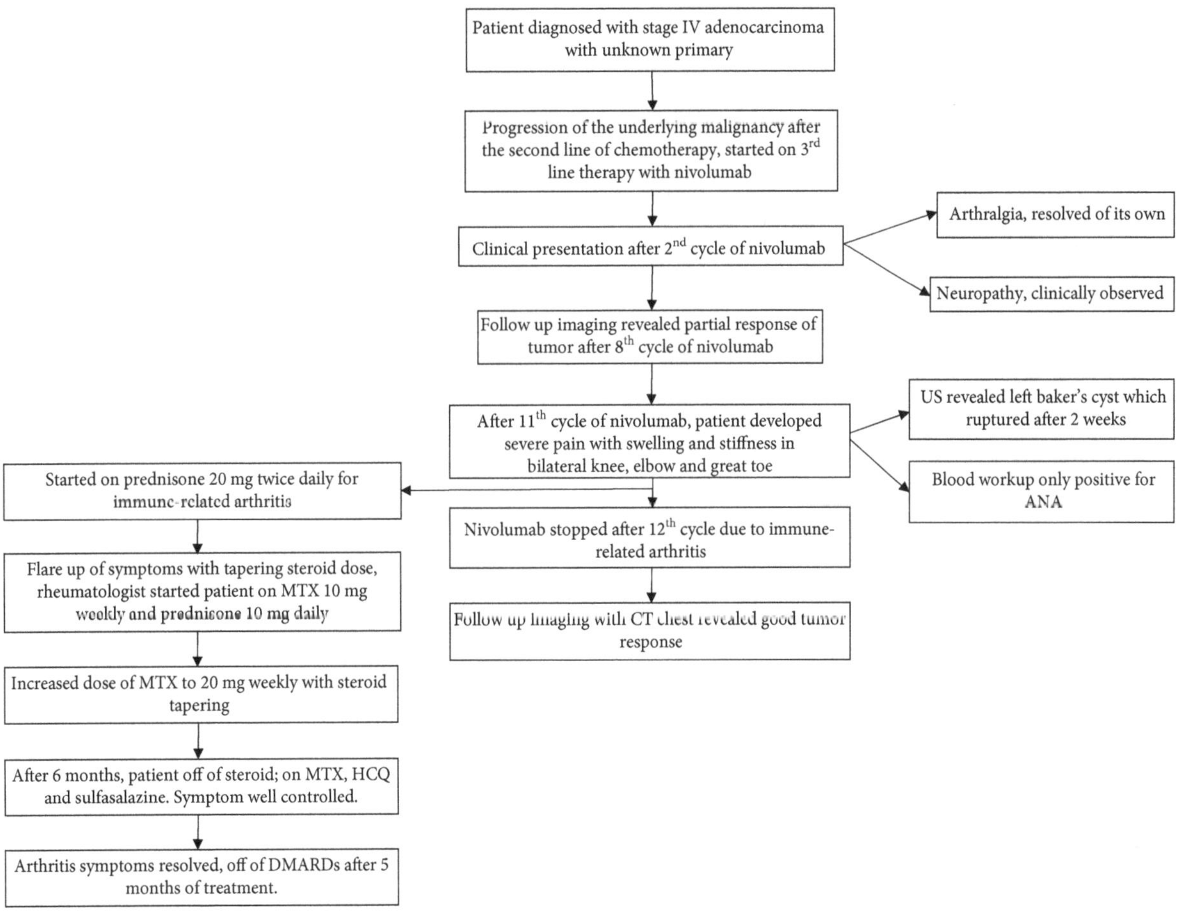

Figure 4: Flowchart illustrating the complete clinical course of the patient. ANA: antinuclear antibody, US: ultrasound, MTX: methotrexate, HCQ: hydroxychloroquine, DMARDs: disease-modifying antirheumatic drugs.

irAEs required biological DMARDs and, in some cases, anti-IL-6 or tumor necrosis factor inhibitor alfa (TNF) with improvement in symptoms [13, 14, 24]. Patients with PMR responded well to steroids with rapid improvement but required TNF alfa inhibitors in one of the cases [14].

Our patient's tumor responded to nivolumab (Figure 3); however, ICI was discontinued due to immune-related arthritis. Most of the cases in th epublished literature did not require discontinuation of the ICIs [26, 32, 33, 34]; in fact, it has been proposed that MSK irAEs are associated with better tumor outcomes from ICI. Kostine et al. reported the incidence of rheumatic irAEs of 6.6% [32] andthe authors also observed higher tumor response in a patient who had rheumatic irAEs and emphasized the continuation of ICIs rather than discontinuation for management of MSK irAEs.

Rheumatic irAEs are different in that they may be chronic in up to one-third of the patients after cessation requiring long-term management [4, 15, 36]. Corticosteroid

Table 2: Summary of published case series or case report on rheumatologic/musculoskeletal immune-related adverse effects (irAEs).

Case series/ report(s)	Number of patients	Immune-checkpoint inhibitor	Primary malignancy	Pattern	Joint involvement	Symmetrical/ Asymmetrical	Axial/ appendicular	Clinical diagnosis	Serology	Therapy	Steroid dose (for arthritis patients only)	Response	ICI status
Chan et al. [17]	2	Anti-PD1: 2	Melanoma: 2	Seronegative arthritis: 2	Polyarthritis: 2	NA	None	Inflammatory arthritis	RF: −ve, anti-CCP: −ve, ANA: −ve	Opioid analgesics: 1, pamidronate, NSAIDs and DMARDs (sulfasalazine, HCQ): 1	Steroid not used	Improvement: 2	Continued: 1, held: 1
Law-Ping-Man et al. [22]	1	Anti-PD1	NSCLC	Psoriatic arthritis	Oligoarthritis	Asymmetrical	None	Inflammatory arthritis	RF: −ve, anti-CCP: −ve, ANA: −ve	Steroid, DMARDs (MTX)	Prednisone (15 mg/day)	Improvement	Continued
Ruiz-Bañobre et al. [23]	1	Anti-PD1	NSCLC	Psoriatic arthritis	Polyarthritis	NA	NR	Inflammatory arthritis	RF: −ve, anti-CCP: −ve, ANA: −ve	IA steroid, steroid, NSAIDs, DMARDS (MTX, sulfasalazine)	Methylprednisone (4 mg/day)	Improvement	Continued
Kim et al. [24]	3	Anti-PD1: 1, anti-PD1 and anti-CTLA-4: 2	Melanoma: 3	Seronegative arthritis: 3	Polyarthritis: 3	Symmetrical: 3	None	Arthritis	RF: −ve, anti-CCP Ab: −ve, ANA: 1	Prednisone and anti-IL-6 Ab: 2, anti-IL-6 Ab (tocilizumab): 1	Prednisone (40 mg/day)	Improvement: 3	NR
Kuswanto et al. [19]	4	Anti-PD1: 4	RCC: 4	Seronegative arthritis: 3, PMR: 1	Polyarthritis: 3	Symmetrical: 2	Pelvic girdle: 1	Inflammatory arthritis	RF: NA, anti-CCP Ab: NA, ANA: NA	Steroid: 1, steroid and IA steroid: 1, steroid and DMARDs (MTX): 1, infliximab: 1	Prednisone (50–20 mg/day)	Improvement: 4	Held: 3
Cappelli et al. [25]	9	Anti-PD1: 2, anti-PD1 and anti-CTLA-4: 7	RCC: 1, small cell lung cancer: 1, melanoma: 3, NSCLC: 4	Seronegative arthritis: 9	Polyarthritis: 8, oligoarthritis: 1	NR	Back pain: 1	Inflammatory arthritis	RF: −ve, anti-CCP Ab: −ve, ANA: 1	Prednisone: 1, dexamethasone: 1, NSAIDs and IA steroid: 1, prednisone and TNF alfa inhibitor: 2, prednisone, DMARDs (MTX, infliximab, etanercept) and IA steroid: 2, prednisone and IA steroid: 2	Prednisone (40–10 mg/day), 120 mg for 1 patient	Improvement: 7, partial response: 1, NR: 1	NR

Table 2: Continued.

Case series/ report(s)	Number of patients	Immune-checkpoint inhibitor	Primary malignancy	Pattern	Joint involvement	Symmetrical/ Asymmetrical	Axial/ appendicular	Clinical diagnosis	Serology	Therapy	Steroid dose (for arthritis patients only)	Response	ICI status
Calabrese et al. [20]	10	Anti-PD1: 1, anti-PD1 and anti-CTLA-4: 6	NSCLC: 1, RCC: 2, melanoma: 4	Seronegative arthritis: 7, PMR: 3	Polyarthritis: 7	Symmetrical: 6, asymmetrical: 1	None	Arthritis	RF: 1, anti-CCP Ab: −ve, ANA: 1	Prednisone: 6, prednisone and DMARDs (HCQ, MTX, infliximab, etanercept, adalimumab): 4	Prednisone (40–15 mg/day)	Significant improvement: 4, moderate improvement: 4, minimal improvement: 2	Held: 4, continued: 3
Belkhir et al. [26]	10	Anti-PD1/PD-L1: 9, anti-PD1 and anti-CTLA-4: 1	Melanoma: 3, lung adenocarcinoma: 2, endometrial adenocarcinoma: 1, squamous cell carcinoma of the vagina: 1, mesothelioma: 1, colon adenocarcinoma: 1, gastric adenocarcinoma: 1	RA: 6, PMR: 4	NR	NR	NR	Inflammatory arthritis	RF: 4, anti-CCP Ab: 6, ANA: 1	Steroid: 7, NSAIDs: 1, NSAIDs and DMARDs (MTX, HCQ): 2	Prednisone (20–10 mg/day) 60 mg for 1 patient	Improvement: 10	Continued: 9
Le Burel et al. [27]	17	Anti-PD1/PD-L1: 15, anti-PD1 and anti-CTLA-4: 2	Melanoma: 3, RCC: 2, lung adenocarcinoma: 3, pleural mesothelioma: 1, endometrioid carcinoma: 1, colon adenocarcinoma: 1, vaginal squamous cell carcinoma: 1, lung squamous carcinoma: 1, urothelial bladder cancer: 1, glioblastoma: 1, renal epithelioid angiomyolipoma: 1, gastric adenocarcinoma: 1	RA: 3, PMR: 4, psoriatic arthritis: 3, seronegative arthritis: 7	Polyarthritis: 13	Symmetrical: 11, asymmetrical: 1	NR	Inflammatory arthritis	RF: 3, anti-CCP Ab: 3, ANA: 1	Steroids: 14, steroid and DMARDs (MTX): 2	NA	Improvement: 9, resolution: 7, stable: 1	NA
Le Bakhaya et al. [28]	26	Anti-PD1: 23, anti-PD1 and anti-CTLA-4: 3	Melanoma: 25, Merkel cell carcinoma: 1	Arthritis: 10, activated osteoarthritis: 5, arthralgia (not specified): 11	Polyarthritis: 7, oligoarthritis: 19	Symmetrical: 16	NR	Arthralgia	RF: 2, anti-CCP ab: 1, ANA: 1	NSAIDs: 19, steroid: 5, DMARDs (sulfasalazine, HCQ): 2	Prednisone (5–10 mg/day)	Complete response: 4, partial response: 15, stable disease: 5	Held: 2

Table 2: Continued.

Case series/ report(s)	Number of patients	Immune-checkpoint inhibitor	Primary malignancy	Pattern	Joint involvement	Symmetrical/ Asymmetrical	Axial/ appendicular	Clinical diagnosis	Serology	Therapy	Steroid dose (for arthritis patients only)	Response	ICI status
Ngo et al. [29]	1	Anti-PD1	Melanoma	Seronegative arthritis	Polyarthritis	Symmetrical	None	Inflammatory arthritis	RF: −ve, anti-CCP: −ve, ANA: −ve	Steroid	Prednisone (40 mg/day)	Improvement	Continued
Haikal et al. [21]	1	Anti-PD1	Melanoma	Seronegative arthritis	Polyarthritis	Symmetrical	None	Arthritis	RF: −ve, anti-CCP: −ve	Steroid and DMARDs (HCQ)	Low-dose steroid	Improvement	NR
Inamo et al. [18]	3	Anti-PD1: 3	Lung adenocarcinoma: 1, lung squamous cell carcinoma: 1, ovarian cancer: 1	Seronegative arthritis: 3	Polyarthritis: 2, oligoarthritis: 1	Symmetrical: 3	None	Inflammatory arthritis	RF: −ve, Anti-CCP Ab: −ve, ANA: −ve	NSAIDs: 1, opioid: 1, NSAIDs and prednisone: 1	Prednisone (20 mg/day) for 1 patient only	Improvement: 3	NR
Smith and Bass [30]	10	Anti- PD1: 3, anti-PD-1 and anti-CTLA-4: 7	Melanoma: 4, lung adenocarcinoma: 2, RCC: 1, Merkel: 1, anal cancer: 1, cervical cancer: 1	RA: 3, PMR: 1, others: 6	Polyarthritis: 4, oligoarthritis: 4, tenosynovitis: 2	NA	NA	Inflammatory arthritis	RF: NA, anti-CCP Ab: 2, ANA: 6	Steroid: 6, steroid and DMARDs (HCQ, sulfasalazine, MTX, mycophenolate mofetil): 4	Prednisone (20–10 mg/day)	Improvement: 4, resolution: 6	Held: 1
Lidar et al. [31]	12	Anti-PD1: 8, anti-CTLA 4: 1, anti-PD1 and anti-CTLA-4: 3	Melanoma: 10, sinonasal carcinoma: 1, endometrial carcinoma: 1	Seronegative arthritis: 12	Polyarthritis: 10, oligoarthritis: 1, monoarthritis: 1	NR	None	Inflammatory arthritis	RF: −ve, anti-CCP Ab: none, ANA: −ve	NSAIDs, steroid: 5, steroid and MTX: 2, NSAIDs, steroid, MTX: 5	Prednisone (>20 mg/day)	Improvement: 11, unknown: 1	Held: 3, continued: 3, off therapy: 6
Kostine et al. [32]	35	Anti-PD1/PD-L1: 33, anti-CTLA-4: 1, anti-PD-L1 and anti-CTLA- 4: 1	Melanoma: 16, lung cancer: 12, RCC: 6, Merkel cell carcinoma: 1	RA: 7, PMR: 11, psoriatic arthritis: 2, others: 15	Mostly polyarthritis: exact no. not reported	Mostly symmetrical	Back pain: 10	Inflammatory and noninflammatory arthritis	RF: −ve, anti-CCP Ab: 1, ANA: 4	Steroid: 18, NSAIDs: 5, steroid and DMARDs (MTX): 2, intraarticular steroid: 1	Prednisone (mean dose 15 mg)	Improvement: 35	Continued: 34
Leipe et al. [33]	14	Anti-PD1: 10, anti-PD1 and anti-CTLA4: 4	Melanoma: 10, NSCLC: 5	Arthritis: 14, PMR: 5, Sicca syndrome: 2, myositis: 1	Polyarthritis: 2, oligoarthritis: 5, monoarthritis: 7	NR	NA	New-onset arthralgia and arthritis	RF: 5, anti-CCP: 1, ANA: 9	Steroid: 3, steroid and DMRDs (MTX): 6, NSAIDs: 2, IA steroid: 8	NR	Improvement: 13	Continued: 14
Narváez et al. [34]	11	Anti-PD1/PD-L1: 10, anti-PD1 and anti-CTLA4: 1	Lymphoma: 2, lung cancer: 4, RCC: 1, epithelioid mesothelioma: 1, pancreatic neuroendocrine cancer: 1, melanoma: 1, urothelial carcinoma: 1	Seronegative arthritis: 5, PMR: 1, Sicca syndrome: 2, inflammatory myositis with fasciitis: 2, paraneoplastic acral vascular syndrome: 1	Polyarthritis: 4, oligoarthritis: 1	Mostly symmetrical	None	Arthritis	RF: −ve, anti-CCP: −ve, ANA: −ve	Steroid: 4, NSAIDs: 1, steroid and DMARDs (HCQ): 3	Prednisone (cobra light schedule): 2 patients, prednisone 60 mg daily for 1 patient and methylprednisone 20 mg daily for 1 patient	Improvement: 10	Continued: 6

is the mainstay of treatment for immune-related arthritis; however, in refractory cases, it is recommended to consider either synthetic or biologic DMARDs [4, 37]. Besides, it is also recommended to stop ICIs in severe cases of inflammatory arthritis and permanently discontinue ICIs in grade 4 toxicities [4, 15, 37]. In our case, the patient had refractory severe immune-mediated inflammatory arthritis requiring to stop ICI, and he achieved remission on the initiation of DMARD during the course of the treatment. Interestingly, the clinical course was further complicated by ruptured Baker's cyst. Although the underlying mechanism for the rupture of Baker's cyst in our patient is unknown; however, nivolumab could be the possible reason based on clinical presentations and temporal relationships. Nevertheless, seronegative rheumatological workup and nonspecific positivity of ANA is consistent with previously published literature.

In conclusion, musculoskeletal irAEs are relatively common. Most patients on ICIs experience mild symptoms which often resolve with glucocorticoids alone. However, immune-related inflammatory arthritis requiring conventional or biologic DMARD therapy remains a clinical challenge. It is of utmost importance to recognize these cases and manage in collaboration with a rheumatologist to improve the clinical outcome and quality of life.

Abbreviations

PD1:	Programmed cell death protein 1
CTLA-4:	Cytotoxic T-lymphocyte-associated protein 4
NSCLC:	Non-small cell lung cancer
RCC:	Renal cell carcinoma
RA:	Rheumatoid arthritis
PMR:	Polymyalgia rheumatica
RF:	Rheumatoid factor
Anti-CCP Ab:	Anti-cyclic citrullinated peptide antibody
ANA:	Antinuclear antibodies
−ve:	Negative
NA:	Not available
NR:	Not reported
DMARDs:	Disease-modifying antirheumatic drugs
MTX:	Methotrexate
HCQ:	Hydroxychloroquine
NSAIDs:	Nonsteroidal anti-inflammatory drug
IA steroid:	Intra-articular steroid.

References

[1] J. Dine, R. Gordon, Y. Shames, M. Kasler, and M. Barton-Burke, "Immune checkpoint inhibitors: an innovation in immunotherapy for the treatment and management of patients with cancer," *Asia-Pacific Journal of Oncology Nursing*, vol. 4, no. 2, pp. 127–135, 2017.

[2] P. Sharma and J. P. Allison, "The future of immune checkpoint therapy," *Science*, vol. 348, no. 6230, pp. 56–61, 2015.

[3] S. C. Wei, C. R. Duffy, and J. P. Allison, "Fundamental mechanisms of immune checkpoint blockade therapy," *Cancer Discovery*, vol. 8, no. 9, pp. 1069–1086, 2018.

[4] L. H. Calabrese, C. Calabrese, and L. C. Cappelli, "Rheumatic immune-related adverse events from cancer immunotherapy," *Nature Reviews Rheumatology*, vol. 14, no. 10, pp. 569–579, 2018.

[5] M. A. Postow, R. Sidlow, and M. D. Hellmann, "Immune-related adverse events associated with immune checkpoint blockade," *New England Journal of Medicine*, vol. 378, no. 2, pp. 158–168, 2018.

[6] T. Pincus, C. J. Swearingen, M. Bergman, and Y. Yazici, "RAPID3 (Routine Assessment of Patient Index Data 3), a rheumatoid arthritis index without formal joint counts for routine care: proposed severity categories compared to disease activity score and clinical disease activity index categories," *The Journal of Rheumatology*, vol. 35, no. 11, pp. 2136–2147, 2008.

[7] I. Puzanov, A. Diab, K. Abdallah et al., "Managing toxicities associated with immune checkpoint inhibitors: consensus recommendations from the society for immunotherapy of cancer (SITC) toxicity management working group," *Journal for ImmunoTherapy of Cancer*, vol. 5, no. 1, p. 95, 2017.

[8] G. D. Velasco, Y. Je, D. Bossé et al., "Comprehensive meta-analysis of key immune-related adverse events from CTLA-4 and PD-1/PD-L1 inhibitors in cancer patients," *Cancer Immunology Research*, vol. 5, no. 4, pp. 312–318, 2017.

[9] B. Thapa, J. Roopkumar, A. S. Kim et al., "Incidence and clinical pattern of immune related adverse effects (irAE) due to immune checkpoint inhibitors (ICI)," *Journal of Clinical Oncology*, vol. 37, no. 15_suppl, p. e14151, 2019.

[10] J. M. Michot, C. Bigenwald, S. Champiat et al., "Immune-related adverse events with immune checkpoint blockade: a comprehensive review," *European Journal of Cancer*, vol. 54, pp. 139–148, 2016.

[11] J. J. Moslehi, J.-E. Salem, J. A. Sosman, B. Lebrun-Vignes, and D. B. Johnson, "Increased reporting of fatal immune checkpoint inhibitor-associated myocarditis," *The Lancet*, vol. 391, no. 10124, p. 933, 2018.

[12] J. Chahine, B. Thapa, C. K. Ala et al., "Immune checkpoint inhibitors associated with cardiotoxicity in cancer patients: a large single-center experience," *Journal of Cardiac Failure*, vol. 25, no. 8, p. S63, 2019.

[13] L. C. Cappelli, A. K. Gutierrez, C. O. Bingham, and A. A. Shah, "Rheumatic and musculoskeletal immune-related adverse events due to immune checkpoint inhibitors: a systematic review of the literature," *Arthritis Care & Research*, vol. 69, no. 11, pp. 1751–1763, 2017.

[14] M. E. Suarez-Almazor, S. T. Kim, N. Abdel-Wahab, and A. Diab, "Review: immune-related adverse events with use of checkpoint inhibitors for immunotherapy of cancer," *Arthritis & Rheumatology*, vol. 69, no. 4, pp. 687–699, 2017.

[15] K. Ohnuma, R. Hatano, N. H. Dang, and C. Morimoto, "Rheumatic diseases associated with immune checkpoint inhibitors in cancer immunotherapy," *Modern Rheumatology*, vol. 29, no. 5, pp. 721–732, 2019.

[16] K. Syrigos, S. Tsagouli, and D. Grapsa, "Nivolumab-induced recurrence of rheumatoid arthritis in a patient with advanced non-small cell lung cancer: a case report," *Annals of Internal Medicine*, vol. 165, no. 12, p. 894, 2016.

[17] M. M. K. Chan, R. F. Kefford, M. Carlino, A. Clements, and N. Manolios, "Arthritis and tenosynovitis associated with the anti-pd1 antibody pembrolizumab in metastatic melanoma," *Journal of Immunotherapy*, vol. 38, no. 1, pp. 37–39, 2015.

[18] J. Inamo, Y. Kaneko, and T. Takeuchi, "Inflammatory tenosynovitis and enthesitis induced by immune checkpoint in-

hibitor treatment," *Clinical Rheumatology*, vol. 37, no. 4, pp. 1107–1110, 2018.

[19] W. F. Kuswanto, L. A. MacFarlane, L. Gedmintas, A. Mulloy, T. K. Choueiri, and B. L. Bermas, "Rheumatologic symptoms in oncologic patients on PD-1 inhibitors," *Seminars in Arthritis and Rheumatism*, vol. 47, no. 6, pp. 907–910, 2018.

[20] C. Calabrese, E. Kirchner, A. Kontzias, V. Velcheti, and L. H. Calabrese, "Rheumatic immune-related adverse events of checkpoint therapy for cancer: case series of a new nosological entity," *RMD Open*, vol. 3, no. 1, Article ID e000412, 2017.

[21] A. Haikal, E. Borba, T. Khaja, G. Doolittle, and P. Schmidt, "Nivolumab-induced new-onset seronegative rheumatoid arthritis in a patient with advanced metastatic melanoma: a case report and literature review," *Avicenna Journal of Medicine*, vol. 8, no. 1, pp. 34–36, 2018.

[22] S. Law-Ping-Man, A. Martin, E. Briens, L. Tisseau, and G. Safa, "Psoriasis and psoriatic arthritis induced by nivolumab in a patient with advanced lung cancer," *Rheumatology*, vol. 55, no. 11, pp. 2087–2089, 2016.

[23] J. Ruiz-Bañobre, E. Pérez-Pampín, J. García-González et al., "Development of psoriatic arthritis during nivolumab therapy for metastatic non-small cell lung cancer, clinical outcome analysis and review of the literature," *Lung Cancer*, vol. 108, pp. 217–221, 2017.

[24] S. T. Kim, J. Tayar, V. A. Trinh et al., "Successful treatment of arthritis induced by checkpoint inhibitors with tocilizumab: a case series," *Annals of the Rheumatic Diseases*, vol. 76, no. 12, pp. 2061–2064, 2017.

[25] L. C. Cappelli, A. K. Gutierrez, A. N. Baer et al., "Inflammatory arthritis and sicca syndrome induced by nivolumab and ipilimumab," *Annals of the Rheumatic Diseases*, vol. 76, no. 1, pp. 43–50, 2017.

[26] R. Belkhir, S. L. Burel, L. Dunogeant et al., "Rheumatoid arthritis and polymyalgia rheumatica occurring after immune checkpoint inhibitor treatment," *Annals of the Rheumatic Diseases*, vol. 76, no. 10, pp. 1747–1750, 2017.

[27] S. Le Burel, S. Champiat, C. Mateus et al., "Prevalence of immune-related systemic adverse events in patients treated with anti-programmed cell death 1/anti-programmed cell death-ligand 1 agents: a single-centre pharmacovigilance database analysis," *European Journal of Cancer*, vol. 82, pp. 34–44, 2017.

[28] K. Buder-Bakhaya, K. Benesova, C. Schulz et al., "Characterization of arthralgia induced by PD-1 antibody treatment in patients with metastasized cutaneous malignancies," *Cancer Immunology, Immunotherapy*, vol. 67, no. 2, pp. 175–182, 2018.

[29] L. Ngo, E. Miller, P. Valen, and E. Gertner, "Nivolumab induced remitting seronegative symmetrical synovitis with pitting edema in a patient with melanoma: a case report," *Journal of Medical Case Reports*, vol. 12, no. 1, p. 48, 2018.

[30] M. H. Smith and A. R. Bass, "Arthritis after cancer immunotherapy: symptom duration and treatment response," *Arthritis Care & Research*, vol. 71, no. 3, pp. 362–366, 2019.

[31] M. Lidar, E. Giat, D. Garelick et al., "Rheumatic manifestations among cancer patients treated with immune checkpoint inhibitors," *Autoimmunity Reviews*, vol. 17, no. 3, pp. 284–289, 2018.

[32] M. Kostine, L. Rouxel, T. Barnetche et al., "Rheumatic disorders associated with immune checkpoint inhibitors in patients with cancer-clinical aspects and relationship with tumour response: a single-centre prospective cohort study," *Annals of the Rheumatic Diseases*, vol. 77, no. 3, pp. 393–398, 2018.

[33] J. Leipe, L. A. Christ, A. P. Arnoldi et al., "Characteristics and treatment of new-onset arthritis after checkpoint inhibitor therapy," *RMD Open*, vol. 4, no. 2, Article ID e000714, 2018.

[34] J. Narváez, P. Juarez-López, J. LLuch et al., "Rheumatic immune-related adverse events in patients on anti-PD-1 inhibitors: fasciitis with myositis syndrome as a new complication of immunotherapy," *Autoimmunity Reviews*, vol. 17, no. 10, pp. 1040–1045, 2018.

[35] S.-T. Liao, C.-S. Chiou, and C.-C. Chang, "Pathology associated to the Baker's cysts: a musculoskeletal ultrasound study," *Clinical Rheumatology*, vol. 29, no. 9, pp. 1043–1047, 2010.

[36] T. J. Braaten, J. R. Brahmer, P. M. Forde et al., "Immune checkpoint inhibitor-induced inflammatory arthritis persists after immunotherapy cessation," *Annals of the Rheumatic Diseases*, 2019.

[37] J. R. Brahmer, C. Lacchetti, B. J. Schneider et al., "Management of immune-related adverse events in patients treated with immune checkpoint inhibitor therapy: American Society of Clinical Oncology clinical practice guideline," *Journal of Clinical Oncology*, vol. 36, no. 17, pp. 1714–1768, 2018.

9

An Elderly Gentleman with Acute Lupus Pneumonitis as the Initial Manifestation of Systemic Lupus Erythematosus

Gina Ferrero,[1] **Kate Chernow**,[2,3] **Marissa Karpoff**,[1] **Pamela Traisak**,[1] **David Feinstein**,[1] **and Hala Eid**[1]

[1]*Cooper University Hospital, Camden, NJ, USA*
[2]*Einstein Medical Center Montgomery, East Norriton, PA, USA*
[3]*Abington Lansdale Hospital, Lansdale, PA, USA*

Correspondence should be addressed to Gina Ferrero; ferrero-gina@cooperhealth.edu

Academic Editor: Tsai Ching Hsu

Systemic lupus erythematosus is a systemic autoimmune disease, with presentations that vary within a population and across the lifespan of an individual. The disease afflicts childbearing women more than men and uncommonly presents in the geriatric population. Lupus pneumonitis is rare, with a reported incidence of 1–4%. Herein, we discuss the case report of an elderly gentleman with biopsy-proven acute lupus pneumonitis (ALP) as an initial presentation of lupus. After starting high-dose steroids, the patient initially improved, though unfortunately endured a non-ST elevation myocardial infarction and recurrent gastrointestinal bleeding. Despite multiple interventions and a prolonged hospital course, his gastrointestinal bleeding persisted. He elected to go on home hospice and ultimately passed away due to ongoing gastrointestinal bleeding. As with our patient, elderly patients can pose a diagnostic dilemma with regard to late-onset lupus; multiple comorbidities and growing evidence that late-onset lupus may manifest with distinct clinical patterns from younger cohorts complicate diagnosis in these patients. It is critical to maintain a broad differential, which includes unusual rheumatic manifestations when management of common comorbidities fails to alleviate symptoms for an elderly patient. Failure to do so may result in delayed diagnosis of rheumatic disease and increased side effects related to treatment. Additionally, this case serves as a reminder that due to the complexity of rheumatic disease and the additional challenge of older patients with baseline comorbidities, sometimes palliative care options may be appropriate.

1. Introduction

Systemic lupus erythematosus (SLE) is a chronic, systemic autoimmune disease that is characterized by disease "flares" and immunologic abnormalities such as antinuclear antibodies. The disease more frequently plagues women of childbearing age than men or elderly. SLE is an enigma, in that we have not fully elucidated all genetic and environmental triggers that lend to the disease. Nevertheless, the typical clinical manifestations, which may vary dramatically from patient to patient, are well-described. We discuss an unusual case of SLE manifesting with acute lupus pneumonitis in an elderly gentleman. Elderly onset lupus is rare; moreover, an initial presentation of lupus pneumonitis is less common but does occur [1]. Of the lupus pulmonary manifestations, lupus pneumonitis is rare even across all demographics with an incidence of 1–4% [2, 3].

2. Case Description

The patient is an 86-year-old male farmer who presented with several months of intermittent nonmassive hemoptysis and a one-week history of progressively worsening dyspnea and fatigue. The patient's medical history was significant for recently diagnosed transfusion-dependent myelodysplastic syndrome, coronary artery disease requiring stenting, atrial fibrillation, and interstitial lung disease attributed to amiodarone requiring 2 L/min oxygen at home. His home medications were pantoprazole 40 mg daily, zolpidem 5 mg nightly, and furosemide 20 mg daily. His hemoptysis had persisted despite discontinuing his dual antiplatelet therapy for his coronary stents. Additionally, the patient's anemia required frequent transfusions to an extent which did not correlate with the mild degree of myelodysplastic syndrome. Therefore, further investigation was warranted.

On the initial physical exam, our patient was afebrile and hemodynamically stable with an oxygen saturation of 94% on 2 L/min oxygen. Breath sounds were notable for fine bibasilar crackles. He exhibited bilateral lower extremity pitting edema. Exam was otherwise unremarkable. Basic laboratory tests were significant for leukocytosis with a left shift noted with a white blood count 21.14 10*3/uL (4.5–11*3/uL) and a microcytic anemia noted with a hemoglobin level 7.8 g/dL (14–18 g/dL). He had a mildly elevated creatinine to 1.31 mg/dl (0.6–1.2 mg/dl). NT-proBNP was 5,375 pg/ml (0–852 pg/ml). Erythrocyte sedimentation rate was greater than 100 mm/hr (0–15 mm/hr), and C-reactive protein was 23.21 mg/dl (<0.5 mg/dl). Imaging with computed tomography (CT) chest demonstrated bilateral diffuse ground glass opacities with central predominance and a mild right-sided effusion (Figure 1).

He was initially treated with diuresis, as there was concern that his pulmonary findings were related to volume overload in the setting of a recent blood transfusion. He was also treated empirically with broad spectrum antibiotics. Despite these efforts, our patient's respiratory status progressively worsened with increasing oxygen requirements to 6 L/min nasal cannula. Arterial blood gas was collected at that time which showed significant hypoxia with arterial PO_2 38 mm (Hg) (86–100 mm (Hg)). Due to his clinical presentation and progressive symptoms, further workup was warranted. A rheumatologic workup was completed. When questioned, the patient endorsed late-onset Raynaud's symptoms, occasional arthralgias without swelling or morning stiffness, and oral sicca symptoms. He denied any history of alopecia, photosensitivity, rashes, oral or nasal ulcers, skin thickening, dysphagia, or reflux disease. He noted that his sister has SLE. Laboratory tests were significant for positive antinuclear antibodies with a 1 : 160 titre in homogenous pattern, C4 complement was decreased to 14 mg/dL (20–59 mg/dl), and C3 complement was normal. Anti-DNA was elevated at 194 IU/ml (<100 IU/ml). Anti-Ro (SSA) was positive at 6.0 (<1.0) and anti-La (SSB) was positive at >8.0 (<1.0). Other rheumatological laboratory tests were negative including anti-Smith antibody, anti-RNP antibody, antichromatin, proteinase 3 antibody, myeloperoxidase antibody, and glomerular basement membrane antibody.

Our patient underwent bronchoscopy and transbronchial biopsy. The bronchoscopy and bronchoalveolar lavage (BAL) showed no findings of diffuse alveolar hemorrhage (DAH) on lavage aliquots. BAL demonstrated 165 cells/uL, 85% segmented neutrophils, 1% lymphocytes, 8% mono/macrophages, and 4% eosinophils. Blood cultures and BAL cultures, including fungal cultures, were negative for infection. The BAL acid-fast bacillus culture grew no acid-fast organisms after six weeks. Cytology was negative

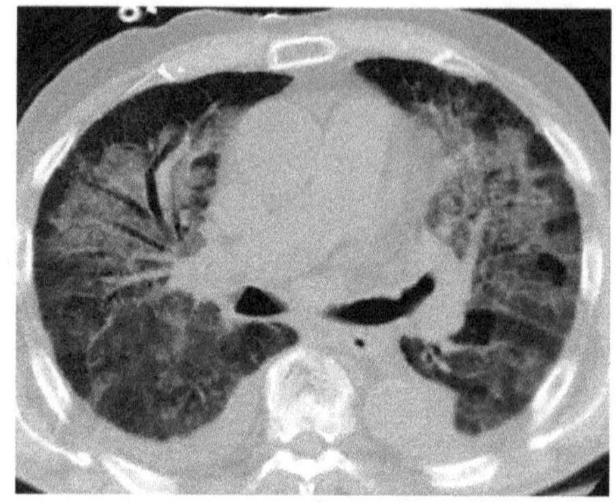

Figure 1: CT chest demonstrating diffuse ground glass opacities bilaterally, central predominant, no focal infiltrates.

for malignant cells. Transbronchial biopsies showed chronic hemorrhage (hemosiderin-laden macrophages), septal acute inflammatory cells with thickening of the alveolar septae, and type II pneumocyte hyperplasia consistent with capillaritis (Figure 2). Given lack of exposure to medications known to cause capillaritis (such as hydralazine, propylthiouracil, phenytoin, retinoic acid, or illicit drugs) in combination with positive ANA, low C4, and high titre anti-DNA, our patient was diagnosed with acute lupus pneumonitis.

3. Treatment and Outcome

Our patient was started on methylprednisolone 60 mg IV daily for acute lupus pneumonitis. Within twenty-four hours of initiating steroids, the patient's respiratory status improved; he was able to converse without dyspnea and was able to ambulate short distances with 2 L/min nasal cannula. Unfortunately, a few days later, he suffered a non-ST elevation myocardial infarction (NSTEMI) for which he underwent cardiac catheterization and coronary stenting. He started back on antiplatelet therapy. The hospital course was further complicated by an upper gastrointestinal bleed secondary to a duodenal ulcer resulting in hypotension requiring vasopressors. Methylprednisolone had to be discontinued temporarily until his gastrointestinal bleed was controlled. Methylprednisolone was ultimately restarted after which the patient endured additional gastrointestinal bleeding. Nevertheless, antiplatelet therapy was continued given the high risk for in-stent thrombosis. Over the course of three weeks, our patient required three esophagogastroduodenoscopies with clipping as well as one coil embolization at the gastroduodenal artery and a later coil embolization at the pancreaticoduodenal artery. In light of stressful repeat procedures and a prolonged hospital course, the patient and family elected to focus on comfort. In the case of further gastrointestinal bleeding, he did not desire further invasive procedures. His goal was to be with his family. He ultimately passed away six days after hospital discharge due to recurrent gastrointestinal bleeding in the company of his loving family.

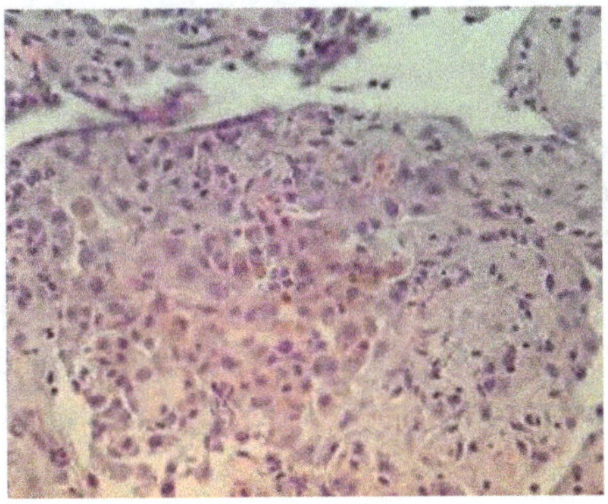

FIGURE 2: Lung parenchyma showing chronic hemorrhage (hemosiderin macrophages), septal acute inflammatory cells with thickening of the alveolar septae, and type II pneumocyte hyperplasia.

4. Discussion

Lupus pneumonitis, one of several respiratory complications of SLE, is rare, with a reported incidence of 1–4% [2, 3]. Furthermore, lupus pneumonitis is uncommon as an initial presentation of SLE; a registry report released in 2018 of 3,215 lupus patients showed only 4% of cases had pulmonary disease of any kind upon initial presentation of SLE, with rates of lupus pneumonitis likely much lower [2]. It should be noted, however, that for late-onset SLE (lupus diagnosed after the age of fifty), the incidence of pulmonary manifestations appears to be increased compared to the younger population (pulmonary involvement (21.2% vs. 11.3%) [4]. Therefore, despite its rarity, lupus pneumonitis as an initial presentation of SLE in the elderly does occur (in this case and in others [1]) and warrants diagnostic consideration.

The constellation of symptoms suggestive of acute lupus pneumonitis is as follows: dyspnea, pleuritic chest pain, cough, fevers, and less occasionally, hemoptysis. [5–7] Hypoxemia is invariably present. Bloodwork is typically significant for high anti-DNA titres [5, 7]. As exemplified in our patient, many previously described patients with lupus pneumonitis have anti-SSA antibodies (up to 82%) [7–9]. Radiographically, we see diffuse ground glass opacities and areas of consolidation suggestive of acinar filling. These findings tend to be in the bilateral lower lobes with or without pleural effusion [5, 10]. As a diagnosis of exclusion, lupus pneumonitis requires evaluation by bronchoscopy with BAL. BAL is primarily used to exclude infectious etiologies and DAH. Biopsy is rarely required to confirm diagnosis.

Historically, there has been debate about the histopathology of lupus pneumonitis and even its existence. Complicating this, the pathological finding of pulmonary fibrosis to suggest acute or chronic lupus pneumonitis is infrequent, though clinical descriptions of lupus pneumonitis are more easily found in literature [11]. One necropsy series explained each case of clinically diagnosed lupus pneumonitis by other processes such as infection, aspiration, heart failure, or uremia [12]. It is important to emphasize that our patient fit not only the clinical picture of lupus pneumonitis but also had consistent biopsy characteristics without another explanation. Both diffuse alveolar damage (DAD) and capillaritis were evident in our patient. DAD refers to hyaline membranes with cellular interstitial infiltrates that result in alveolar edema. Capillaritis occurs in the setting of complement and immunoglobulin protein deposition and characteristic neutrophilic infiltrates in the alveolar interstitium. The process results in injury and necrosis of capillary walls, disruption of the epithelial-endothelial alveolar basement membrane, and subsequent extravasation of neutrophils and red blood cells into the alveolar space. As demonstrated in our patient, hemosiderin-laden macrophages secondary to erythrophagocytosis and interstitial hemosiderin implied a chronic pathological process [13].

The diagnosis of lupus pneumonitis was not initially at the top of our differential, particularly given the patient's demographic and comorbidities. He was initially treated preemptively for volume overload and an infectious process. Unique aspects of the case bring to mind additional differentials. The patient's occupation as a farmer makes subacute hypersensitivity pneumonitis a potential cause, though such a patient would not present with hemoptysis. CT chest in this case would be expected to show centrilobular nodules, mid-to-upper lobe predominant ground glass opacities, and evidence of air trapping. In a patient with myelodysplastic syndrome, paraneoplastic autoimmune syndromes may be considered. Regarding the patient's history of amiodarone-induced interstitial lung disease (ILD), we were unable to obtain records from the period of the diagnosis and therefore cannot comment on whether or not the patient presented in the typical manner. If the diagnosis of amiodarone-induced lung toxicity was not straightforward, the new diagnosis of lupus pneumonitis brings to light the possibility that the gentleman had chronic SLE-associated ILD, particularly given his autoantibodies specific for SLE and CT changes. Similarly, the presence of SSA and SSB antibodies raises the possibility of Sjögren's syndrome complicated by ILD. Ultimately, the patient's acute clinical decline in addition to biopsy findings were consistent with an acute process as opposed to an insidious ILD. Though biopsy is typically not required to diagnose ILD, one would expect to find chronic infiltrate such as lymphocytes or plasma cells, as opposed to acute inflammatory cells (as in our patient) and possibly fibrosis [7]. Ultimately DAD and capillaritis were found on biopsy, and given concomitant serology, a positive ANA, low C4, and high titre anti-DNA, our patient was diagnosed with acute lupus pneumonitis.

Once our biopsy was reviewed, DAH remained high on the differential. It is important to note that both DAD and capillaritis may be seen in DAH in addition to ALP. In fact, DAD and ALP may be thought of as two processes on the same disease spectrum [10]. Additionally, our patient's clinical presentation of hemoptysis in conjunction with ground glass opacities on CT scan makes DAH a consideration. Nevertheless, the case is most consistent with ALP given lack of hemorrhagic aliquots on BAL in addition to biopsy findings. While biopsy findings are not specific to ALP versus DAH, the pattern found in our patient supports

ALP. ALP may be used in reference to DAD without hemorrhage, while DAH demonstrates gross alveolar hemorrhage and less commonly shows DAD [3, 10]. Though DAH may present with capillaritis, the common pattern is "bland" DAH (DAH without capillaritis), which was not our patient's finding [7, 10].

Given that acute lupus pneumonitis has been thought of as a mild form of the same respiratory disease process that includes DAH, it is not surprising that treatment is similar [10]. Unfortunately, there are no controlled studies for treatment. Rheumatologists are guided based on approach to other well studied complications of SLE such as nephritis, insights into treatment for acute interstitial pneumonia, and case reports. Once infection is ruled out in the setting of acute lupus pneumonitis with BAL, antibiotics may be discontinued and steroids, the mainstay of treatment, initiated. Prednisone is used at a dose of 1–1.5 mg/kg bodyweight/day [7, 14]. If there is significant tachypnea or hypoxemia warranting intensive care unit level of care, methylprednisolone pulse treatment with 1 g/day for 3 days should be administered. Steroid sparing immunosuppressive therapy should be used when feasible. Cyclophosphamide is commonly prescribed for patients with inadequate response to steroids [3, 7]. Alternatively, azathioprine, rituximab, and intravenous immune globulin have been used with variable response [7, 15–17]. The prognosis of lupus pneumonitis is poor. The mortality rate is estimated to be 40–50% during the acute episode. Of the patients who survive lupus pneumonitis, 50% will have persistent interstitial infiltrates and lung function abnormalities suggesting progression of chronic interstitial pneumonitis [17]. While it is promising that our elderly patient initially improved with methylprednisolone, he eventually succumbed to complications of various disease processes and their competing treatments.

It is important to note that the 2019 European League Against Rheumatism/American College of Rheumatology classification criteria for SLE does not include pulmonary manifestations outside of serosal involvement [18]. Thus, given our patient's lack of other clinical criteria of SLE, he does not fit classification criteria. While classification criteria are excellent at describing a homogenous group of individuals for research purposes, they often fall short for the diagnostic use in more atypical cases such as our patient. This case report echoes Boddaert et al.'s epidemiological findings regarding late-onset SLE [4]. Patients with late-onset lupus were significantly more likely to have pulmonary complications, whereas they were less likely to demonstrate a number of findings of the classification criteria including photosensitivity, alopecia, nephritis, and malar rashes [4]. A number of other studies have also found that malar rashes and photosensitivity are significantly less common in elderly onset disease, whereas sicca symptoms are more common [19–21].

This case is a reminder that severe organ and life-threatening initial presentations of lupus occur in the elderly population and that vigilance is necessary to recognize these cases, particularly in light of other comorbidities that may cloud atypical presentations. The heterogeneous nature of lupus presentations is further compounded by the variable signs noted in elderly cohort studies. Knowing this, it is important for clinicians to be on guard against allowing improbable presentations of SLE to slip out of their differentials. In this case, diagnosis of SLE was not the only challenge. High-dose steroids are difficult for elderly patients to tolerate. Methylprednisolone likely contributed to our patients NSTEMI and recurrent GI bleeding. Therefore, in cases of elderly lupus patients requiring steroids, a thorough risk and benefit discussion with the patient and family members is prudent.

References

[1] K. Ikeda, T. Ishibashi, H. Noji et al., "A 92-year-old man with systemic lupus erythematosus who developed acute lupus pneumonitis," *The Journal of Rheumatology*, vol. 27, no. 1, pp. 234–237, 2000.

[2] J. Narváez, F. Sánchez-Alonso, H. Borrell et al., "Primary respiratory disease in patients with systemic lupus erythematosus: data from the Spanish rheumatology society lupus registry (RELESSER) cohort," *Arthritis Research & Therapy*, vol. 20, no. 1, p. 1, 2018.

[3] M. P. Keane and J. P. Lynch, "Rare diseases bullet 7: pleuropulmonary manifestations of systemic lupus erythematosus," *Thorax*, vol. 55, no. 2, pp. 159–166, 2000.

[4] J. Boddaert, D. L. T. Huong, Z. Amoura, B. Wechsler, P. Godeau, and J.-C. Piette, "Late-onset systemic lupus erythematosus," *Medicine*, vol. 83, no. 6, pp. 348–359, 2004.

[5] R. A. Matthay, M. I. Schwarz, T. L. Petty et al., "Pulmonary manifestations of systemic lupus erythematosus: review of twelve cases of acute lupus pneumonitis," *Medicine*, vol. 54, no. 5, pp. 397–410, 1975.

[6] G. S. Cheema and F. P. Quismorio, "Interstitial lung disease in systemic lupus erythematosus," *Current Opinion in Pulmonary Medicine*, vol. 6, no. 5, pp. 424–429, 2000.

[7] G. Aguilera-Pickens and C. Abud-Mendoza, "Manifestaciones pulmonares en lupus eritematoso sistémico: afección pleural, neumonitis aguda, enfermedad intersticial crónica y hemorragia alveolar difusa," *Reumatología Clínica*, vol. 14, no. 5, pp. 294–300, 2018.

[8] M. T. Hedgpeth and D. W. Boulware, "Interstitial pneumonitis in antinuclear antibody-negative systemic lupus erythematosus: a new clinical manifestation and possible association with anti-Ro (SS-A) antibodies," *Arthritis & Rheumatism*, vol. 31, no. 4, pp. 545–548, 1988.

[9] T. Mochizuki, S. Aotsuka, and T. Satoh, "Clinical and laboratory features of lupus patients with complicating pulmonary disease," *Respiratory Medicine*, vol. 93, no. 2, pp. 95–101, 1999.

[10] J. J. Swigris, A. Fischer, J. Gilles, R. T. Meehan, and K. K. Brown, "Pulmonary and thrombotic manifestations of systemic lupus erythematosus," *Chest*, vol. 133, no. 1, pp. 271–280, 2008.

[11] S. Quadrelli, C. Alvarez, S. Arce et al., "Pulmonary involvement of systemic lupus erythematosus: analysis of 90 necropsies," *Lupus*, vol. 18, no. 12, pp. 1053–1060, 2009.

[12] H. M. Haupt, G. W. Moore, and G. M. Hutchins, "The lung in systemic lupus erythematosus," *The American Journal of Medicine*, vol. 71, no. 5, pp. 791–798, 1981.

[13] H. R. Collard, T. E. King, and M. I. Schwarz, *Alveolar Hemorrhage and Rare Infiltrative Diseases in: Murray and Nadel's Textbook of Respiratory Medicine*, Elsevier, Amsterdam, Netherlands, 6th edition, 2016.

[14] B. Crestani, "The respiratory system in connective tissue disorders," *Allergy*, vol. 60, no. 6, pp. 715–734, 2005.

[15] G. Chetan, S. Mahadevan, K. Sulanthung, and P. Narayanan, "Intravenous immunoglobulin therapy of lupus pneumonitis," *The Indian Journal of Pediatrics*, vol. 74, no. 11, pp. 1032-1033, 2007.

[16] S. W. Lim, D. Gillis, W. Smith, P. Hissaria, H. Greville, and C. A. Peh, "Rituximab use in systemic lupus erythematosus pneumonitis and a review of current reports," *Internal Medicine Journal*, vol. 36, no. 4, pp. 260–262, 2006.

[17] S. A. Wan, C. L. Teh, and A. T. Jobli, "Lupus pneumonitis as the initial presentation of systemic lupus erythematosus: case series from a single institution," *Lupus*, vol. 25, no. 13, pp. 1485–1490, 2016.

[18] M. Aringer, "European league against rheumatism/American college of rheumatology classification criteria for systemic lupus erythematosus," *Arthritis & Rheumatology (Hoboken, N.J.)*, vol. 71, no. 9, pp. 1400–1412, 2019.

[19] J. L. Medlin, K. E. Hansen, S. R. Fitz, and C. M. Bartels, "A systematic review and meta-analysis of cutaneous manifestations in late- versus early-onset systemic lupus erythematosus," *Seminars in Arthritis and Rheumatism*, vol. 45, no. 6, pp. 691–697, 2016.

[20] L. J. Catoggio, E. R. Soriano, P. M. Imamura et al., "Late-onset systemic lupus erythematosus in Latin Americans: a distinct subgroup?" *Lupus*, vol. 24, no. 8, pp. 788–795, 2015.

[21] A. Tomic-Lucic, R. Petrovic, M. Radak-Perovic et al., "Late-onset systemic lupus erythematosus: clinical features, course, and prognosis," *Clinical Rheumatology*, vol. 32, no. 7, pp. 1053–1058, 2013.

10

Combined Left Central Retinal Artery Occlusion and Bilateral Anterior Ischemic Optic Neuritis: A Rare Presentation of Giant Cell Arteritis

Anne D. D. Joseph,[1] **Jebananthy Anandaselvam Pradeepan**,[1] **Thirunavukarasu Kumanan**,[1] **and Muthusamy Malaravan**[2]

[1]*University Medical Unit, Teaching Hospital Jaffna, Jaffna, Sri Lanka*
[2]*Department of Ophthalmology, Teaching Hospital Jaffna, Jaffna, Sri Lanka*

Correspondence should be addressed to Anne D. D. Joseph; anne.rajendrenjoseph@yahoo.com

Academic Editor: Constantine Saadeh

Giant cell arteritis, a large vessel vasculitis is characterized by headache, visual impairment, constitutional symptoms, and increased inflammatory markers. Visual involvement in giant cell arteritis ranges from amaurosis fugax to permanent visual loss, and extensive bilateral visual impairment is a rare presentation. We hereby report a case of combined left central retinal artery occlusion and bilateral anterior ischemic optic neuritis in a patient who poorly responded to standard corticosteroid therapy.

1. Introduction

Giant cell arteritis (GCA), also known as temporal arteritis, is the most common systemic vasculitides in older adult populations [1, 2]. It is a disease often observed in the age group of more than 50 years with the peak incidence in the seventh decade. Many of the symptoms and signs of the GCA are due to the involvement of the cranial branches of arteries that originate from the arch of the aorta, but the vascular involvement can be widespread.

The most common symptom of GCA is a new onset headache, usually around the temporal region. Abrupt onset of visual disturbances, in particular transient monocular visual loss, jaw claudication, unexplained fever, fatigue, anemia, or other constitutional symptoms and signs with high erythrocyte sedimentation rate (ESR) and/or high serum C-reactive protein (CRP) are the common observations at presentation. Simultaneous onset of bilateral visual loss is an unusual clinical entity.

2. Case Presentation

A 75-year-old lady, known patient with optimally controlled hypertension with amlodipine monotherapy for 5 years duration, presented with sudden painless onset of visual blurring involving the left eye for 3 days duration which was progressed to the level of perception of light (Pl) on the same side. Approximately 24 hours later, she developed gradual blurring of vision in the right eye too. She had left-sided intermittent jaw pain for a week prior to the onset of visual symptoms; however, she did not have a history of fever, frontotemporal headache, malaise, or constitutional symptoms. Past ophthalmological history included bilateral uncomplicated cataract extraction two years prior to the current presentation, and her visual acuity was 6/12 in the left eye and 6/12 in the right eye prior to the admission.

On examination, she was oriented and alert with the Glasgow Coma Scale (GCS) of 15 out of 15, was afebrile, and had tenderness over the left temporal region, but no thickening of the temporal artery was noted. Ophthalmic examination showed her visual acuity in the left eye Pl; in right eye, it was 1/10 with complete ocular motility. Other system examinations including the neurological examination were unremarkable.

Detailed examination of the eyes by the ophthalmology team revealed both pseudophakic eyes with normal intraocular

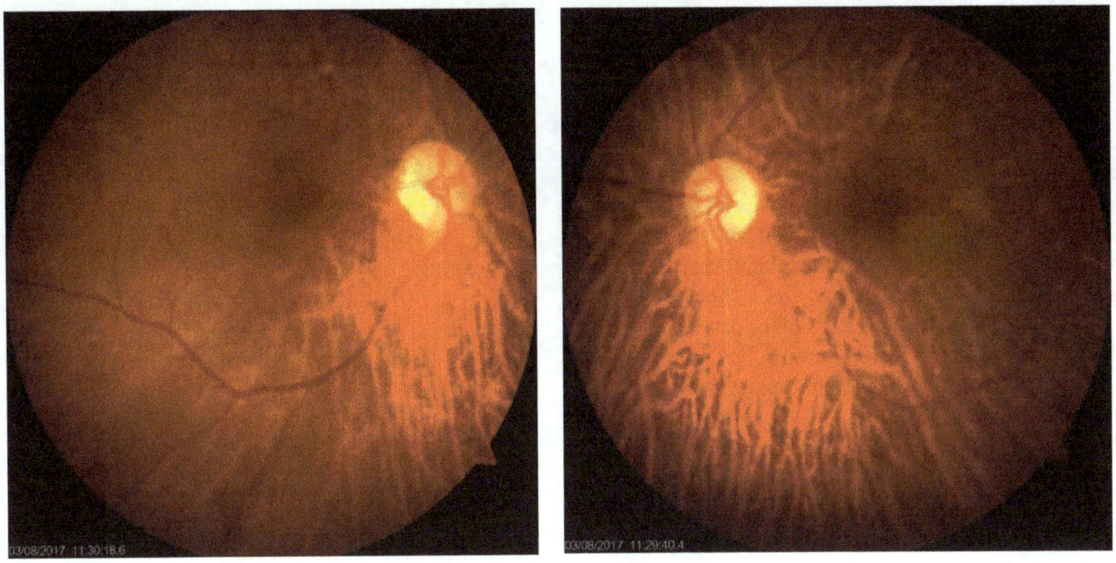

(a) (b)

FIGURE 1: Fundus photograph of the right (a) and left (b) eyes. The right eye shows a pale disc, and the left eye shows a pale disc and cherry red spot.

pressures in each eye (right eye 12 mm·Hg and left eye 14 mm·Hg). She had a bilateral pale disc and evidence of central retinal artery occlusion in the left eye (Figure 1).

Investigations revealed ESR 130 mm/1st hour, CRP 101 mg/L, white blood cell count 9560/mm^3 with neutrophil predominance, haemoglobin 9.7 g/dL with normochromic normocytic cells, and platelets 350000/mm^3 Her urine analysis, renal, and liver profile were normal. Chest radiograph, electrocardiogram, and 2D echocardiogram were unremarkable. As she had visual impairment, a magnetic resonance imaging (MRI) of the brain was performed, which also was unremarkable.

A clinical diagnosis of giant cell arteritis was made and was proceeded with a left side temporal artery biopsy which confirmed the diagnosis of giant cell arteritis. She was initiated on intravenous methylprednisolone 1 g daily for 3 days on presumptive diagnosis, while the histological confirmation was awaited and followed by 40 mg prednisolone (1 mg/kg) oral daily for four weeks.

A negative result obtained in aetiology directed investigations including anti-nuclear antibodies (ANA), venereal disease research laboratory (VDRL), retroviral screening, and tuberculosis quantiferon gold test.

After continuation of tapering dose of glucocorticoids for a period of 6 months, she noted to have no significant improvement of vision in both eyes. But her vision was not deteriorated after the steroid therapy.

3. Discussion

Giant cell arteritis is a large vessel vasculitis. It mainly involves the aorta and its branches. Visual impairment in GCA can be transient described as amaurosis fugax or permanent. Bilateral visual impairment is a rare presentation in this spectrum [2–4].

Even with the prompt corticosteroid therapy, permanent, complete, or partial visual loss in one or both eyes is reported to be 15 to 20%, and involvement of both eyes is rare and the incidence is less than 1% [3, 5]. Common fundoscopic finding in GCA is anterior ischemic optic neuropathy (AION), and also they can have central retinal artery occlusion, central retinal vein occlusion, or branch artery occlusion [3, 5]. This is the first case reported from Sri Lanka that describes a bilateral AION and central retinal artery occlusion which is an unusual extensive ophthalmic involvement of GCA [3, 5].

Even though the onset of headache is a striking feature, this particular patient had neither headache nor significant constitutional symptoms at presentation. She had biopsy-proven GCA, supported with clinical features such as age more than 50 years, elevated ESR (>50), and tenderness over the temporal artery region. The presentation itself is 93.5% sensitive and 91.2% specific to diagnose GCA according to the American College of Rheumatology (ACR) criteria. She had jaw claudication which is considered as an additional adverse prognostic marker that predicts visual impairment [5]. Additional aetiology-directed investigations were done to exclude the other possible causes of central retinal artery occlusion.

With the initial presentation of visual loss, the standard therapy recommended is high-dose steroids of intravenous methylprednisolone 500 mg–1 g daily for three days followed by oral prednisolone in a dose of 1 mg/kg/day (maximum 60 mg/day) [6, 7]. The blindness caused by GCA is preventable in the majority of cases when diagnosis is made early in the course of the disease [8] as the delay in diagnosis or treatment of GCA can cause several serious consequences, including irreversible visual loss.

However, in this case immediate high-dose steroid therapy was initiated ahead of temporal artery biopsy, but did not result in a favorable outcome in terms of vision though no progressive visual deterioration was noted after initiation of treatment as described in some studies [5, 8, 9].

In conclusion, this case demonstrates an extremely rare spectrum of clinical presentation with an ophthalmic involvement of giant cell arteritis. Even with standard glucocorticoid therapy, the outcome in terms of vision was minimal in this particular patient. When an elderly individual presents with striking symptoms of transient visual loss, headache, and jaw claudication, GCA should be considered as an important differential diagnosis to prevent undue delay in initiating steroid therapy. Jaw claudication was the only initial symptom of this patient which was overlooked by the patient and resulted in a preventable serious lifelong disability.

References

[1] C. Salvarani, F. Cantini, and G. G. Hunder, "Polymyalgia rheumatica and giant-cell arteritis," *The Lancet*, vol. 372, no. 9634, pp. 234–245, 2008.

[2] B. T. Horton, T. B. Magath, and G. E. Brown, "Arteritis of the temporal vessels: a previously undescribed form," *Archives of Internal Medicine*, vol. 53, no. 3, pp. 400–409, 1934.

[3] C. Font, M. C. Cid, B. Coll-Vinent, A. Lopez-Soto, and J. M. Grau, "Clinical features in patients with permanent visual loss due to biopsy- proven giant cell arteritis," *Rheumatology*, vol. 36, no. 2, pp. 251–254, 1997.

[4] I. Vodopivec and J. F. Rizzo, "Ophthalmic manifestations of giant cell arteritis," *Rheumatology*, vol. 57, no. 2, pp. ii63–ii72, 2018.

[5] A. G. Singh, T. A. Kermani, C. S. Crowson et al., "Visual manifestations in giant cell arteritis: trend over 5 decades in a population-based cohort," *The Journal of Rheumatology*, vol. 42, no. 2, pp. 309–315, 2015.

[6] B. Dasgupta, F. A. Borg, N. Hassan et al., "BSR and BHPR guidelines for the management of giant cell arteritis," *Rheumatology*, vol. 49, no. 8, pp. 1594–1597, 2010.

[7] N. G. P. Ferreira, L. M. Falcão, A. T. Alves, and F. Campos, "Giant cell arteritis: a closer look at its ophthalmological manifestations," *BMJ Case Report*, vol. 2015, bcr2015210995, 2015.

[8] S. S. Hayreh, P. A. Podhajsky, and B. Zimmerman, "Ocular manifestations of giant cell arteritis," *American Journal of Ophthalmology*, vol. 125, no. 4, pp. 509–520, 1998.

[9] P. D. Aiello, J. C. Trautmann, T. J. McPhee, A. R. Kunselman, and G. G. Hunder, "Visual prognosis in giant cell arteritis," *Ophthalmology*, vol. 100, no. 4, pp. 550–555, 1993.

11

Tonsillitis-Related Arthritis: Advanced Understandings of Tonsillitis and Sterile Inflammatory Arthritis

Shigeto Kobayashi,[1] **Issei Kida**,[1] **Yuuki Makiyama**,[2] **Yoshinori Taniguchi**,[3] **Kurisu Tada**,[4] **and Naoto Tamura**[4]

[1]*Department of Internal Medicine and Rheumatology, Juntendo University Koshigaya Hospital, Koshigaya, Saitama 343-0032, Japan*
[2]*Department of Otolaryngology, Yokohama City Minato Red Cross Hospital, Yokohama, Kanagawa 231-8682, Japan*
[3]*Department of Endocrinology, Metabolism,Nephrology and Rheumatology, Kochi Medical School Hospital, Kochi University, Nankoku, Kochi 783-8505, Japan*
[4]*Department of Internal Medicine and Rheumatology, Juntendo University School of Medicine, Tokyo 13-8421, Japan*

Correspondence should be addressed to Shigeto Kobayashi; shigeto@juntendo.ac.jp

Academic Editor: Gregory J. Tsay

A 49-year-old man developed acute aseptic arthritis of the nonmigratory and asymmetrical type in his knee, ankle, and bilateral metatarsal joints 13 days after treatment with antibiotics for acute tonsillitis. He was diagnosed with tonsillitis-related arthritis after other rheumatic diseases were ruled out. Treatment with salazosulfapyridine, methotrexate, and methylprednisolone for 3 months did not completely improve. Then, tonsillectomy was undertaken and arthritis rapidly improved. *Finegoldia magna* (previously *Peptostreptococcus magnus*) was cultured from the microabscesses of the resected tonsils. After outpatient follow-up, the patient did not experience a relapse of arthritis for more than 2.7 years without any treatment. Poststreptococcal reactive arthritis (PSRA) is well described. However, up to 40% of patients with tonsillitis-related arthritis did not demonstrate evidence of streptococcal infection. It is noted that tonsillectomy is necessary to remove the tonsillar microabscesses and eradicate bacterial infection of the tonsils, especially for patients with a prolonged and/or recurrent course of PSRA and/or tonsillitis-related arthritis.

1. Introduction

Reactive arthritis (ReA) is sterile arthritis that occurs in genetically predisposed individuals who have human leukocyte antigen- (HLA-) B27 secondary to an extra-articular infection, usually of the gastrointestinal or genitourinary tract. *Salmonella, Shigella, Yersinia,* and *Chlamydia* are the bacteria involved in this disease [1, 2]. On the other hand, sterile arthritis following group A β-hemolytic streptococcal tonsillitis or upper respiratory tract infection is described as poststreptococcal ReA (PSRA) [3, 4]. Compared with acute rheumatic fever (ARF), PSRA is characterized by a latent period of around 10 days between the antecedent streptococcal infection and the development of nonmigratory arthritis, which is shorter in 7–10 days than that in 10–28 days' period seen in ARF; longer duration of arthritis, which is more than 2 months longer than 2 to 3 weeks in ARF; poor response to aspirin; the absence of carditis; the marked severity of arthritis; and a tendency for recurrence and persistence of arthritis [3–6].

We previously reported on adult patients with PSRA and/or tonsillitis-related arthritis, some of whom were resistant to antibiotics and nonsteroidal anti-inflammatory drugs (NSAIDs) underwent tonsillectomy: viable bacteria in microabscesses from the resected palatine tonsils were demonstrated; moreover, arthritis completely disappeared by the removal of the infected tonsils [7, 8], and no one experienced a recurrence of arthritis. Herein, we describe the case of a patient with tonsillitis-related arthritis in whom streptococcal infection was not found and whose arthritis was resistant to NSAIDs, salazosulfapyridine (SASP), methotrexate (MTX), and glucocorticoid treatment for 3 months. Then, tonsillectomy was undertaken, and after removal of tonsillar microabscesses, his arthritis rapidly disappeared.

2. Case Presentation

A 49-year-old man was hospitalized at a local district for severe sore throat and fever (temperature, 40°C) that persisted for several days. He was diagnosed with acute tonsillitis and treated with antibiotics. The microbiological examination was not performed at that time before the administration of antibiotics, and elevated levels of anti-streptokinase (ASK) and anti-streptolysin O (ASO) antibodies were not observed at the hospital. On his 13th day of confinement, the patient rapidly developed arthritis in his right foot and left knee, and his C-reactive protein level increased to 10.13 mg/dl (normal, <0.3 mg/dl). His otorhinolaryngologist could not associate his tonsillitis with arthritis, and the patient read our article on tonsillitis-related arthritis. He then consulted an orthopedic doctor, who, in turn, referred him to our clinic for specialist assessment.

Upon presentation, the patient was walking very slowly on a cane, was afebrile, and had arthritis of both knees and both ankles, as well as the second to fourth metatarsal joints of both feet. Inflamed joints were found predominantly on his left knee and right ankle (Figure 1). A knee aspirate was completed: no crystal was found in the synovial fluid, and no bacteria were cultured.

The patient had no history of skin and eye involvement or gastrointestinal and urinary tract infections. He has had episodes of recurrent tonsillitis since he was 12 years old. His C-reactive protein level was 5.36 mg/dl. The serum level of uric acid was within the normal level. Rheumatoid factor and other autoantibodies were negative, as were ASK and ASO antibodies. Human lymphocyte antigen- (HLA-) B27 was not demonstrated.

He was diagnosed with tonsillitis-related arthritis and recommended the removal of his palatine tonsils as written in our article. Although, the treatments of NSAIDs (SASP) (1 g/d, which is the maximum dose approved in Japan) and MTX (12 mg/week; maximum dose approved in Japan, 16 mg/week) for more than 3 months and intramuscular methylprednisolone (3 injections of 40 mg) did not completely improve the patient's arthritis. Therefore, tonsillectomy was undertaken, and *Finegoldia magna* (previously *Peptostreptococcus magnus*) was demonstrated in the resected tonsils. A slight contracture on the patient's left knee, but no arthritis, was found 1 month after the surgery as we expected. The patient did not experience a relapse of arthritis for more than 2.7 years without any medication (Figure 2).

3. Discussion

PSRA is widely understood to be distinct from acute rheumatic fever (ARF). Diagnostic criteria for PSRA include persistent, additive, nonmigratory acute arthritis in one or more joints, evidence of prior group A β-hemolytic streptococcal infection, and the lack of other major criteria for ARF [3–9]. However, it is not always easy to diagnose PSRA since it needed to be distinguished from viral arthritis, septic arthritis, and diseases of peripheral spondyloarthritis [4], and the spectrum of this disease is wide and significantly heterogeneous [10, 11].

In our old series of adult patients, only 62% of patients were positive for ASO and/or ASK, and only 57% of throat cultures for group A streptococcus were revealed to be positive [7, 8]. This may be due to the reason that some of our adult patients had a long period and recurrent history of chronic tonsillitis and subsequent arthritis [8]. Moreover, it was reported that 20–40% of patients were unable to demonstrate evidence of streptococcal infection [7, 8, 12]. *Pseudomonas aeruginosa, Klebsiella oxitosa, Chlamydia trachomatis, Staphylococcus, Serratia,* group B *Streptococcus, Staphylococcus aureus,* and *Peptostreptococcus* were isolated from throat swabs of our patients who were not demonstrated evidence of infection of *Streptococcus* [7, 11]. Our patient in this case report had a history of recurrent tonsillitis, and it may be possible that *Streptococcus* was replaced by other bacteria such as *F. magna* which are resistant to antibiotics and/or phagocytosis.

Therefore, clinicians should understand that not only *Streptococcus* but also other bacteria will induce sterile arthritis similar to that of PSRA, although its clinical manifestations do not differ from those of PSRA. In addition, many bacteria have been reported to be involved in a disorder of "widely interpreted ReA" [13]. Since evidence of streptococcal infection was not found in the case described herein, we prefer to use the term "tonsillitis-related arthritis" in diagnosis but not PSRA, based on the definition of the criteria proposed by the Fourth International Workshop of Reactive Arthritis in 1999 [14]. The term "ReA" could be used only if the clinical picture and the microbes involved are associated with HLA-B27 and spondyloarthritis [8, 14].

Most patients, especially children with PSRA or tonsillitis-related arthritis, respond well to antibiotics and NSAIDs and resolve within 8 weeks [9]. However, it is noted that 77% of adult patients with PSRA did not resolve arthritis within 6 weeks [11]. The bacteria involved in classical ReA reside intracellularly in host cells. However, *Streptococcus* and *F. magna* are extracellular bacteria, some of which can produce biofilm patches around them that are capable of not only escaping contact with antibiotics but also avoiding phagocytosis and/or autophagy inside the macrophages/monocytes [15]. Therefore, it is essential to understand that microabscesses existing inside the palatine tonsils are the real foci of bacterial infection, especially in patients who are resistant to antibiotics. In our old study, the mean duration of arthritis before diagnosis was much longer in 8 patients (38.6 ± 47.0 months; mean ± standard deviation) who had undertaken tonsillectomy than that of 13 patients (13.0 ± 17.9 months) who were not undertaking tonsillectomy (data not shown) [8, 16].

Moreover, tonsils have been widely understood as the pathogen reservoir, which indicates that infection of the tonsils has multiple foci, the microbiome is polymicrobial, and bacteria are present throughout the tissue [15].

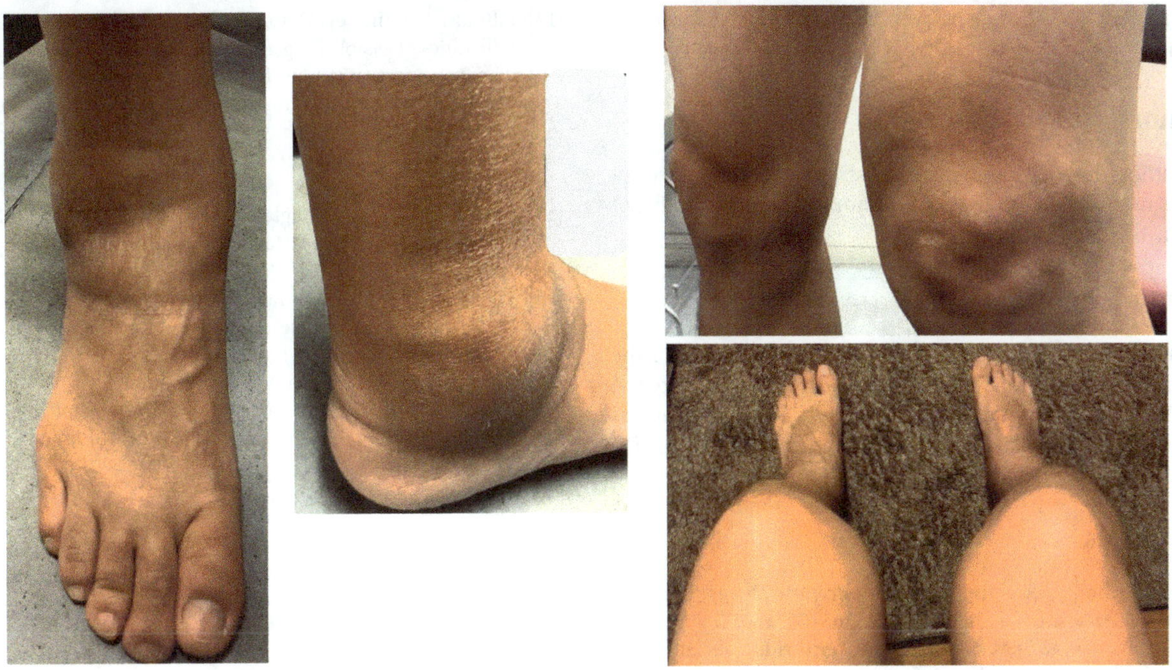

FIGURE 1: Case presentation. The patient presented with inflamed joints of the left ankle and right knee when he was referred to our hospital.

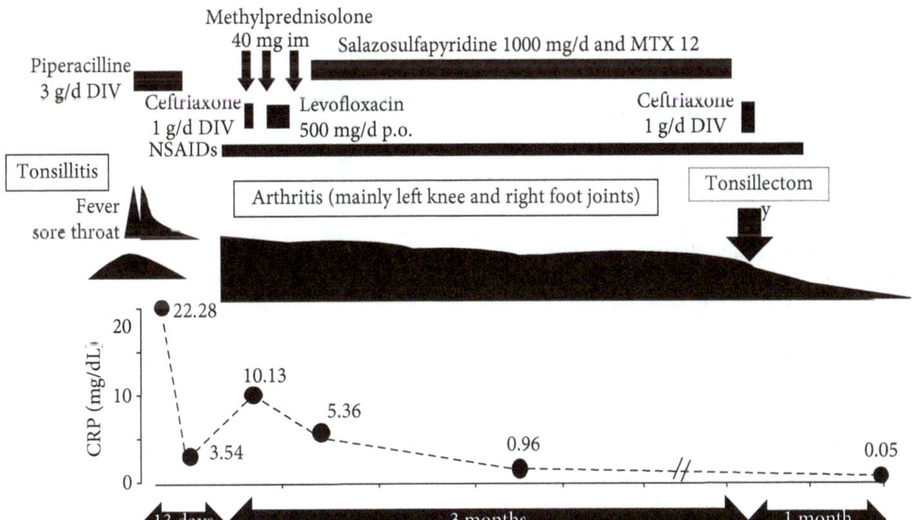

FIGURE 2: Clinical course. Since arthritis was not improved with the treatments for more than 3 months, tonsillectomy was undertaken. No arthritis was demonstrated 1 month after the surgery, and no recurrence of arthritis was found for more than 2.7 years without any treatment.

Therefore, the persistence of viable *Streptococcus* and other extracellular bacteria in the CD14+ cells of the tonsils would allow for their movement to the joints and induce aseptic arthritis as we previously demonstrated the fragments of *Streptococcus* in a patient's synovial fluid cells [7].

Therefore, viable bacteria persistently exist in the tonsils for a long period, and this might be an explanation why frequent recurrence and/or long-period treatment were experienced in adult patients with PSRA/tonsillitis-related arthritis [7, 8, 11].

4. Conclusions

Our case demonstrates that tonsillectomy is effective for the treatment of tonsillitis-related arthritis to eradicate the bacterial infection in the tonsils. If arthritis does not respond to prolonged treatment with antibiotics and NSAIDs and if, especially, patients have a history of recurrent tonsillitis, tonsillectomy is recommended for preventing comorbidities such as toxic shock syndrome [8, 17]. General practitioners, especially otorhinolaryngologists, orthopedic doctors, and rheumatologists, should be well aware of this disorder to diagnose appropriately and treat it efficiently.

Authors' Contributions

All authors have discussed the questions in the manuscript and agree to the content. The authors played a significant role in this paper.

Acknowledgments

The authors are grateful to Prof. Yasuaki Harabuchi of the Department of Otolaryngology Head & Neck Surgery, Asahikawa Medical University, for providing medical advice. The authors thank Enago (https://www.enago.com/) for the English language review of this manuscript.

References

[1] S. K. Schmitt, "Reactive arthritis," *Infectious Disease Clinics of North America*, vol. 31, no. 2, pp. 265–277, 2017.

[2] P. Ahvonen, K. Sievers, and K. Aho, "Arthritis associated with *Yersinia enterocolitica* infection," *Acta Rheumatologica Scandinavica*, vol. 15, no. 1-4, pp. 232–253, 1969.

[3] C. Deighton, "β Haemolytic streptococci and reactive arthritis," *Annals of the Rheumatic Diseases*, vol. 52, no. 6, pp. 475–482, 1993.

[4] M. H. Arnold and A. Tyndall, "Poststreptococcal reactive arthritis," *Annals of the Rheumatic Diseases*, vol. 48, no. 8, pp. 686–688, 1989.

[5] Y. Uziel, L. Perl, J. Barash, and P. J. Hashkes, "Post-streptococcal reactive arthritis in children: a distinct entity from acute rheumatic fever," *Pediatr Rheumatology Online Journal*, vol. 9, no. 1, p. 32, 2011.

[6] H. Pathak and T. Marshall, "Post-streptococcal reactive arthritis: where are we now," *BMJ Case Reports*, vol. 2016, 1996.

[7] S. Kobayashi, N. Tamura, T. Akimoto et al., "Reactive arthritis induced by tonsillitis," *Acta Otolaryngology*, vol. 523, pp. 206–211, 1996.

[8] Y. Taniguchi, H. Nishikawa, T. Yoshida et al., "Expanding the spectrum of reactive arthritis (ReA): classic ReA and infection-related arthritis including poststreptococcal ReA, poncet's disease, and iBCG-induced ReA," *Rheumatology International*, vol. 41, no. 8, pp. 1387–1398, 2021.

[9] C. Chun and D. J. Kingsbury, "Poststreptococcal reactive arthritis: diagnostic challenges," *Perm Journal*, vol. 23, no. 18, p. 304, 2019.

[10] P. Padhan and D. Danda, "Clinical spectrum of post-streptococcal reactive arthritis (PSRA) revisited: juvenile versus adult-onset disease," *International Journal of Rheumatic Diseases*, vol. 22, no. 4, pp. 750-751, 2019.

[11] S. L. Mackie and A. Keat, "Poststreptococcal reactive arthritis: what is it and how do we know?" *Rheumatology*, vol. 43, no. 8, pp. 949–954, 2004.

[12] A. E. Muşetescu, M. Florea, M. C. ForŢofoiu et al., "Streptococcal tonsillitis related reactive arthritis-clinical, ultrasound imaging and immunohistochemical study," *Romanian Journal of Morphology and Embryology*, vol. 58, no. 3, pp. 801–807, 2017.

[13] H. Zeidler and A. P. Hudson, "Reactive arthritis update: spotlight on new and rare infectious agents implicated as pathogens," *Current Rheumatology Reports*, vol. 23, no. 7, p. 53, 2021.

[14] J. Braun, G. Kingsley, D. van der Heijde, and J. Sieper, "On the difficulties of establishing a consensus on the definition of and diagnostic investigations for reactive arthritis. Results and discussion of a questionnaire prepared for the 4th international workshop on reactive arthritis, Berlin, Germany, July 3–6, 1999," *Journal of Rheumatology*, vol. 27, no. 9, pp. 2185–2192, 2000.

[15] J. J. Johnston and R. Dauglas, "Adenotonsillar microbiome: an update," *Postgraduate Medical Journal*, vol. 94, no. 1113, pp. 398–403, 2018.

[16] S. Kobayashi, N. Tamura, G. Ichikawa, Y. Takasaki, and H. Hashimoto, "Reactive arthritis induced by *Pseudomonas aeruginosa*," *Clinical Rheumatology*, vol. 15, pp. 516-517, 1996.

[17] T. P. Brito, I. M. Hazboun, and F. L. Fernandes, "Deep neck abscesses: study of 101 cases," *Brazilian Journal of Otorhinolaryngology*, vol. 83, no. 3, pp. 341–348, 2017.

12

A Case of Heparin-Induced Thrombocytopenia that Developed in the Therapeutic Course of Anti-Neutrophil Cytoplasmic Antibody-Associated Vasculitis

Taketoshi Nonaka,[1] Makoto Harada,[1] Masahiko Sumi,[2] Wataru Ishii,[3] Tohru Ichikawa,[1] and Mamoru Kobayashi[1]

[1]*Department of Nephrology, Nagano Red Cross Hospital, 5-22-1 Wakasato, Nagano 380-8582, Japan*
[2]*Department of Hematology, Nagano Red Cross Hospital, 5-22-1 Wakasato, Nagano 380-8582, Japan*
[3]*Department of Rheumatology, Nagano Red Cross Hospital, 5-22-1 Wakasato, Nagano 380-8582, Japan*

Correspondence should be addressed to Makoto Harada; tokomadaraha724@gmail.com

Academic Editor: Tsai-Ching Hsu

Background. Heparin-induced thrombocytopenia (HIT) causes thrombocytopenia via an immunological mechanism, resulting in severe organ injury due to arterial-venous thrombosis. HIT often develops in hemodialysis patients owing to heparin use. Anti-neutrophil cytoplasmic antibody-associated vasculitis (AAV) is a systemic vasculitis, and cases of AAV complicated with HIT are rare. In addition, it mostly occurs in patients undergoing hemodialysis. *Case Presentation.* An 87-year-old woman presented with rapidly progressive renal failure and severe leg edema. She was diagnosed with AAV and treated with glucocorticoid and heparin calcium to prevent deep vein thrombosis. Eight days after the start of heparin calcium, her platelet count decreased and the anti-platelet factor 4-heparin complex antibody was strongly positive (>5.0 U/mL; the cutoff point of the anti-platelet factor 4-heparin complex antibody evaluated by the latex turbidity assay is 1.0 U/mL). She was diagnosed with HIT and treated with argatroban. Subsequently, her platelet counts increased gradually. *Conclusion.* We encountered a case of HIT that developed prior to the induction of hemodialysis in the clinical course of AAV. When AAV clinical course presents thrombocytopenia, the possibility of HIT should be considered.

1. Introduction

Heparin-induced thrombocytopenia (HIT) causes thrombocytopenia and develops a severe arterial-venous thrombosis via the immunological mechanism, which produces antibodies targeting the platelet factor 4 (PF4) complex with heparin [1]. Argatroban is usually used as an initial therapy [1]. It has been reported that patients who undergo hemodialysis and patients with autoimmune disorders are significantly associated with developing HIT [2, 3]. The reasons are as follows: most patients undergoing hemodialysis are treated with heparin in the hemodialysis session, and autoimmune disorders may be the risk factor in the abnormal production of the antigen-antibody complex [2, 3].

Anti-neutrophil cytoplasmic antibody-associated vasculitis (AAV) is a systemic vasculitis characterized by the presence of anti-neutrophil cytoplasmic antibodies (ANCAs) [4]. AAV often causes severe organ injury such as alveolar hemorrhage, interstitial pneumonia, and a rapid progressive glomerulonephritis resulting in dialysis [4].

Cases of coexistence of AAV and HIT are rare, but several cases do exist [5–8]. Most of these coexistent cases developed HIT after initiating hemodialysis due to AAV-induced renal failure. However, herein, we present a case of HIT that developed prior to the induction of hemodialysis in the clinical course of AAV and report the details of the clinical course and discuss the association between AAV and HIT.

Table 1: Main clinical data of the current case at hospital admission.

Urinalysis	
Protein	2+ 7.08 g/gCr
Hematuria	3+ 10–19 HPF
Blood analysis	
WBC	9500 μL
Neut	80%
Lym	11.6%
Mono	7.6%
Eos	0.6%
Baso	0.2%
Hb	7.2 g/dL
Plt	431,000 μL
Total protein	4.3 g/dL
Albumin	1.3 g/dL
BUN	37.4 mg/dL
Cr	2.25 mg/dL
UA	6.1 mg/dL
Na	135 mEq/L
K	4.4 mEq/L
Cl	106 mEq/L
AST	15 U/L
ALT	4 U/L
LDH	157 U/L
ALP	153 U/L
γGT	20 U/L
T. bil	0.4 mg/dL
RF	72 IU/mL
ANA (homogeneous)	×20
C3	98 mg/dL
C4	31 mg/dL
CH50	42.8 U/mL
MPO-ANCA	147 U/mL
PR3-ANCA	<1.0 U/mL
Anti-GBM antibody	<2.0 U/mL

WBC, white blood cells; Hb, hemoglobin; Plt, platelet; BUN, blood urea nitrogen; Cr, creatinine; UA, uric acid; Na, sodium; K, potassium; Cl, chloride; AST, aspartate aminotransferase; ALT, alanine aminotransferase; LDH, lactate dehydrogenase; ALP, alkaline phosphatase; γGT, gamma-glutamyl transpeptidase; T. bil, total bilirubin; RF, rheumatoid factor; ANA, antinuclear antibody; C3, complement 3; C4, complement 4; CH50, complement hemolytic activity assay; MPO-ANCA, myeloperoxidase-anti-neutrophil cytoplasmic antibody; PR3-ANCA, proteinase 3-anti-neutrophil cytoplasmic antibody; anti-GBM antibody, anti-glomerular basement membrane antibody.

2. Case Presentation

An 87-year-old woman who presented with appetite loss and leg edema was admitted for evaluation. Blood examination revealed an inflammatory response (C-reactive protein level was 7.85 mg/dL), kidney dysfunction (blood urea nitrogen was 37.4 mg/dL, and the serum creatinine level was 2.25 mg/dL), and hypoalbuminemia. Urinary examination revealed severe proteinuria (7.05 g/gCr) and hematuria. In addition, the patient was positive for myeloperoxidase-ANCA (147 U/mL). The main laboratory data are presented in Table 1.

According to these results, she was diagnosed with AAV and glucocorticoid therapy was started (an oral dose of prednisolone 40 mg/day). The patient was considered to be at a high risk of deep vein thrombosis; therefore, heparin calcium therapy was also administered. Although the systemic inflammation improved after glucocorticoid therapy, the leg edema and hypoalbuminemia did not improve. Her body weight steadily increased, and leg edema worsened 14 days after hospitalization; she received hemodialysis therapy. Although the baseline platelet count was 400,000 to 500,000/μL, 8 days after the start of heparin calcium therapy, her platelet count gradually decreased. In addition, blood examination performed 26 days after hospitalization revealed that the platelet count was 81,000/μL, the fibrinogen level was low at 138 mg/dL, and the FDP-D-dimer level was high at 18.2 μg/mL (Figure 1). According to the 4Ts scoring, reduction of 50% or more of the platelet count and a platelet decrease between 5 and 10 days after using heparin are consistent. Additionally, because the FDP-D-dimer was high, she might have had thrombosis. Other causes of thrombocytopenia were not detected. Therefore, it was highly possible that she developed HIT. In addition, the patient was strongly positive for the anti-PF4-heparin complex antibody (the titer of the anti-platelet factor 4-heparin complex antibody evaluated by the latex turbidity assay was more than 5.0 U/mL). The titer measurement result was extremely high because the cutoff point of the anti-platelet factor 4-heparin complex antibody evaluated by the latex turbidity assay is 1.0 U/mL. These results were the basis of the HIT diagnosis. We performed Doppler echography for her legs to evaluate deep vein thrombosis 28 days after hospitalization. However, deep vein thrombosis was not detected. Because we expected her renal function to recover at that time, enhanced computed tomography to evaluate systemic thrombosis was not performed. Heparin was discontinued 29 days after hospitalization, and argatroban therapy was administered, following which warfarin therapy was administered. After starting argatroban therapy, her platelets count gradually increased (Figure 1). Fortunately, no symptoms due to arterial or venous thrombosis presented in her clinical course. Fifty-two days after her hospitalization, the platelet count improved to 200,000/μL. Because her AAV activity was well controlled and the titer of MPO-ANCA was reduced, the dose of prednisolone was decreased. However, because kidney function was not recovered, she was administered maintenance hemodialysis therapy.

3. Discussion

In the current case, heparin therapy was administered because of a high risk for developing deep vein thrombosis and HIT developed prior to hemodialysis. Concerning the clinical course of the current case, 8 days after the start of heparin calcium therapy, her platelet count gradually decreased. This would be consistent with HIT. In addition, heparin was used in the hemodialysis session until 29 days after hospitalization. This is the reason the platelet count continued to decrease. In the current case, the titer of the anti-platelet factor 4-heparin complex antibody was extremely high at more than 5.0 U/mL (the cutoff point by the latex turbidity assay is 1.0 U/mL). It is thought that a high

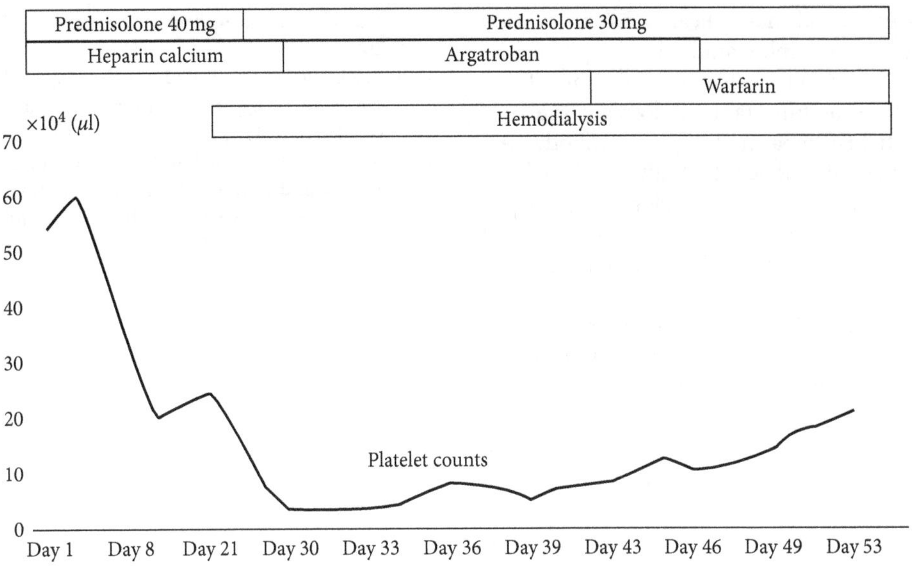

FIGURE 1: Clinical course of the platelet count in the current patient. Eight days after the start of heparin calcium, the platelet count gradually decreased.

TABLE 2: Clinical characteristics of previously published four coexisting cases of anti-neutrophil cytoplasmic antibody-associated vasculitis and heparin-induced thrombocytopenia.

	Sex	Age	Type of ANCA	Type of organ injury	Treatment	Onset of HIT and type of heparin
Roe et al. [5]	M	65	PR3	Crescentic glomerulonephritis, pulmonary hemorrhage	mPSL pulse, PSL, CY, hemodialysis	9 days after the start of hemodialysis, unfractionated heparin
Kaneda et al. [6]	F	91	MPO	Kidney dysfunction, pulmonary hemorrhage	mPSL pulse, PSL, hemodialysis	13 days after the start of hemodialysis, unfractionated heparin
Mandai et al. [7]	M	40	MPO	Crescentic glomerulonephritis, interstitial pneumonia	mPSL pulse, PSL, CY, PE, hemodialysis	5 days after the start of hemodialysis, unfractionated heparin
Thong et al. [8]	M	71	PR3	Kidney dysfunction	mPSL pulse, PSL, CY, hemodialysis	15 days after the start of hemodialysis, unfractionated heparin and dalteparin

ANCA, anti-neutrophil cytoplasmic antibody; CY, cyclophosphamide therapy; F, female; HIT, heparin-induced thrombocytopenia; M, male; MPO, myeloperoxidase; mPSL, methylprednisolone; PE, plasma exchange therapy (including double filtration plasmapheresis); PR3, proteinase 3; PSL, prednisolone.

titer of the anti-platelet factor 4-heparin complex antibody is the reason why the recovery of the platelet count from argatroban therapy was slow.

Kato et al. have noted that hemodialysis, autoimmune diseases, gout, and heart failure were significantly correlated with HIT in their retrospective observational study. Most patients undergoing hemodialysis are treated with heparin in their dialysis session, and cases of HIT are often reported [2]. A previous study from Japan reported that the incidence of HIT in patients undergoing hemodialysis was 3.9% [2]. Kato et al. have performed a multivariate analysis of 55 cases of in-hospital HIT and concluded that there is a significant association between HIT and autoimmune diseases [3]. There are rare but several cases of HIT in the clinical course of AAV [5–8]. We present the clinical characteristics of previously published four coexisting cases of AAV and HIT (Table 2) [5–8].

The age range was 40 to 91 years; the ratio of MPO-to-proteinase 3 ANCA was 1:1, and male-to-female ratio was 3:1. These cases showed severe organ injury, a systemic severe kidney injury requiring hemodialysis and an acute lung injury due to alveolar hemorrhage, and bronchiolitis obliterans resulting in pneumonia. Four cases were treated with methylprednisolone pulse therapy (250 to 1,000 mg) and a high dose of prednisolone, two were treated with cyclophosphamide, and one was treated with plasma exchange therapy. All cases developed HIT after the start of these immunosuppressive therapies and hemodialysis. Even with strong immunosuppressive therapy, the production of antibodies targeting the PF4 complex with heparin may not be suppressed. The previous reports of treating HIT by immunosuppressive therapy are really limited. Although Schell et al. treated HIT by plasma exchange and rituximab, the patient required bilateral limb amputation [9]. Previous research using murine models has indicated that production of the anti-PF4-heparin complex antibody is regulated by not only B cells but also CD4 T cells [10]. Therefore, T-cell suppression may be also important to decrease the production of the anti-PF4-heparin complex antibody. Although all these cases developed HIT after the start of hemodialysis, the patient in our case developed HIT before the initiation of hemodialysis. There was no relationship between the HIT occurrence and hemodialysis in the current case. AAV may be associated with the development of HIT. In addition, patients with AAV are likely to be treated with heparin because patients with AAV often require plasma exchange therapy and/or hemodialysis and AAV is a high risk factor for deep vein thrombosis [1, 11]. Therefore, we should consider the possibility of HIT when patients with AAV develop thrombocytopenia. However, because coexisting cases of AAV and HIT are uncommon, further studies of these types of cases are required to determine the significant association between both diseases.

In conclusion, we should consider the possibility of HIT when patients with AAV develop thrombocytopenia after the start of heparin use.

References

[1] J. Hirsh, N. Heddle, and J. G. Kelton, "Treatment of heparin-induced thrombocytopenia," *Archives of Internal Medicine*, vol. 164, no. 4, pp. 361–369, 2004.

[2] S. Yamamoto, M. Koide, M. Matsuo et al., "Heparin-induced thrombocytopenia in hemodialysis patients," *American Journal of Kidney Diseases*, vol. 28, no. 1, pp. 82–85, 1996.

[3] S. Kato, K. Takahashi, K. Ayabe et al., "Heparin-induced thrombocytopenia: analysis of risk factors in medical inpatients," *British Journal of Haematology*, vol. 154, no. 3, pp. 373–377, 2011.

[4] C. Pagnoux, "Updates in ANCA-associated vasculitis," *European Journal of Rheumatology*, vol. 3, no. 3, pp. 122–133, 2016.

[5] S. Roe, M. Cassidy, A. Haynes, and J. Byrne, "Heparin-induced thrombocytopenia (HIT) and thrombosis syndrome in a haemodialysis-dependent patient with systemic vasculitis," *Nephrology Dialysis Transplantation*, vol. 13, no. 12, pp. 3226–3229, 1998.

[6] K. Kaneda, N. Fukunaga, A. Kudou et al., "Heparin-induced thrombocytopenia (HIT) in an acute uremic patient with ANCA-associated glomerulonephritis," *Nihon Toseki Igakkai Zasshi*, vol. 42, no. 6, pp. 453–458, 2009.

[7] S. Mandai, K. Nagahama, Y. Tsuura et al., "Recovery of renal function in a dialysis-dependent patient with microscopic polyangiitis and both myeloperoxidase anti-neutrophil cytoplasmic antibodies and anti-glomerular basement membrane antibodies," *Internal Medicine*, vol. 50, no. 15, pp. 1599–1603, 2011.

[8] K. M. Thong, P. Toth, and A. Khwaja, "Management of heparin-induced thrombocytopenia (HIT) in patients with systemic vasculitis and pulmonary haemorrhage," *Clinical Kidney Journal*, vol. 6, no. 6, pp. 622–625, 2013.

[9] A. M. Schell, M. Petras, Z. M. Szczepiorkowski, and D. L. Ornstein, "Refractory heparin induced thrombocytopenia with thrombosis (HITT) treated with therapeutic plasma exchange and rituximab as adjuvant therapy," *Transfusion and Apheresis Science*, vol. 49, no. 2, pp. 185–188, 2013.

[10] Y. Zheng, M. Yu, A. Padmanabhan et al., "Critical role of CD4 T cells in PF4/heparin antibody production in mice," *Blood*, vol. 125, no. 11, pp. 1826–1829, 2015.

[11] A. Kang, M. Antonelou, N. L. Wong et al., "High incidence of arterial and venous thrombosis in antineutrophil cytoplasmic antibody-associated vasculitis," *Journal of Rheumatology*, vol. 46, no. 3, pp. 285–293, 2019.

13

Coexistence of Relapsing Polychondritis and Sickle Cell Disease in a Child

Bernard Ofoe Tetteh,[1] **Florence-Barbara Yebuah**,[2] **Maame-Boatemaa Amissah-Arthur**,[1,3] and **Dzifa Dey**[1,3]

[1]*Rheumatology Unit, Department of Internal Medicine and Therapeutics, Korle-Bu Teaching Hospital, Accra, Ghana*
[2]*Ophthalmology Department, Korle-Bu Teaching Hospital, Accra, Ghana*
[3]*Rheumatology Unit, Department of Internal Medicine and Therapeutics, University of Ghana Medical School, Accra, Ghana*

Correspondence should be addressed to Bernard Ofoe Tetteh; tetteh.ofoe.bernard@gmail.com

Academic Editor: Remzi Cevik

Relapsing polychondritis (RP) is a rare, severe connective tissue disease of unknown etiology affecting cartilaginous and proteoglycan-rich structures in an episodic and inflammatory manner. Approximately a third of RP cases occur in conjunction with another disease usually systemic autoimmune rheumatic disease, or myelodysplastic syndrome. Sickle cell disease (SCD) is a common inherited hematologic condition characterized by the inheritance of two abnormal hemoglobins, of which one is a hemoglobin S, presenting with severe acute and chronic complications from vaso-occlusive phenomena, which can be difficult to differentiate from RP. The pathogenesis of RP is poorly understood but suggests an autoimmune mechanism with a link to sickle cell disease yet to be established. Treatment is empiric with steroids, anti-inflammatory, and disease-modifying antirheumatic drugs being the mainstay of therapy. Severe complications occur despite treatment, with respiratory involvement being the most catastrophic. This case report reviews a complex case of RP in an 11-year-old girl with sickle cell disease (SF genotype) presenting with bilateral red painful eyes, a painful swollen left ear, and knee pain. Laboratory findings revealed elevated inflammatory markers with negative immune serology. A diagnosis of RP was made based on the patient's symptomatology, presentation, and fulfillment of 5 out of the 6 clinical features using McAdam's criteria. Management was instituted with a myriad of conventional and biologic DMARDs and other anti-inflammatory medications with no significant improvement and the development of complications of airway obstruction from disease activity and osteoporotic fracture from steroid therapy and underlying hemoglobinopathy. In children, the diagnosis of RP is delayed or overlooked due to its low incidence, variability in clinical symptoms, or sharing similar clinical features with other coexisting disease entities. This article reports its occurrence in the pediatric population and highlights the difficulty in managing such cases as there are no defined standard treatment protocols.

1. Introduction

Relapsing polychondritis (RP) is a rare, severe connective tissue disease with an episodic and progressive inflammatory nature involving cartilaginous structures, mainly the ear, nose, and laryngotracheobronchial tree. The disease also affects the joints, sclera, and various proteoglycan-rich tissues including the media of arteries [1].

Sickle cell disease (SCD) refers to a group of disorders of hemoglobin in which the sickle mutation is coinherited with a mutation at the other beta globin allele that reduces normal beta globin production. These include sickle cell anemia, sickle cell thalassemia, hemoglobin SC disease, and hemoglobin SF disease, which our patient had. SCD presents with severe acute and chronic complications involving many organs in the form of acute pain episodes, anemia, recurrent infections, and chronic end organ damage [2].

RP is common in patients aged 40–50 years but may occur at any age with a genetic link suggested by a significantly higher frequency of HLA-DR4 in patients with RP than in healthy individuals [1] and shows various immune responses directed against type 2 collagen and matrilin-1 [3].

Approximately 30% of RP cases coexist with other autoimmune inflammatory disorders with a small percentage being associated with nonrheumatic conditions [4]. However, the coexistence of RP and SCD has not been reported, and the management of such cases remains uncertain.

RP is thought to be very rare among individuals of African descent with the majority of patients being of Caucasian origin [5]. Pediatric RP accounts for less than 5% of the cases reported, and it is characterized by frequent hospitalizations and emergency room visits, missed school attendance, and significant disability [6].

The most common clinical features of RP are chondritis and polyarthritis.

Bilateral auricular chondritis is the most common feature observed in 90% of cases during the course of the disease, and this presents as painful, red, violaceous edema confined to the cartilaginous part of the ear. This leads to deformation of the ear following repeated flares and resembles the cauliflower ear of professional boxers. They can also present with either conductive or sensorineural hearing loss, saddle nose deformity, and laryngotracheobronchial involvement. Nonerosive asymmetric arthritis, ocular manifestations such as episcleritis, scleritis, uveitis, retinopathy, and conjunctivitis are also features of the disease [7]. Less frequently, patients can present with neurological involvement in the form of headaches, vasculitis, meningitis, and cerebral infarction, with IgA nephropathy, tubulointerstitial nephritis, and glomerulonephritis being some of the renal manifestations [7].

The diverse and nonspecific clinical features of RP alongside its relative rarity frequently lead to a diagnostic delay [8] which is associated with the lack of ear, nose, or joint involvement but presents with early signs of intermittent arthritis or eye involvement in such cases [4]. RP patients may develop significant disabilities during the course of the disease such as hearing and visual impairments, and 30–50% of patients suffer pulmonary complications [9, 10].

The diagnosis of RP is mainly clinical using a classification criteria developed by McAdam and later expanded on by Damiani-Levine and Michet, which includes recurrent inflammation of both auricular, nasal, laryngeal and tracheal cartilages, noninflammatory arthritis, inflammation of ocular structures, and cochlear or vestibular damage [4]. The diagnosis can also be made from a positive biopsy of the ear, nasal, or respiratory cartilage [4, 7]. There are no laboratory investigations specific for the diagnosis of RP and laboratory findings may be suggestive of ongoing inflammation or organ damage revealing the presence of anemia, thrombocytosis, leukocytosis, or a derangement in renal function or urinalysis signifying renal impairment [7]. In RP, serological tests such as the rheumatoid factor, antinuclear antibodies (ANA), complement levels, extractable nuclear antibodies (ENA), and antiphospholipid antibodies are usually negative, but may be positive in the presence of other associated autoimmune conditions [11]. ANA is usually negative and can occur in low titers. The presence of significant titers of ANA in a patient with RP connotes a possibility of an associated autoimmune disorder [7]. Antineutrophil cytoplasmic antibodies (ANCA) may be present in about 25% of patients with RP which can be an incidental finding or the presence of an ANCA-associated vasculitis or herald the beginning of one [3].

The management of RP is mainly empirical as there are no evidence-based guidelines for treatment. The aim of therapy is to reduce inflammation through immunosuppression and prevent multiorgan damage to cartilaginous structures [7]. Mild disease is treated with low dose steroids, NSAIDs, colchicine, and dapsone while high dose steroids and conventional DMARDs such as methotrexate, azathioprine cyclophosphamide, or mycophenolate mofetil are employed in severe life-threatening flares [4]. Biologic therapy agents such as infliximab, etanercept, and adalimumab appear to show efficacy in the treatment of RP that is resistant to conventional DMARDs [12].

The disease entity continues to baffle the scientific community because of its rarity, unknown etiopathogenesis, clinical diversity, unpredictable progression, and uncodified treatment [1]. Coexistence of SCD and RP, an autoimmune disorder, poses a diagnostic and therapeutic challenge as patients with these conditions can present with symptoms that are similar in both conditions, for instance, fever, polyarthritis, and multiorgan involvement. Therefore, early diagnosis of RP is important to define the best treatment modality which may include targeted biological therapy [13].

RP in the setting of sickle cell disease can be difficult to diagnose as a result of the nonspecific nature of symptoms and presentation; therefore, a high index of suspicion is needed to make the diagnosis early and institute treatment to prevent the significant morbidity and mortality associated with the disease, especially in the pediatric group.

The purpose of this article is to highlight the fact that the disease can occur in the pediatric population and also in association with sickle cell disease. It also aims to reiterate the difficulty in managing such cases as there are no written protocols in the treatment of RP and that medications used in the treatment of RP can worsen SCD and its complications.

We describe a case of relapsing polychondritis in an 11-year-old girl with sickle cell disease (SF genotype) who suffered severe respiratory tract involvement, which posed a considerable management challenge. This case is of significant interest due to the rarity of the condition, the young age of our patient, and the association with sickle cell disease; previously unreported in the literature compared to the known coexistence with autoimmune conditions such as vasculitis, systemic lupus erythematosus, and rheumatoid arthritis, and the hurdles encountered during treatment.

2. Case Report

A 9-year-old young girl was referred to the rheumatology clinic from the ophthalmology unit as a case of systemic vasculitis with episcleritis. She presented with recurrent bilateral red painful eyes, a painful swollen left ear, and left knee pain in the preceding 10 months. A month prior to the presentation, she had developed an intermittent fever and reduced hearing. Three months prior to this, she had been admitted with painful swelling of the left knee and a fever, for which she was treated for septic arthritis of the left knee. Two years preceding the visit to the rheumatology clinic, she had also presented to the otorhinolaryngology unit on several occasions with complaints of hearing difficulty and was diagnosed with otitis externa. She has sickle cell disease-genotype SF and is a regular attendant at the pediatric sickle cell clinic. She did not suffer from an autoimmune condition, but had a first-degree cousin with systemic lupus erythematosus. She is the first of 2 children (her younger sibling is well) and has been unable to attend school due to arthralgia and difficulty hearing.

2.1. Clinical and Laboratory Findings. On examination, there was mild pallor, axillary lymphadenopathy, and bilateral conjunctival injection with proptosis. The pinnae were swollen, erythematous, and tender, resembling "cauliflower ears" (Figure 1). The cardiorespiratory system examination was normal. There was acute synovitis of both knees with an old arthrotomy scar on the left (Figure 2).

Results from a previous synovial biopsy showed moderate, chronic inflammatory infiltrates composed of lymphocytes and plasma cells with stromal edema and congested vessels, but no malignant cells were seen, in keeping with chronic synovitis. The audiology assessment confirmed bilateral sensorineural hearing loss, worse in the left ear.

Laboratory investigations showed the following: Hb 10.7 g/dl (11–18 g/dl): microcytic, hypochromic pattern; WBC 15.7×10^9/L ($2.5–8.5 \times 10^9$); and platelets 688×10^9/L ($150–450 \times 10^9$). Erythrocyte sedimentation rate (ESR) and C reactive protein (CRP) were elevated at 96 mm/hr (0–15 mm/hr) and 143.7 mg/l (<5 mg/l), respectively. Hep atitis B, hepatitis C, and retroviral screens were negative. Hb electrophoresis–Hb A2–3%, Hb F–38.8%, Hb S–57.7%. The rheumatoid factor, ANA, and ENA panel were negative.

The initial diagnoses considered were juvenile idiopathic arthritis, septic arthritis of the left knee, systemic vasculitis, relapsing polychondritis (RP), and Cogan's syndrome, but the condition was subsequently confirmed to be RP with inflammatory arthritis based on the diagnostic criteria by McAdam et al. She initially fulfilled 4 out of the 6 features which are as follows: recurrent chondritis of both auricles, nonerosive inflammatory arthritis, inflammation of ocular structures, and bilateral sensorineural hearing loss, and later went on to develop an additional feature of chondritis of laryngeal and or tracheal cartilages as outlined below.

2.2. Clinical Course. She was admitted and started on intravenous (IV) clindamycin 180 mg 6 hourly and IV ciprofloxacin 200 mg 12 hourly for septic arthritis; oral ibuprofen 200 mg 12 hourly, oral paracetamol 250 mg 8 hourly, and prednisolone 15 mg daily to which she showed initial signs of response. The steroids and analgesia were started to help control the inflammation and pain associated with the disease. However, her disease flared up again with significant knee pain and swelling, a left conjunctival injection associated with pain, and high inflammatory markers. Prednisolone was increased from 15 mg to 20 mg daily, and oral methotrexate 7.5 mg weekly and folic acid 5 mg weekly were introduced. The inflammation in the eye persisted, though there was a reduction in inflammatory markers (ESR 70 mm/hr., CRP 111.7 mg/l) at subsequent reviews. The methotrexate dose was titrated up to 10 mg weekly, and the prednisolone dose was further increased to 30 mg daily. Two months after initiation of therapy, she had resolution of the auricular inflammation and a reduction in intermittent eye inflammation. Her knee swelling and tenderness had improved (Figure 2(c)), with a significant decline in her inflammatory markers (ESR-34 mm/hr, CRP 42.7 mg/l). The dose of methotrexate was increased further from 10 mg to 15 mg weekly. This was to provide steroid-sparing treatment, as she still had significant symptoms despite the higher doses of steroids used for control of inflammation. Despite the increase in the methotrexate dose, there was still significant disease activity after 2 months which signified some degree of corticosteroid dependence. The dose of prednisolone was tapered gradually at a dose of 5 mg weekly anytime there was a decrease in inflammatory markers, suggesting a reduction in inflammation.

Due to failure to respond adequately to methotrexate, as evidenced by the frequency of disease flares and worsening of her eye symptoms, she also developed cataracts due to the high doses of steroids used. This led to the introduction of infliximab 10 months into treatment. She received the loading course of 100 mg of intravenous infliximab at 0, 2, and 6 weeks, but was unable to continue with the maintenance therapy of 8-weekly infusions due to financial constraints. Despite the short course of infliximab, clinical benefits such as reduction in arthritis and eye inflammation were noted. Six weeks after her last infliximab infusion, she developed difficulty breathing.

This progressed, leading to her presenting in the emergency room with signs of respiratory distress. On examination, she had audible inspiratory stridor, tachypnea, inspiratory rhonchi, and a slight reduction in breath sounds bilaterally, though vesicular in nature.

Lateral cervical X-ray showed partial narrowing in the region of the cricoid cartilage (Figure 3). A diagnosis of upper airway obstruction (subglottic) secondary to perichondritis of the cricoid cartilage with respiratory fatigue was made upon review by the otorhinolaryngologist and pulmonologist. Treatment ensued with intravenous dexamethasone 2 mg 8 hourly, nebulized Pulmicort 500 mcg 12 hourly, and salbutamol 2.5 mg 4 hourly, and she was transferred to the intensive care unit. An emergency tracheostomy to relieve the subglottic stenosis was performed. She recovered well and was discharged on day 4 of admission.

Her medications were reviewed, taking into account the financial challenges to include oral colchicine 500 mcg twice daily, oral methotrexate 15 mg weekly and oral prednisolone 40 mg daily which was to be tapered gradually. Knee synovitis persisted, requiring intra-articular injections of 80 mg of methylprednisolone acetate into each joint.

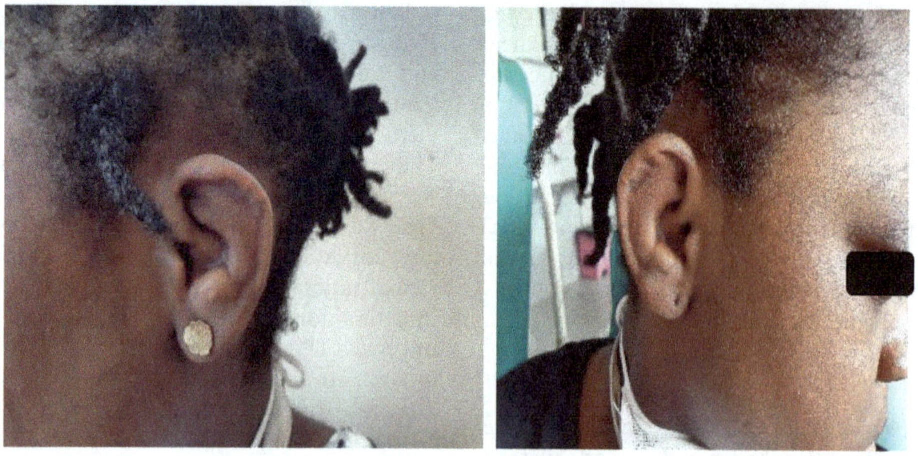

Figure 1: Swollen erythematous right and left ears with shriveled up outer ears resembling cauliflower ears.

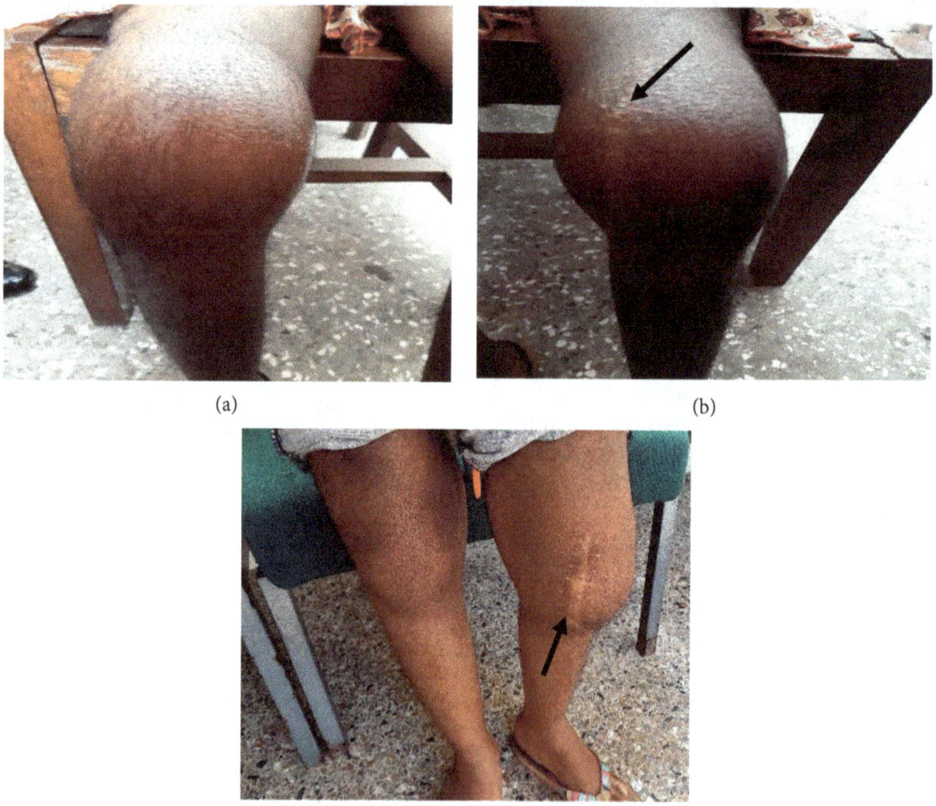

(a) (b)

(c)

Figure 2: (a, b) Synovitis of the right and left knees when the patient was first seen at the outpatients' department. (c) A significant decrease in knee synovitis 2 months into treatment, with an old arthrotomy scar (arrowed).

Tracheostomy care was carried out regularly at the otorhinolaryngology department, and close vigilance for infection was maintained.

A year and a half from the start of her treatment, she developed mid- to low-back pain. An X-ray of the lumbosacral spine showed a vertebral collapse at the L1 vertebra. A compression fracture was confirmed on MRI, with similar but less pronounced changes seen in T11, L3, and L4 vertebrae, suggestive of a bone softening process in keeping with glucocorticoid-induced osteoporosis and underlying hemoglobinopathy (Figure 4).

Steroid dose reduction continued and bisphosphonate therapy with alendronate 35 mg weekly was introduced. Oral dapsone 25 mg daily was added to her treatment for disease

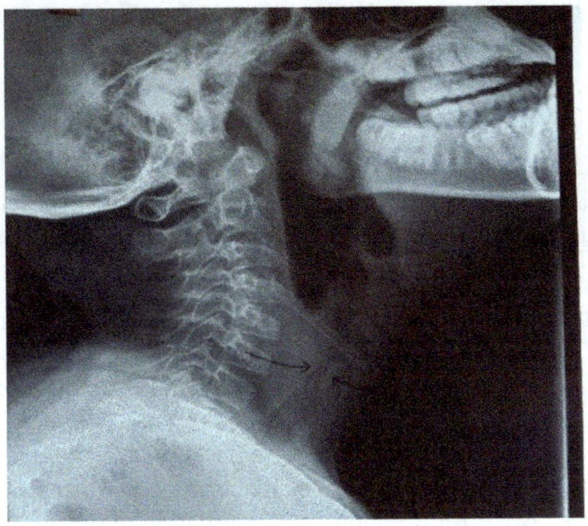

FIGURE 3: Lateral cervical X-ray showed partial narrowing in the region of the cricoid cartilage (arrowed).

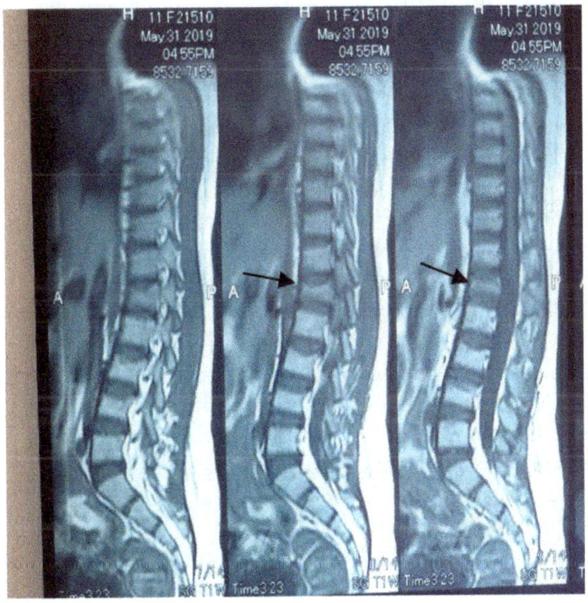

FIGURE 4: Compression fracture at the L1 vertebra (arrowed), with similar but milder changes in the T11, L3, and L4 vertebrae suggestive of a bone softening process due to glucocorticoid-induced osteoporosis and underlying hemoglobinopathy a year and a half into the treatment of her condition.

control due to its immunosuppressive and anti-inflammatory properties, but she continues to have remitting and relapsing disease.

3. Discussion

Relapsing polychondritis is an uncommon disorder of unknown cause characterized by inflammation of cartilage predominantly affecting the ears, nose, and laryngotracheobronchial tree which is among the most serious though less common manifestations of RP [14]; all of which manifested in the 11-year-old child as above mentioned. Other features she had were scleritis, sensorineural hearing loss, and arthritis.

RP can cause cardiac abnormalities such as valvular regurgitation, aneurysms, pericarditis, myocarditis, coronary vasculitis, and conduction abnormalities. Skin lesions such as purpura, erythema nodosum or multiforme, urticaria, livedo reticularis, and panniculitis can also occur in patients with RP with renal disease manifesting in the form of mesangial expansion or segmental necrotising glomerulonephritis [15].

The peak age of incidence is between the fourth and the fifth decade of life, but relapsing polychondritis may affect children and the elderly alike [8] and occurs with similar frequency in both genders although a slight female predominance has been cited. RP has documented cases in all ethnic groups, but most cases appear to be of Caucasian origin with no apparent familial tendency [5].

Pediatric RP represents less than 5% of the cases reported, with the age at onset varying from 1.7 months to 17 years. The clinical presentation is similar to that of adults, but there is a higher rate of severe airway disease in the pediatric population, and it commonly affects females [14]. About 30% of patients with RP will also have another rheumatologic disorder, the most frequent being systemic vasculitis, followed by rheumatoid arthritis and systemic lupus erythematosus. Children with RP frequently have a family history of autoimmunity and usually do not have associated autoimmune diseases [4], as is seen in our patient.

Nonrheumatic conditions such as inflammatory bowel disease, myelodysplastic syndrome, and Grave's disease have been associated with RP, and these conditions may predate the appearance of RP by months or years or can occur concurrently [1]. There are currently no reports of sickle cell disease associated with RP as our patient had, and whether it is part of the group of nonrheumatic diseases is yet to be established.

Vaso-occlusive crises (VOC) of SCD can mimic RP arthritis and the two can be particularly difficult to distinguish clinically since both SCD and RP have involvement of the small and large joints; however, patients with RP usually have asymmetric nonerosive intermittent arthritis of these joints with axial sparing [15]. SCD arthritis is usually

Table 1: Diagnostic criteria for RP according to McAdam et al. [9], and the observed frequencies of clinical presentation in patients, during the course of the disease [7].

1. Recurrent chondritis of both auricles (90%)
2. Chondritis of nasal cartilage (53%)
3. Nonerosive inflammatory arthritis (50–85%)
4. Chondritis of laryngeal and or tracheal cartilages (50%)
5. Inflammation of ocular structures, including conjunctivitis, keratitis, scleritis/episcleritis, and/or uveitis (50–60%)
6. Cochlear and or vestibular (6%) damage manifested by neurosensory hearing loss (46%), tinnitus, and/or vertigo

symmetric, with over 60% of cases having a preference for large joints and the lower extremity bones [16].

With the coexistence of these two disease entities in the setting of developing arthritis, determining whether it is RP arthritis or a VOC with superimposed inflammation resulting from local phagocytosis of sickled erythrocytes can be challenging. This phenomenon may drive the development of inflammatory arthritis in that synovial ischemia can lead to the release of synovial antigens into circulation and subsequently lead to the activation of autoantibodies against the synovium of the SCD patient, leading to inflammatory arthritis. Recurrent VOC in SCD can lead to a continuous inflammatory response that shares many characteristics and cytokines with arthritis of inflammatory origin, an example being interleukin 1 and 6, which are common to both of them [17].

The diagnosis of RP is a real challenge for physicians because of its diverse nature and insidious onset. The multiple clinical presentations and episodic nature of RP cause a significant delay in diagnosis, ranging from 1.9 to 10 years, with an average of five physicians being consulted before diagnosis, particularly in the pediatric population [8]. This delay is even more significant in patients with SCD, as they share some nonspecific symptoms such as arthralgia, fever, and multiorgan involvement. In addition, the poor knowledge of this condition by pediatricians may account for a mean delay of five years [14]. It is therefore recommended to have a sturdy respiratory and cardiovascular surveillance plan in all patients with early or associated pulmonary features to help delay disease progression [15] and reduce morbidity and mortality.

The diagnosis is certain when three or more of the clinical features listed in Table 1 are present along with a positive biopsy from the ear, nasal, or respiratory cartilage. A positive biopsy is only necessary when the clinical features are not typical.

The diagnosis can also be made when one or more of the above features and a positive biopsy are present, or when two or more separate sites of cartilage inflammation are present and respond to steroids or dapsone; or when three or more of the above features are present according to Damiani and Levine [18].

From Table 1, recurrent chondritis of both auricles is the most common feature of RP, being present in up to 90% of patients during the course of the disease, with nonerosive inflammatory arthritis being the second most common feature. Clinicians can therefore look out for chondritis of the ear in the early phase of the condition with repeated flares leading to severe destruction of the cartilage and subsequent loss of normal morphology of the pinna. This deformity resembles the "cauliflower ear" of professional boxers in a small percentage of patients [7].

The presence of inflammation in 2 or 3 cartilages of either the auricular, nasal, or laryngotracheal structures confirms the diagnosis of RP, or the confirmation of inflammation in one of the above listed cartilages plus 2 other minor criteria, namely, hearing loss, ocular inflammation, vestibular dysfunction, or seronegative arthritis, clinches the diagnosis of RP [19]. These criteria were used to finalize the diagnosis of RP in the case presented, as she had 5 out of the 6 diagnostic criteria according to McAdam.

This young patient with RP exhibited significant disease activity and severity with complex presentations which has led to management challenges with no breakthrough in therapies administered. The management of RP is mainly empirical due to the lack of understanding of the etiopathogenesis, absence of clinical trials or validated treatment recommendations, and the rarity of the disease entity [1]. First-line therapy involves the use of corticosteroids, dapsone, colchicine, and nonsteroidal anti-inflammatory drugs. Steroid-sparing medications such as methotrexate, cyclophosphamide, azathioprine, chlorambucil, mycophenolate mofetil, minocycline, and leflunomide may be used as second-line therapy and have been shown to be effective in some patients with steroid-resistant or steroid-dependent and/or life-threatening disease. They are also used to decrease the adverse effects of excessive steroid therapy [1, 15]. From the case discussion, our patient was started on most of the medications aforementioned with methotrexate being the only steroid-sparing medication used as some of the others were either expensive (mycophenolate) or not available in the country (leflunomide) with no notable improvement in disease condition with significant steroid dependence occurring in an attempt to control the disease. The refractory nature of the disease had resulted in persistently high doses of prednisolone being used, leading to complications of steroid-induced cataracts, osteoporosis, and vertebral fracture developing. Patients with SCD have decreased bone density due to erythroid hyperplasia from increased hematopoietic activity in bone resorption which invariably leads to generalized osteoporosis and cortical thinning [16]. This was further worsened with resultant vertebral fracture in our patient who needed high dose steroids to control her disease state. Biologics seem to be the new artillery in the war against autoimmune rheumatic disorders, like RP [7, 15] with case reports supporting its use in treating young patients with episcleritis and tracheal chondritis [20].

The most common biologic prescribed in the management of RP is infliximab, with adalimumab and tocilizumab being the next most prescribed in second and third place, respectively. Other biologics that have been used include rituximab, etanercept, and anakinra [7, 12]. The effectiveness of biologic therapy in RP is mixed, spanning from a good response to a complete lack of efficacy [12]; some patients with RP may have resolution of symptoms with biologics, while others will not. Infliximab, which has been used as a third-line agent [15], could not be pursued for this patient due to significant financial constraints, even though it showed a significant response. Colchicine and dapsone were started as a result of their reported efficacy in RP management [1] and were the next cheapest and readily available agents in our setting as the patient could not afford continuation of biologic therapy with Infliximab. In resource-limited areas such as in our setting, a few conventional and biologic DMARDs are available; namely, methotrexate, azathioprine, mycophenolate mofetil, and cyclophosphamide, with infliximab, rituximab, and only recently, tocilizumab, as the biologic artillery.

4. Conclusion

RP is an infrequent multisystemic, potentially lethal autoimmune condition of unknown etiology, affecting cartilaginous and proteoglycan-rich tissues in an episodic pattern with treatment being empiric. Though rare, especially in the young, we report on an unusually young patient who had sickle cell disease as a comorbidity and an aggressive clinical course of RP, with complications due to both disease and treatment. Diagnostic delays increase morbidity and mortality associated with both diseases; hence, early recognition and diagnosis are paramount to enable prompt treatment for improved clinical outcomes. The concomitant use of steroids in the management of RP though beneficial worsened severe SCD associated complications which justified the need for other therapies with cost being a significant limitation.

Further studies are needed to determine the prevalence of RP in patients with SCD and any pathophysiological links and also to define therapeutic options or modalities in managing patients with both conditions.

References

[1] F. Kemta Lekpa and X. Chevalier, "Refractory relapsing polychondritis: challenges and solutions," *Open Access Rheumatology Research and Reviews*, vol. 10, 2018.

[2] E. V. Asare, I. Wilson, A. A. Benneh-Akwasi Kuma, Y. Dei-Adomakoh, F. Sey, and E. Olayemi, "Burden of sickle cell disease in Ghana: the Korle-Bu experience," *Advances in hematology*, vol. 2018, Article ID 6161270, 2018.

[3] I. File, "Relapsing polychondritis with p-ANCA associated vasculitis: which triggers the other?" *World Journal of Clinical Cases*, vol. 2, no. 12, 2014.

[4] S. Rednic, L. Damian, R. Talarico, C. A. Scirè, A. Tobias, and N. Costedoat-Chalumeau, "Relapsing polychondritis: State of the art on clinical practice guidelines," *RMD Open*, vol. 4, 2018.

[5] L. Longo, A. Greco, A. Rea, V. R. Lo Vasco, A. De Virgilio, and M. De Vincentiis, "Relapsing polychondritis: A clinical update," *Autoimmunity Reviews*, vol. 15, 2016.

[6] C. A. Rimland, M. A. Ferrada, N. Sinaii et al., "Patient-perceived burden of disease in pediatric relapsing polychondritis," *Journal of Rheumatology*, vol. 46, no. 12, pp. 1627–1633, 2019.

[7] F. Borgia, F. Giuffrida, F. Guarneri, and S. P. Cannavò, "Relapsing polychondritis: An updated review," *Biomedicines*, vol. 6, 2018.

[8] N. Hazra, A. Dregan, J. Charlton, M. C. Gulliford, and D. P. D'Cruz, "Incidence and mortality of relapsing polychondritis in the UK: A population-based cohort study," *Rheumatology*, vol. 54, no. 12, pp. 2181–7, 2015.

[9] L. P. McAdam, M. A. O'Hanlan, R. Bluestone, and C. M. Pearson, "Relapsing polychondritis: Prospective study of 23 patients and a review of the literature," *Medicine (United States)*, vol. 55, no. 3, 1976.

[10] C. Yu and S. A. Joosten, "Relapsing polychondritis with large airway involvement," *Respirology Case Reports*, vol. 8, no. 1, Article ID e00501, 2020.

[11] A. R. Fonseca, S. K. De Oliveira, M. C. Rodrigues, I. L. Aymoré, R. C. Domingues, and F. R. Sztajnbok, "Relapsing polychondritis in childhood: three case reports, comparison with adulthood disease and literature review," *Rheumatology International*, vol. 33, no. 7, pp. 1873–8, 2013.

[12] F. Kemta Lekpa, V. B. Kraus, and X. Chevalier, "Biologics in relapsing polychondritis: A literature review," *Seminars in Arthritis and Rheumatism*, vol. 41, no. 5, 2012.

[13] V. Li-Thiao-Te, F. Uettwiller, P. Quartier, F. Lacaille, B. Bader-Meunier, and V. Brousse, "Coexistent sickle-cell anemia and autoimmune disease in eight children: pitfalls and challenges," *Pediatric Rheumatology*, vol. 16, no. 1, 2018.

[14] J. T. Alqanatish and J. R. Alshanwani, "Relapsing polychondritis in children: A review," *Modern Rheumatology*, vol. 30, no. 5, pp. 788–798, 2020.

[15] J. Kingdon, J. Roscamp, S. Sangle, and D. D'Cruz, "Relapsing polychondritis: A clinical review for rheumatologists," *Rheumatology*, vol. 57, 2018.

[16] R. Vaishya, A. K. Agarwal, E. O. Edomwonyi, and V. Vijay, "Musculoskeletal manifestations of sickle cell disease: A review," *Cureus*, 2015.

[17] I. M. McFarlane, D. J. Ozeri, Y. Saperstein, M. R. Alvarez, S. Z. Leon, K. Koci et al., "Rheumatoid Arthritis in sickle-cell population: Pathophysiologic insights, clinical evaluation and management," *Rheumatology: Current Research*, vol. 07, no. 03, 2017.

[18] J. M. Damiani and H. L. Levine, "Relapsing polychondritis—report of ten cases," *The Laryngoscope*, vol. 89, no. 6, 1979.

[19] C. J. Michet, C. H. McKenna, H. S. Luthra, and W. M. O'Fallon, "Relapsing polychondritis. Survival and predictive role of early disease manifestations," *Annals of Internal Medicine*, vol. 104, no. 1, pp. 74–8, 1986.

[20] V. M. Navarrete, C. V. Lebrón, F. J. De Miera, C. P. Candau, and F. N. Sarabia, "Sustained remission of pediatric relapsing polychondritis with adalimumab," *Journal of Clinical Rheumatology: Practical Reports on Rheumatic & Musculoskeletal Diseases*, vol. 20, no. 1, pp. 45–6, 2014.

14

Nephrotic Syndrome due to Focal Segmental Glomerulosclerosis Complicating Sjögren's Syndrome: A Case Report and Literature Review

Shigekazu Kurihara,[1] Makoto Harada,[1,2] Tohru Ichikawa,[1] Takashi Ehara,[3] and Mamoru Kobayashi[1]

[1]*Department of Nephrology, Nagano Red Cross Hospital, 5-22-1 Wakasato, Nagano 380-8582, Japan*
[2]*Department of Nephrology, Shinshu University School of Medicine, 3-1-1 Asahi, Matsumoto 390-8621, Japan*
[3]*Graduate School of Health Sciences, Matsumoto University, 2095-1 Niimura, Matsumoto 390-1241, Japan*

Correspondence should be addressed to Makoto Harada; tokomadaraha724@gmail.com

Academic Editor: Gregory J. Tsay

Background. Renal tubular acidosis and tubulointerstitial nephritis constitute the primary renal complications associated with Sjögren's syndrome (SjS), and glomerulonephritis and nephrotic syndrome are rare. *Case Presentation.* A 79-year-old Japanese woman presented with bilateral leg edema and weight gain and was diagnosed with nephrotic syndrome. In addition, she reported a 5-year history of dryness of mouth and was diagnosed with SjS. Renal biopsy revealed segmental glomerulosclerosis, with some specimens showing collapse of the glomerular capillary loops, proliferation of glomerular epithelial cells, and sclerotic lesions at the tubular poles, without spike formation, double contour lesions, or any other changes of the glomerular basement membrane. Immunofluorescence staining showed no immune complex (immunoglobulin IgG, IgA, or IgM) or complement (C3) deposition in the glomerular capillary walls. Based on these findings, she was diagnosed with focal segmental glomerulosclerosis (FSGS). The administration of steroid and cyclosporine achieved complete remission of nephrotic syndrome. *Conclusion.* Although glomerular diseases are rare, a variety of glomerular lesions including FSGS are reported in patients with SjS. Therefore, renal biopsy is warranted in patients with SjS presenting with severe urinary abnormalities.

1. Introduction

Sjögren's syndrome (SjS) is a complicated chronic systemic inflammatory disorder of the exocrine glands. This autoimmune disease is characterized by sialadenitis, dacryoadenitis, hypergammaglobulinemia, and positive results with tests for various autoantibodies [1]. Tubulointerstitial nephritis (TIN) and renal tubular acidosis constitute the typical renal complications associated with SjS. Glomerular diseases presenting with nephrotic syndrome are extremely rare in these patients [2, 3]. Reportedly, a variety of glomerular lesions occur in patients with SjS [4]. We describe the case of an elderly woman with nephrotic syndrome secondary to focal segmental glomerulosclerosis (FSGS) complicating SjS. Owing to the rarity of the condition, we have described the clinical course and histopathological findings in detail. In addition, we have discussed various glomerular diseases complicating SjS.

2. Case Report

A 79-year-old Japanese woman presented with bilateral leg edema and reported a weight gain of 7 kg over a month before admission. Urinary examination revealed increased urinary protein levels, and blood tests revealed hypoalbuminemia; thus, she was diagnosed with nephrotic syndrome. She reported a history of liver disorder diagnosed 10 years earlier along with an approximately 5-year history of dryness of mouth. Physical examination revealed attenuated breath sounds in the left lower lung field without pulmonary adventitious sounds. Examination of the bilateral lower extremities revealed pitting edema. Laboratory data are shown in Table 1. Urinary examination revealed urinary protein levels of 5711 mg/day, hematuria (20–29 red blood cells/high-power field), and urinary *N*-acetyl-beta-D-glucosaminidase and β2-microglobulin levels were elevated at 129.3 U/L and 2539 U/L, respectively. Blood tests revealed the following results: total protein 6.3 g/dL, serum albumin 1.7 g/dL, blood urea nitrogen 14.9 mg/dL, creatinine 0.65 mg/dL, aspartate aminotransferase 65 U/L, alanine aminotransferase 33 U/L, lactate dehydrogenase 392 U/L, alkaline phosphatase 1235 U/L, and gamma-glutamyl-transferase 664 U/L. Anti-SS-A and anti-SS-B antibody test results were negative; however, the salivary glands showed reduced secretory activity, and the Saxon test results were positive. The Schirmer test also showed a positive test result. A lip biopsy revealed lymphocytic infiltration. Tests for anti-nuclear antibody and rheumatoid factor showed positive results. Salivary gland scintigraphy was not performed. Based on the American College of Rheumatology criteria determined from Sjögren International Collaborative Clinical Alliance data, she was diagnosed with SjS [5, 6]. In addition, her hepatobiliary enzyme level was elevated. Although a liver biopsy was not performed, she was clinically diagnosed with primary biliary cholangitis (PBC) based on her chronic liver disorder and positive results with anti-mitochondrial M2 antibody testing [7].

A kidney biopsy was performed, and the specimen included 33 glomeruli, with 1 showing global sclerosis and 3 showing segmental glomerulosclerosis, with a few showing collapse of the glomerular capillary loops, proliferation of glomerular epithelial cells, and sclerotic lesions identified at the tubular poles. Spike or double contour lesions were not detected in the glomerular basement membrane. Notably, histopathological findings of TIN were not detected in the specimens (Figure 1). There was one glomerulus in the immunofluorescence specimen. Immunofluorescence staining showed no glomerular deposition of immunoglobulin (IgG, IgA, and IgM), C3, or fibrinogen. Based on these findings, she was diagnosed with FSGS. Unfortunately, the specimen used for electron microscopy did not include any glomeruli. The current patients did not show any electrolyte disturbances in the blood or excess electrolyte excretion in the urine. The blood pH level of the patient did not show the acidemia. In addition, the ability to concentrate urine was normal. Concerning the pathological findings of the tubular interstitial area, it was only slight lymphocytic infiltration, and the patient did not develop obvious tubulointerstitial nephritis. Unfortunately, urinary amino acid analysis was not conducted, or titratable acid levels were not evaluated. According to these results, we considered that the current case did not have the clinical manifestations of renal tubular disease.

Steroid therapy was initiated (oral prednisolone at a dose of 40 mg/day). Four weeks after initiation of steroid therapy, the proteinuria was not sufficiently decreased; hence, we added cyclosporine therapy (oral dose at 50 mg/day). Her blood cyclosporine level 2 hours after the oral administration of cyclosporine was controlled at 800 ng/mL. Angiotensin II receptor blocker (irbesartan) was added to her regimen after which her urinary protein level gradually decreased with an increase in serum albumin levels. Complete remission was achieved on day 269 after treatment initiation. The urinary protein/urinary creatinine ratio was 0.09 g/g Cr, her serum albumin level increased to 3.7 g/dL, and her leg edema disappeared (Figure 2).

3. Discussion

In the current case, the patient developed nephrotic syndrome over the clinical course of SjS and PBC. Glomerular diseases rarely complicate SjS. Goules et al. and Maripuri et al. have reported only 5 cases of severe or nephrotic-range proteinuria in 60 patients with SjS in whom a kidney biopsy was performed [2, 3] allowing for the detection of glomerular lesions. Notably, 9 previous studies have reported renal biopsy findings in patients with SjS [2, 3, 5–11]. Table 2 shows a summary of these studies. The incidence rate of TIN was high at 37.1 to 97.9%, and glomerular diseases were rare. Glomerular diseases primarily included mesangial proliferative glomerulonephritis (including IgA nephropathy), membranous nephropathy, membranoproliferative glomerulonephritis (MPGN), FSGS, and minimal change disease. The incidence rate of FSGS was reportedly 1.6 to 8.3%.

Reportedly, renal amyloidosis [12], podocytic infolding glomerulopathy [13], lupus-associated lesions [4], and anti-neutrophil cytoplasmic antibody-associated nephritis are known to occur in patients with SjS [4]. Treatment for renal involvement primarily includes the administration of corticosteroid, and a few patients receive other immunosuppressants such as cyclosporine, cyclophosphamide, mycophenolate mofetil, and rituximab. Limited data are available regarding renal prognosis in these patients. Jasiek et al. and Ren et al. reported that 5 cases of 95 patients and 4 cases of 130 patients developed end-stage renal disease, respectively [7, 10]. There is lack of data comparing renal prognosis based on the histopathological findings of renal biopsy specimens. Notably, Kidder et al. reported that patients with SjS with glomerular diseases showed higher mortality rates than those with TIN [5]. Infectious diseases are a common cause of death in patients with SjS showing renal involvement [9]. Thus, although glomerular diseases are less common in patients with SjS, various renal lesions are known to develop. In addition, the treatment strategy differs based on the results of histopathological diagnosis. Therefore, renal biopsy is warranted in patients with SjS with significant urinary abnormalities, such as severe proteinuria and/or hematuria.

In the current case, the patient developed nephrotic syndrome secondary to FSGS. Although secondary FSGS could be attributed to several etiopathogenetic factors such as familial, viral, drug-induced, structural, and functional responses (nephron depletion and hemodynamic changes) [14], this patient showed no obvious findings that could have resulted in secondary FSGS. Therefore, we could not conclusively establish an association between SjS and FSGS. However, a causal association between these diseases and FSGS could be deduced based on the fact that this patient developed both, SjS and PBC (which are rare conditions manifesting with immunological abnormalities), and the

Table 1: Main laboratory data of the current case.

Blood analysis					
WBC	8190	/μL	C3	67	mg/dL
RBC	4100000	/μL	C4	15	mg/dL
Hb	12.3	g/dL	CH50	34.1	U/mL
Plt	208000	/μL	CRP	0.43	mg/dL
TP	6.3	g/dL	IgG	1440	mg/dL
ALB	1.7	g/dL	IgA	415	mg/dL
ChE	369	U/L	IgM	1565	mg/dL
T.Ch	323	mg/dL	Cryoglobulins	(-)	
TG	233	mg/dL	Serum immunofixation M protein	(-)	
AST	65	U/L	pH	7.48	
ALT	33	U/L	PaCO2	30.3	mmHg
LDH	392	U/L	PaO2	59.8	mmHg
ALP	1235	U/L	Bicarbonate	22.3	mmol/L
γ-GT	664	U/L	Osmolarity	292	mOsm/kg
BUN	14.9	mg/dL	Anti-nuclear antibody	2560	(speckled)
Cr	0.65	mg/dL	Anti-mitochondria M2 antibody	20.6 (+)	
UA	5.7	mg/dL	Anti-double stranded DNA antibody	(-)	
Na	140	mmol/L	Anti-ribonucleoprotein antibody	(-)	
K	3.9	mmol/L	Anti-SS-A/Ro antibody	(-)	
Cl	110	mmol/L	Anti-SS-B/La antibody	(-)	
Ca	7.5	mg/dL	Anti-scleroderma-70 antibody	(-)	
iP	3.7	mg/dL	Anti-Jo-1 antibody	(-)	
Mg	2.5	mg/dL	Anti-centromere antibody	(-)	
Urinalysis					
pH	6.0		UUA	62.6	mg/dL
UP	(3+)		UNa	39	mEq/L
OB	(-)		UK	34	mEq/L
NAG	129.3	U/L	UCl	38	mEq/L
β2-MG	2539	U/L	UCa	1.0	mg/dL
Osmolarity	408	mOsm/kg	UiP	47.6	mg/mL
UUN	579.3	mg/dL			
UCr	116.9	mg/dL			

WBC: white blood cells; RBC: red blood cells; Hb: hemoglobin; Plt: platelet; TP: total protein; ALB: albumin; ChE: cholinesterase; T.Ch: total cholesterol; TG: triglycerides; AST: aspartate aminotransferase; ALT: alanine aminotransferase; LDH: lactate dehydrogenase; ALP: alkaline phosphatase; γ-GT: gamma-glutamyltransferase; BUN: blood urea nitrogen; Cr: creatinine; UA: uric acid; Na: sodium; K: potassium; Cl: chloride; Ca: calcium; iP: inorganic phosphorus; Mg: magnesium; C3: complement 3; C4: complement 4; CH50: 50% hemolytic complement activity; CRP: C-reactive protein; IgG: immunoglobulin G; IgA: immunoglobulin A; IgM: immunoglobulin M; UP: urinary protein; OB: occult blood; NAG: *N*-acetyl-beta-D-glucosaminidase; β2-MG: beta-2-microglobulin; UUN: urine urea nitrogen; UCr: urine creatinine; UUA: urine uric acid; UNa: urine sodium; UK: urine potassium; UCl: urine chloride; UCa: urine calcium; UiP: urine inorganic phosphorus.

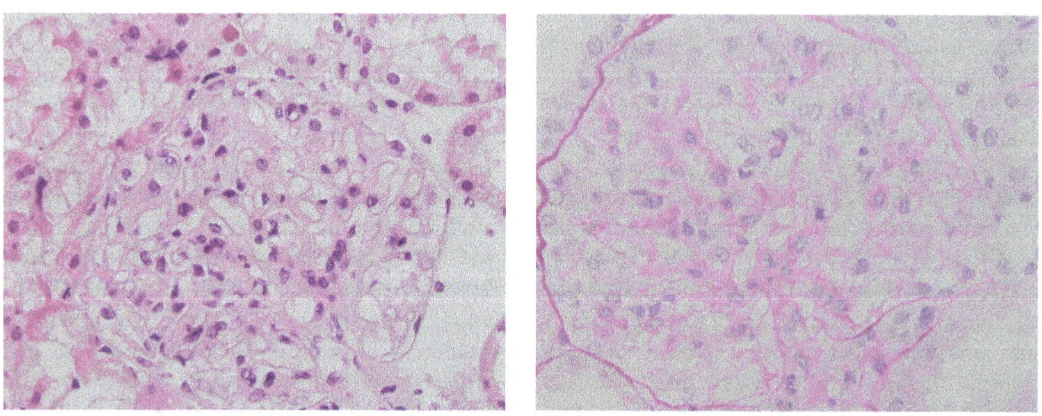

(a) (b)

Figure 1: Continued.

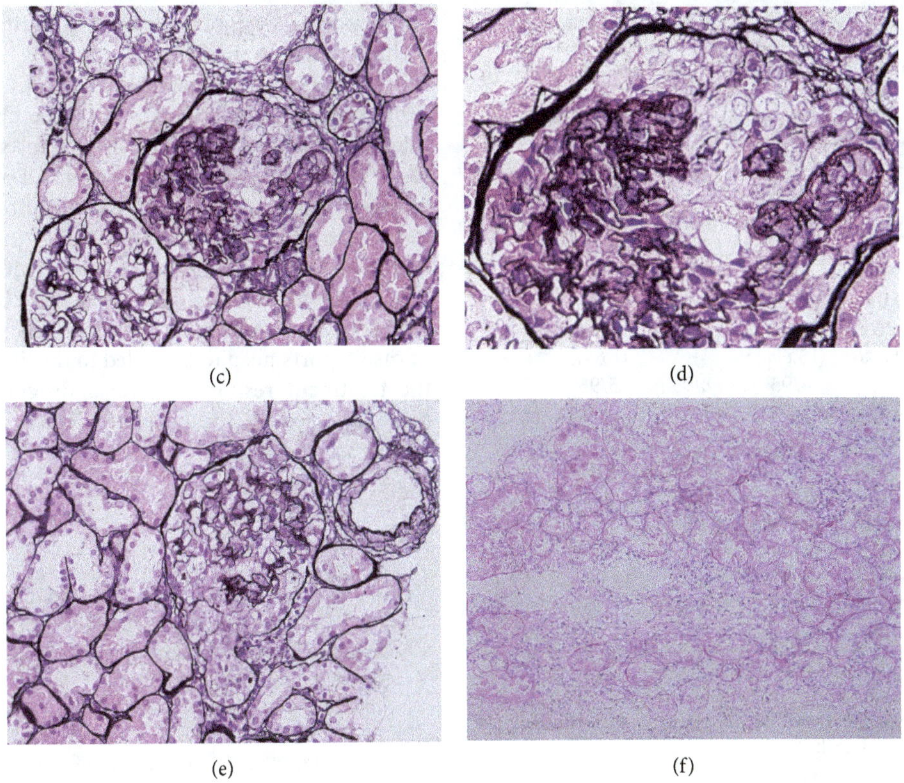

FIGURE 1: Histopathological findings in a kidney biopsy specimen showing collapse of capillary loop and segmental sclerosis with proliferation of glomerular epithelial cells. (a) Hematoxylin-eosin staining, high magnification. Intraluminal cell proliferation or necrotizing crescentic formation is not shown. (b) Periodic acid-Schiff staining, high magnification. Mesangial matrix proliferation or mesangial cell proliferation is not shown. (c) Periodic acid-methenamine-silver staining, low magnification. (d) Periodic acid-methenamine-silver staining, high magnification. A segmental lesion is observed at the tubular pole. (e) Periodic acid-methenamine-silver staining, low magnification. (f) Periodic acid-Schiff staining. Although there was slight lymphocytic infiltration in the tubulointerstitial area, obvious tubulointerstitial nephritis was not detected.

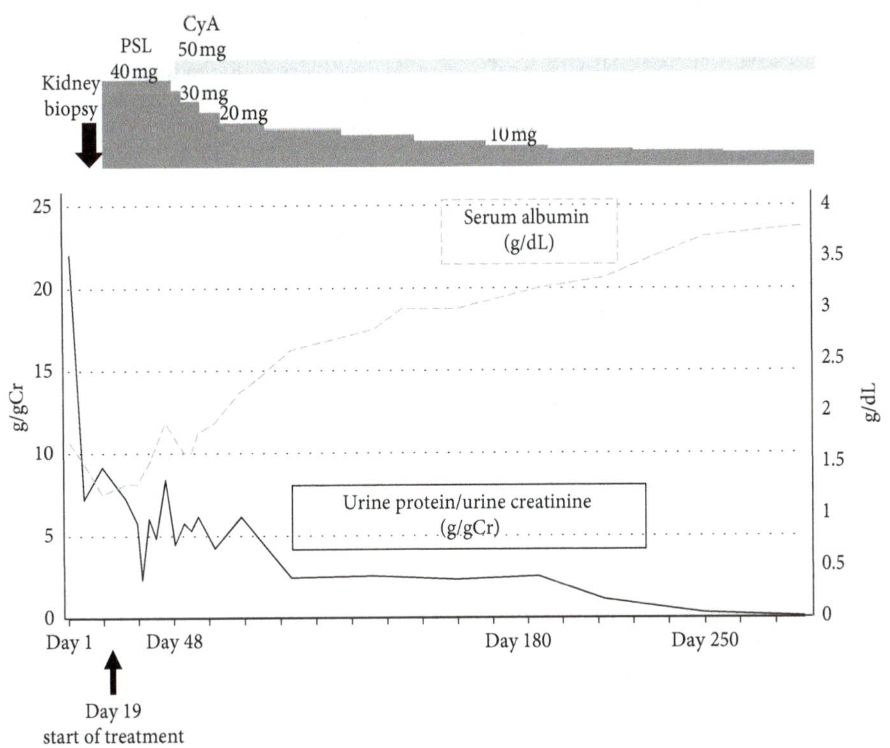

FIGURE 2: Patient's clinical course. The patient was treated with PSL and CyA. The urine protein/urine creatinine ratio gradually decreased until complete remission (urine protein excretion <0.3 g/gCr) was achieved. CyA: cyclosporine; PSL: prednisolone.

Table 2: Summary of renal biopsy findings of previous studies.

	Renal biopsy findings and frequency (positive biopsies/ total biopsies)					
	TIN	MesGN	MN	MPGN	FSGS	MCD
[8]	29/35 (82.9%)	2/35 (5.7%)	2/35 (5.7%)	ND	ND	ND
[3]	17/24 (70.8%)	ND	1/24 (4.2%)	2/24 (8.3%)	2/24 (8.3%)	ND
[2]	13/35 (37.1%)	7/35 (20.0%)	2/35 (5.7%)	10/35 (28.6%)	1/35 (2.9%)	ND
[9]	37/64 (57.8%)	21/64 (32.8%)	10/64 (15.6%)	ND	1/64 (1.6%)	ND
[10]	93/95 (97.9%)	ND	4/95 (4.2%)	8/95 (8.4%)	5/95 (5.3%)	2/95 (2.1%)
[11]	9/17 (52.9%)	3/17 (17.6%)	ND	ND	1/17 (5.9%)	ND
[5]	13/25 (52.0%)	1/25 (4.0%)	1/25 (4.0%)	6/25 (24.0%)	ND	1/25 (4.0%)
[6]	53/103 (51.5%)	6/103 (5.8%)	37/103 (35.9%)	ND	3/103 (2.9%)	4/103 (3.9%)
[7]	33/41 (80.5%)	2/41 (4.9%)	1/41 (2.4%)	3/41 (7.3%)	2/41 (4.9%)	ND

FSGS: focal segmental glomerulosclerosis; MCD: minimal change disease; MesGN: mesangial proliferative glomerulonephritis; MN: membranous nephropathy; MPGN: membranoproliferative glomerulonephritis; ND: no data; TIN: tubulointerstitial nephritis.

observation that immunosuppressive therapy with corticosteroid and cyclosporine was effective in this case.

Unfortunately, there have been no investigations or case reports that concern the prognosis and clinical response of the cases with FSGS and SjS. This is the first case report describing the details of the clinical course and treatment response of the case with FSGS and SjS. Therefore, in order to discuss the appropriate treatment or prognosis, further accumulation of similar cases with current patients is necessary. Because there are few cases of glomerular diseases coexisting with SjS, it is difficult to describe the best treatment options in each glomerular disease. However, we summarized and mentioned the treatment options of each representative glomerular disease developed in the patients with SjS as follows: Concerning the treatment options of the cases with SjS and other glomerular diseases, previous studies have reported the treatment and clinical responses [2–4, 7]. MPGN secondary to cryoglobulinemia develops in the cases with SjS. Cases of MPGN secondary to cryoglobulinemia have been treated with steroids (including pulse therapy), immunosuppressants, rituximab, and plasma exchange therapy [2–4, 7]. In fact, steroids alone or steroid and cyclophosphamide therapy have often achieved complete remission of MPGN cases due to SjS-associated cryoglobulinemia [2–4, 7]. Recently, several reports have suggested that rituximab is effective in MPGN and vasculitis due to cryoglobulinemia and systemic manifestation due to SjS [4, 15, 16]. Mesangial proliferative glomerulonephritis in patients with SjS has been treated with steroids alone or steroids and immunosuppressants (methotrexate, cyclophosphamide, or azathioprine) [2, 4, 17]. Membranous nephropathy in patients with SjS has been treated with steroids alone or steroids and immunosuppressants (cyclosporine, cyclophosphamide, and rituximab) [2, 4, 18]. Minimal change disease was successively treated with steroids alone, and another patient was treated with hydroxychloroquine [3, 4, 19]. Although the clinical response to these treatments has been reported to be successful, as these results were cited from case reports and series studies, there may be a publication bias. Clinical studies will be needed to determine the efficacy of various immunosuppressive therapies against glomerular diseases with SjS.

We report this rare case of SjS and PBC complicated by nephrotic syndrome secondary to FSGS. A greater number of case reports need to be added to the literature to establish the treatment response or renal prognosis of glomerular diseases based on the histopathological diagnosis of renal biopsy specimens.

References

[1] K. Asmussen, V. Andersen, G. Bendixen, M. Schiodt, and P. Oxholm, "A new model for classification of disease manifestations in primary Sjögren's syndrome: evaluation in a retrospective long-term study," *Journal of Internal Medicine*, vol. 239, no. 6, pp. 475–482, 1996.

[2] A. V. Goules, I. P. Tatouli, H. M. Moutsopoulos, and A. G. Tzioufas, "Clinically significant renal involvement in primary Sjögren's syndrome: clinical presentation and outcome," *Arthritis & Rheumatism*, vol. 65, no. 11, pp. 2945–2953, 2013.

[3] S. Maripuri, J. P. Grande, T. G. Osborn et al., "Renal involvement in primary Sjögren's syndrome: a clinicopathologic study," *Clinical Journal of the American Society of Nephrology*, vol. 4, no. 9, pp. 1423–1431, 2009.

[4] H. François and X. Mariette, "Renal involvement in primary Sjögren syndrome," *Nature Reviews Nephrology*, vol. 12, no. 2, pp. 82–93, 2016.

[5] D. Kidder, E. Rutherford, D. Kipgen, S. Fleming, C. Geddes, and G. A. Stewart, "Kidney biopsy findings in primary Sjögren syndrome," *Nephrology Dialysis Transplantation*, vol. 30, no. 8, pp. 1363–1369, 2015.

[6] H.-X. Yang, J. Wang, Y.-B. Wen et al., "Renal involvement in primary Sjögren's syndrome: a retrospective study of 103 biopsy-proven cases from a single center in China," *International Journal of Rheumatic Diseases*, vol. 21, no. 1, pp. 223–229, 2018.

[7] H. Ren, W. M. Wang, X. N. Chen et al., "Renal involvement and followup of 130 patients with primary Sjögren's syndrome," *Journal of Rheumatology*, vol. 35, no. 2, pp. 278–284, 2008.

[8] K. Ichikawa, T. Konta, H. Sato, Y. Ueda, and H. Yokoyama, "The clinical and pathological characteristics of nephropathies in connective tissue diseases in the Japan renal biopsy registry (J-RBR)," *Clinical and Experimental Nephrology*, vol. 21, no. 6, pp. 1024–1029, 2017.

[9] D. F. Lin, S. M. Yan, Y. Zhao et al., "Clinical and prognostic characteristics of 573 cases of primary Sjögren's syndrome," *Chinese Medical Journal*, vol. 123, no. 22, pp. 3252–3257, 2010.

[10] M. Jasiek, A. Karras, V. Le Guern et al., "A multicentre study of 95 biopsy-proven cases of renal disease in primary Sjögren's syndrome," *Rheumatology*, vol. 56, no. 3, pp. 362–370, 2017.

[11] A. Jain, B. H. Srinivas, D. Emmanuel, V. K. Jain, S. Parameshwaran, and V. S. Negi, "Renal involvement in primary Sjogren's syndrome: a prospective cohort study,"

Rheumatology International, vol. 38, no. 12, pp. 2251–2262, 2018.

[12] V. Ooms, M. Decupere, E. Lerut, Y. Vanrenterghem, and D. R. J. Kuypers, "Secondary renal amyloidosis due to long-standing tubulointerstitial nephritis in a patient with Sjögren syndrome," *American Journal of Kidney Diseases*, vol. 46, no. 5, pp. e75–e80, 2005.

[13] K. Koike, Y. Utsunomiya, Y. Ito et al., "A case of glomerulopathy showing podocytic infolding in association with Sjögren's syndrome and primary biliary cirrhosis," *Clinical and Experimental Nephrology*, vol. 12, no. 6, pp. 489–493, 2008.

[14] V. D. D'Agati, A. B. Fogo, J. A. Bruijn, and J. C. Jennette, "Pathologic classification of focal segmental glomerulosclerosis: a working proposal," *American Journal of Kidney Diseases*, vol. 43, no. 2, pp. 368–382, 2004.

[15] B. Terrier, D. Launay, G. Kaplanski et al., "Safety and efficacy of rituximab in nonviral cryoglobulinemia vasculitis: data from the French Autoimmunity and Rituximab registry," *Arthritis Care & Research*, vol. 62, no. 12, pp. 1787–1795, 2010.

[16] J.-E. Gottenberg, G. Cinquetti, C. Larroche et al., "Efficacy of rituximab in systemic manifestations of primary Sjögren's syndrome: results in 78 patients of the Autoimmune and Rituximab registry," *Annals of the Rheumatic Diseases*, vol. 72, no. 6, pp. 1026–1031, 2013.

[17] Y. Chen, X. Zhao, D. Tang et al., "IgA Nephropathy in two patients with Sjögren's syndrome: one with concomitant autoimmune hepatitis," *Internal Medicine*, vol. 49, no. 1, pp. 37–43, 2010.

[18] A. Baba, S. Hara, Y. Sato, K. Yamada, S. Fujimoto, and T. Eto, "Three patients with nephrotic syndrome due to membranous nephropathy complicated by Sjögren's syndrome," *Nihon Jinzo Gakkai Shi*, vol. 47, no. 8, pp. 882–886, 2005.

[19] M.-L. Yang, M.-C. Kuo, T.-T. Ou, and H.-C. Chen, "Primary Sjögren's syndrome with minimal change disease—a case report," *The Kaohsiung Journal of Medical Sciences*, vol. 27, no. 5, pp. 190–194, 2011.

15

Acquired Factor VIII Deficiency Presenting as Gross Hematuria in a Hispanic, Pregnant Patient with Previously Undiagnosed Connective Tissue Disease

Christine Loftis[1] **Emilia C. Dulgheru**[2] **and Rosa White**[1]

[1]*University of Texas at Rio Grande Valley, Internal Medicine Department- Doctor Hospital at Renaissance, 5423 S McColl Rd, Edinburg, TX 78539, USA*
[2]*Rheumatology Institute-Doctor Hospital at Renaissance, Edinburg, TX 78539, USA*

Correspondence should be addressed to Christine Loftis; christine.loftis01@gmail.com

Academic Editor: Mario Salazar-Paramo

Acquired factor VIII deficiency is a bleeding disorder caused by the presence of autoantibodies against clotting factor VIII. We report a case of a 24-year-old pregnant woman who presented with gross hematuria secondary to acquired factor VIII deficiency in the presence of a previously undiagnosed connective tissue disease. This article includes a literature review of pregnancy-related cases of acquired factor VIII deficiency. We also reviewed various therapeutic approaches for the management of the acquired factor inhibitor which include achieving hemostasis and elimination of the inhibitor via immunosuppressive agents. This case report describes the rare presentation of acquired factor VIII deficiency related to pregnancy and highlights the importance of considering a factor VIII inhibitor in the differential diagnosis of patients who present with bleeding and prolonged PTT during the peripartum and postpartum periods.

1. Introduction

Acquired factor VIII deficiency is a rare bleeding diathesis caused by the development of autoantibodies against clotting factor VIII [1]. The annual incidence of the disorder is between 1.3 and 1.5 per million [1]. Apart from reproductive-aged women during pregnancy and postpartum periods, acquired factor VIII deficiency typically occurs after the fifth decade of life [2]. Patients affected with acquired factor VIII deficiency present with severe or life-threatening bleeding episodes in the absence of previous bleeding predisposition. Bleeding severity varies ranging from simple dermatological manifestations such as petechiae and ecchymoses to internal bleeding [3] Acquired factor VIII deficiency has been associated with several underlying conditions such as malignancy, immunological disorders, perinatal period, and various medications. Although the association with underlying disorders has been reported, most of the cases remain idiopathic.

2. Case Presentation

A 24-year-old Hispanic pregnant woman, gravida 2 para 1, was admitted for gross hematuria without precipitating factors at 29 weeks of gestation. The patient reported that this was the first episode of hematuria and had no prior history of bleeding during her previous pregnancy or otherwise. The patient's review of systems was significant for an erythematous, maculopapular, nonpruritic rash, occurring intermittently on the lower extremities since age 13. The patient had never been given a formal diagnosis but noted that the rash also occurred during her first pregnancy, resolved spontaneously, and recurred about 2 weeks prior to the current admission. The patient denied family history of hemophilia, von Willebrand disease, or autoimmune conditions such as rheumatoid arthritis, systemic lupus erythematosus, scleroderma, or Hashimoto's thyroiditis. The patient endorsed episodes of photosensitivity but denied constitutional symptoms, arthralgia, oral ulcers, myalgia, pleuritic chest pain, xerostomia, keratoconjunctivitis sicca, or any other significant symptoms. On physical examination, the patient had bilateral upper extremity and lower back large ecchymoses, a palpable purpura on the anterior aspect of the right thigh, bilateral knees, and hips, and postinflammatory hyperpigmentation on the distal aspect of lower extremities. Laboratory tests (Table 1) showed a prolonged PTT of 92.1 s (RI: 24.3–36.7 s). Subsequent workup revealed negative antiphospholipid panel including negative pus anticoagulant, cardiolipin antibodies, and beta-2 glycoprotein 1 antibodies. The von Willebrand factor was present in adequate amounts. There was a significantly decreased factor VIII level of <1% (RI: 50–180%), and PTT failed to correct with the addition of fresh plasma (mixing studies) which suggested the presence of an inhibitor. Bethesda assay was positive at 74.9 U (RI: 0.6 U) which confirmed a high titer factor VIII inhibitor. Further workup revealed a positive antinuclear antibody with high titer by ELISA and positive SS-A and SS-B antibodies. Urinalysis showed proteinuria of 858 mg/24 h. Double-stranded DNA and anti-Smith antibodies were negative. Complement C3 and C4 were present in normal amounts. The patient was diagnosed with acquired factor VIII deficiency and presumed systemic lupus erythematosus (SLE). She was initially treated with DDAVP 30 mcg intranasally along with prednisone 45 mg BID (1 mg/kg a day in divided doses) while in our facility. The patient was transferred to a tertiary center for a higher level of care where she received IVIG (intravenous immune globulin) 1 gm/kg for 2 days along with porcine factor VIII. She was discharged from the hospital on a prednisone taper. The patient was followed closely by a maternal-fetal medicine specialist and a hemophilia specialist. The patient later delivered a healthy baby girl at 36 weeks via vaginal delivery without complications. At the three-year follow-up, the patient remains in remission, and her daughter has been without any cardiac problems or bleeding diathesis. She was advised against future pregnancy.

Table 1: Laboratory results.

Parameter	Patient	Reference range
PT	11.8 s	9.8–12.6 s
INR	1.05	0.87–1.15
PTT	92.1 s	24.3–36.7 s
Coagulation factor VIII activity	<1%	50–180%
Factor VIII inhibitor titer	74.9 BU	<0.6 BU
vWF Ag	190%	50–217%
vWF ristocetin cofactor	122%	42–200%
vWF Ag, multimeric	Normal	
PTT-La screen	80 s	<40 s
Hexagonal phase confirm	Negative	
DRVVT screen	22 s	<45 s
DNA ds Ab	0.9 IU/mL	<10 IU/mL
RNP 70	0.3 U/mL	<7.0 U/mL
Rheumatoid factor quantitative	44.6 IU/mL	<14.0 IU/mL
ANA	>32.0 ratio	>1.0 ratio
Cardiolipin Ab IgG	<14 GPL	< or = 14
Cardiolipin Ab IgM	<12 GPL	< or = 14
B2-glycoprotein IgM Ab	<9 GPL	< or = 20
B2-glycoprotein IgG Ab	<9 GPL	< or = 20
Anticentromere antibody	<0.4 U/mL	<7.0 U/mL
Jo 1 antibody	<0/3 U/mL	<7.0 U/mL
Scl 70 antibody	<0.6 U/mL	<7.0 U/mL
Smith antibody (Sm)	<0.8 U/mL	<7.0 U/mL
SS-A/Ro antibody	>240 U/mL	<7.0 U/mL
SS-B/La antibody	97 U/mL	<7.0 U/mL
U1RNP antibody	0.6 U/mL	<7.0 U/mL
Complement C3	174 mg/dL	87–200 mg/dL
Complement C4	20 mg/dL	19–52 mg/dL
Immunoglobulin A	242 mg/dL	66–443 mg/dL
Antistreptolysin O	<1 IU/mL	<250 IU/mL
ANCA	Negative	
Urine culture	Negative	
Random urine protein/creatinine ratio	858 mg/gm	161 mg/gm

3. Discussion

Acquired factor VIII deficiency associated with pregnancy most commonly occurs during the peripartum and postpartum period and rarely occurs before pregnancy. The cause and timing remain unclear, but many studies speculate that it is due to the complex immunological changes that occur during pregnancy. Some sources have theorized that the development of the inhibitor is due to sensitization of the mother's immune system to fetal factor VIII during previous pregnancies; however, some patients who acquire an inhibitor to factor VIII develop the inhibitor in the first pregnancy (Table 2). The inhibitor autoantibody that is produced in patients with acquired factor VIII deficiency attaches to a specific subunit of factor VIII, the C2 domain, which results in diminished procoagulant activity and subsequent bleeding [16]. This is like the formation of neutralizing antibodies against factor VIII in 25% of patients with hemophilia A who are transfused with plasma-derived or recombinant factor VIII. In the rare event of clinical manifestations during pregnancy, such as in our patient, the presence of factor VIII autoantibodies also puts the fetus at risk of bleeding due to the maternofetal transplacental passage of IgG antibodies. To date, there are less than fifty reported cases of the maternal transplacental passage of the inhibitor resulting in acquired factor VIII deficiency in the fetus. Although rare, it is important to counsel the patient on the possibility of these risks [17]. There is no current accurate way to determine the severity of bleeding in patients with factor inhibitors based solely on titer levels. Studies have shown that inhibitors to factor VIII are cleared in a nonlinear manner, thus resulting in an underestimation of bleeding risk in some patients [18].

Acquired factor VIII deficiency occurs most commonly in primigravid women at 2-3 months postpartum. These patients typically present with soft tissue bleeding; however, vaginal bleeding, hemarthrosis, and hematuria have been the presenting symptoms in 13–18% of the reported cases [3]. Although our patient was gravida 2, she delivered her first child 2.5 months prior to the conception that resulted in her

TABLE 2: Review of the literature.

Article	Citation	Presentation	Findings	Outcome
41	Michiels et al. [4]	37 y/o G1P1 presented 4 months postpartum with bruises and hemarthrosis.	FVIII-0.02 U/mL FVIII inhibitor: 7.9 BU	Treated with prednisone taper of 1 mg/kg with remission within 2 months while on 20 mg/d without recurrence at 5-year f/u.
		22 y/o G3P3 presented 7 months postpartum with menorrhagia and bleeding after tooth extraction.	FVIII: 0.01–0.02 U/mL FVIII inhibitor: 12 BU	Treatment with cyclophosphamide 100 mg/day (0.7 mg/kg/d) without inhibitor disappearance; however, spontaneous remission developed 10 months later after discontinuing medication. Subsequent pregnancy without bleeding diathesis.
		31 y/o G2P2 presented 2 months postpartum with muscle and soft tissue bleeding, menorrhagia, ecchymoses, and hemarthrosis.	FVIII: <0.01 U/mL FVIII inhibitor: 24 BU	Treated with 4000 U human factor VIII, prednisone 1 mg/kg/d for 6 weeks, and cyclophosphamide 2 mg/kg/d concomitantly from the 3rd to 6th week of prednisone treatment, with a 5-day course of high-dose gamma-globulin at 0.5 g/kg/day. Recurrence of the inhibitor with removal of agents resulting in IVIG being initiated. Remission at 28 months.
		24 y/o G2P1A1 presented after delivery of stillborn with PPH and subsequent hemarthrosis.	FVIII: <0.01 FVIII inhibitor: 295–625 BU	Treated with 1 mg/kg prednisone for 3 weeks without remission. Five years later presented with FVIII 600 BU and thus 10K U of cryoprecipitate. At 24 years after treatment, the patient still had not achieved remission.
38	Coller et al. [5]	22 y/o primigravid woman presented with severe vaginal bleeding postpartum day 6.	PT: 12.6/13.0 sec PTT: 74/45 sec FVIII: 8% FIX: 90% FVIII inhibitor: 15 BU von Willebrand factor: 90%	Treated with 60 mg prednisone daily, became free of inhibitor within months, and had a successful second pregnancy without any subsequent bleeding diathesis.
6	Chaari et al. [9]	19 y/o F presented PPD one with large vaginal hematoma.	aPTT: 87/30 sec FVIII: 7% FVIII inhibitor: 64 BU	Treatment began with initial surgical intervention for evacuation of hematoma but was complicated by bleeding into the abdominal cavity and genitalia. The patient was given recombinant FVIIa and activated prothrombin complex concentrates. Due to symptom progression, the patient started on prednisone alone for 3 days followed by cotherapy with cyclophosphamide without symptom improvement. The patient passed away PPD 2/2 hemorrhagic shock.
5	Seethala et al. [7]	36 y/o woman presented with PPH s/p NSVD secondary to acquired factor VIII deficiency.	PTT: 71.7/45 sec PT: 15.9 sec INR: 1.3 FVIII: <1% FVIII inhibitor: >54.3 BU	Received factor VII and desmopressin. Treated with methylprednisolone, cytoxan, and plasmapheresis with appropriate decline in PTT but was discontinued because of sepsis prior to discharge. The patient was readmitted for bacteremia and succumbed to severe sepsis.
4	Kotani et al. [8]	31 y/o G1P1p developed postpartum hemorrhage after delivery. A female neonate developed subcutaneous hemorrhage on dorsum of hand on day 1of life s/p routine blood draw secondary to transplacental transfer of the inhibitor.	PT: 10.6 sec PTT: 76.9 sec FVIII: <1% FVIII inhibitor: 458 BU/mL PT: 14.3 sec PTT: 80.3 sec FVIII: <1% FVIII inhibitor: 199 BU/mL	Treatment for 31 y/o F consisted of 19 U PRBCS, 51 U FFP, steroid pulse therapy, and 3 vials of factor VII during hospital course and discharged on 30 mg/day of prednisolone. 10 months postpartum PTT WNL without any further complications. Neonate required no treatment and factor VIII, and PTT returned to baseline at postnatal month 4.

TABLE 2: Continued.

Article	Citation	Presentation	Findings	Outcome
35	Chaari et al. [6]	31 y/o woman presented with several areas of ecchymoses over lower extremities several days prior to delivery.	FVIII: 18% FVIII inhibitor: 1, 4 BU	Treated with prednisone and rituximab.
8	Porteous et al. [10]	32 y/o primigravid woman developed postpartum hemorrhage hours after delivery.	PTT: 78.2 sec PT: 10.9 sec FVIII: <1% FVIII inhibitor: 15 BU	Treated with 1 mg/kg/day (60 mg) prednisolone, 5 doses of recombinant FVIIa 360 IU, 2 doses of DDAVP 0.3 μg/kg, 20 U PRBCs, tranexamic acid 1 g daily over 20 days with continued bleeding. Bleeding was controlled with bilateral internal pudendal artery embolization. Maintenance therapy was achieved with prednisolone 60 mg and tranexamic acid 500 mg tds.
23	Sebastian et al. [11]	25 y/o F with a history of secondary APS in the setting of SLE and acquired factor VII inhibitor at 10 weeks of gestation developed retroperitoneal bleeding. Prior to current conception, the patient was symptomatic having suffered from several areas of ecchymoses on extremities, episcleritis, and urticaria and having been diagnosed with a PE 6 months prior.	PTT: 94/37 sec FVIII: 1.33% FVIII inhibitor: 614.4 BU C3: 0.57 C4: <0.08 Anti-ANA: 1 : 320 SS-A and Ro52: present Anti-dsDNA: 18.35/ 100 IU/mL	Treatment consisted of methylprednisolone IV, recombinant factor VII, prednisone 1 mg/kg, and cyclosporine 250 mg/day. The patient consented to terminate pregnancy. Continued maintenance therapy with cyclosporine 200 mg/day, chloroquine 250 mg/day, and methylprednisolone.
7	Rodrigues et al. [12]	34 y/o primigravid F presented PPD forty with complaints of spontaneous hematomas on extremities and intramuscular bleeding on the back, forearms, ankle, and thighs.	APTT: 62/<38 sec FVIII: 3.5% FVIII inhibitor: 10 BU FIX: 124% Fibrinogen: 430/ 450 mg/DL	Treated with prednisone 1 mg/kg/d plus tranexamic acid. The patient had remission of the disease with normalization of FVIII without the presence of the inhibitor in ~2 years.
29	Lee et al. [13]	18 y/o F primigravid presented 9 months postpartum with painful swelling of knees and ankles, multiple bruises on hands and feet, and menorrhagia.	PT: 10.2/(10–14 sec) INR: 0.95/1.5 sec APTT: 84.3/40 sec FVIII: 1.4% Anti-FVIII: 28 BU	Treated with activated prothrombin complex concentrate and FEIBA anti-inhibitor coagulant complex at a dose of 50–100 units/kg q12 h. Corticosteroids were considered but not indicated due to remission of symptoms.
39	Azam et al. [14]	26-year-old multiparous woman presented PPD 2 with hemoperitoneum following lower segment C-section.	PTT: 90 sec (0–32 sec) Normal PT/INR FVIII level: 1% Positive inhibitor Normal lupus anticoagulant Normal vWF Normal antiphospholipid IgM and IgG	Treated with prednisone 60 mg/day initially with taper and initiation azathioprine.
2	Qian et al. [15]	35-year-old PPD 48 with chest pain and was found to have pleural hemorrhage.	PT: 15.2 sec PTT: 68.40 sec FVIII inhibitor: positive Inhibitor: 7.4%	Treated with aPCC, human factor VIII concentrates, corticosteroids, and plasma. At 6 months, no recurrence.

current pregnancy. As the immunology of pregnancy poses a conundrum, the presence of an untreated autoimmune condition could have potentially interfered in the dynamic of antibody formation and clearance in our patient.

The isolated elevated PTT that failed to correct with the mixing study in the context of bleeding is suggestive of the inhibitor rather than lupus anticoagulant with latter triggering clotting events. Laboratory testing was negative for the lupus anticoagulant, but factor VIII activity was significantly decreased at less than 1%. Bethesda assay was positive at 74.9 U confirming the presence of an inhibitor to factor VIII. A unique aspect of our case was the importance of recognizing the presentation of a previously undiagnosed connective tissue disorder.

The patient reported intermittent erythematous rash reminding of purpura as well as photosensitivity since age 13, without any formal evaluation or diagnosis. Additional testing during current pregnancy showed the presence of positive ANA, SS-A, and SS-B antibodies in addition to proteinuria, suggesting a diagnosis of SLE [19].

In addition to potential bleeding occurrence in the fetus, the possible passive transplacental transfer of maternal anti-SS-A and SS-B IgG antibodies incurs the risk of neonatal lupus [20]. These presented a double risk for our patient that could have potentially increased morbidity.

The phenomenon that resulted in developing an inhibitor to factor VIII could represent a concerted occurrence of undiagnosed SLE as an autoimmune situation and the short interpregnancy interval between the patient's prior and current pregnancy and the hormonal changes associated. As the development of factor VIII inhibitors typically occurs in the 2-3 postpartum period, the patient became pregnant around the same interval, and the amplification of the process leading to high-titer pathogenic antibodies could have been caused by immunological processes of both undiagnosed SLE and occurrence of subsequent pregnancy. Flares of SLE with the characteristic antibody production that characterize the disease occur frequently in the postpartum period.

The immunology of pregnancy in SLE poses a paradoxical juncture of immune tolerance required to insure the viability of semiallogenic graft and the disturbance of the tolerance characteristic of SLE. The most important immune alteration is related to the function of Treg cells. The number or the functionality of Treg cells is diminished in a disease characterized by loss of immune tolerance such as SLE, whereas the immune tolerance of the fetus is insured by Treg in a normal pregnancy. Tregs' presence is correlated with the pregnancy outcome. Lower Tregs are associated with pregnancy complications. Moreover, the immunological processes of pregnancy are complicated by the confrontation of two separate immune systems—the maternal immune system and the fetal-placental immune system [21].

4. Literature Review

Our literature review identified fifteen cases of acquired factor VIII deficiency associated with pregnancy with patient's ages ranging between 18 and 37 years. The literature indicates that most cases of acquired factor VIII inhibitors develop after the first pregnancy and typically between 2 and 3 months postpartum. Based on our literature review, we did note that several of the patients developed acquired factor VIII inhibitors after delivering their first child; however, most patients developed postpartum hemorrhage within days of delivery [5, 7–10]. There were other primigravid cases where the patient developed acquired factor VIII inhibitors, but symptoms did not manifest until 2-9 months postpartum [4, 12, 15, 22]. Still, there were cases of acquired factor VIII deficiency in women after their second pregnancy [14, 17] and third pregnancy [4]. There did not seem to be any correlation with the gravid status of the patient and clinical outcomes. Of the fifteen cases reviewed, two patients died from complications related directly to the acquired factor deficiency in the setting of hemorrhagic shock [9] and indirectly secondary to sepsis in the setting of immunosuppression for eradication therapy [20]. These two women were aged 19 and 36, respectively, without other comorbid conditions and had initial inhibitor levels within the 50–60 BU range. An important aspect of each of the aforementioned cases is that each patient had significant vaginal bleeding on presentation. In the former case, the patient presented with a large vaginal hematoma with intra-abdominal bleeding, and the latter developed uncontrolled vaginal bleeding for which she delayed treatment for due to travel between the United States and Mexico. It is unclear whether the prompt intervention could have improved outcomes in these patients, but it is important to consider the acquired factor VIII inhibitor as a differential in a patient with persistent vaginal bleeding during or after pregnancy. Of note, there were three patients (including our case) who developed an acquired factor deficiency prior to delivery [6, 11]. As mentioned previously, our patient developed the inhibitor during her second pregnancy. However, she had a short interval between her first and second pregnancy. One of the cases of acquired factor deficiency prior to delivery was in a patient with an underlying diagnosis of SLE [11]. During our literature search, we did not identify other cases reported of concomitant acquired factor deficiency in pregnant patients with underlying connective tissue diseases. As noted, our patient had an eventful delivery; however, the aforementioned patient had to terminate the pregnancy due to retroperitoneal bleeding which increased the risk for mortality for both patient and fetus.

Regarding the titer level and severity of bleeding, there appeared to be a higher requirement for blood products, worsening of bleeding diathesis, and, in some cases, worse outcomes with a Bethesda titer >100 BU [4, 8, 9, 11]. In one of the cases, the patient inhibitor level increased from the initial level of 64 BU to a level as high as 132 BU. As previously mentioned, this patient died due to hemorrhagic shock on postpartum day 8 [9]. Likewise, the case of acquired factor VIII concomitantly with SLE resulted in a massive retroperitoneal bleed. This patient had an initial titer of 614 BU; however, the patient was able to successfully clear the inhibitor although she did have to terminate pregnancy due to the risk of worsening complications if she continued to term [11]. Moreover, Michiels et al. described a case of a young woman who delivered a stillborn and subsequently developed postpartum hemorrhage with titers as high as 625 BU [4]. This patient did not receive remission at follow-up visits 24 years later despite immunosuppressive therapy. Lastly, Kotani et al. described a case of postpartum hemorrhage with an initial titer level of 458 BU. This patient along with her neonate developed complications; however, after the patient received several blood products including nineteen packed red blood cells, fifty-one units of fresh frozen plasma, 4.8 mg of factor VIIa, and pulse steroid therapy, the patient developed remission [8]. Previous studies note that severity of bleeding does not correlate with the titer level; however, our literature review shows that the severity of bleeding is at least correlated with the titer level of the inhibitor level which reaches as high as 100 BU.

Remission was achieved in most patients by a two-step process aimed at controlling the bleeding and eliminating the inhibitor. Our literature review showed that several patients were treated with some combinations of either desmopressin, factor eight inhibitor bypassing activity

(FEIBA), recombinant human factor VIIa, or recombinant porcine factor VIII concentrate, tranexamic acid, or some other blood products including packed red blood cells or fresh frozen plasma. Several agents were used for eradication of the inhibitor including prednisone, methylprednisolone, cyclophosphamide, rituximab, and azathioprine. The European Acquired Hemophilia Registry (EACH 2) reported 42 documented cases of acquired factor VIII deficiency associated with the peripartum period out of the total 501 documented cases. Of the 42 cases, 74% of patients acquired complete remission with first-line immunosuppressive treatment with all women being alive at the last follow-up visit. To date, there has not been a registry developed in the United States.

5. Learning Points

Acquired factor VIII hemophilia secondary to the coagulation factor inhibitor autoantibody is a rare condition that can be associated with pregnancy and the peripartum period. When it does occur during pregnancy, it most often occurs postpartum but can rarely appear before delivery. The patients present with a large sweep of bleeding manifestations that can pose diagnostic and management challenges. Elevated PTT that fails to correct by adding fresh plasma suggests the presence of the inhibitor and should trigger further workup. As cases are extremely rare, increased awareness and further studies are needed so that prompt intervention can be achieved.

Acknowledgments

This study was supported by Doctors Hospital at Renaissance.

References

[1] A. A. Barg, T. Livnat, G. Kenet, and M. D. Gili, "An extra X does not prevent acquired hemophilia - pregnancy-associated acquired hemophilia A," *Thrombosis Research*, vol. 151, pp. S82–S85, 2017.

[2] L. Mo and G. C. Bao, "Acquired factor VIII deficiency: two case reports and a review of literature," *Experimental Hematology & Oncology*, vol. 6, no. 8, 2017.

[3] S. A. Shobeiri, E. C. West, M. J. K. Md, and T. E. Nolan, "Postpartum acquired hemophilia (factor VIII inhibitors): a case report and review of the literature," *Obstetrical and Gynecological Survey*, vol. 55, no. 12, pp. 729–737, 2000.

[4] J. J. Michiels, K. Hamulyak, H. K. Nieuwenhuis, I. Novakova, and H. H. van Vliet, "Acquired haemophilia A in women postpartum: management of bleeding episodes and natural history of the factor VIII inhibitor," *European Journal of Haematology*, vol. 59, no. 2, pp. 105–109, 1997.

[5] B. S. Coller, M. B. Hultin, L. W. Hoyer et al., "Normal pregnancy in a patient with a prior postpartum factor VIII inhibitor: with observations on pathogenesis and prognosis," *Blood*, vol. 58, no. 3, pp. 619–624, 1981.

[6] M. Chaari, M. Sassi, V. Galea, G. T. Gerotziafas, and I. Elalamy, "Hémophilie A acquise découverte au cours de la grossesse à propos d'un cas et revue de la littérature," *La Revue de Medecine Interne*, vol. 33, no. 7, pp. 401–404, 2012.

[7] S. Seethala, S. Gaur, E. Enderton, and J. Corral, "Postpartum acquired hemophilia: a rare cause of postpartum hemorrhage," *Case Reports in Hematology*, vol. 2013, Article ID 735715, 2 pages, 2013.

[8] Y. Kotani, M. Shiota, M. Umemoto, E. Koike, M. Tsuritani, and H. Hoshiai, "Case of acquired hemophilia with factor VIII inhibitor in a mother and newborn," *Journal of Obstetrics and Gynaecology Research*, vol. 37, no. 8, pp. 1102–1105, 2011.

[9] M. Chaari, R. Bouhlel, S. Kallel et al., "Post partum acquired hemophilia A with fatal outcome: a case report," *Annales de Biologie Clinique*, vol. 70, no. 6, pp. 741–746, 2012.

[10] A. O. R. Porteous, D. S. Appleton, F. Hoveyda, and C. C. Lees, "Acquired haemophilia and postpartum haemorrhage treated with internal pudendal embolisation," *BJOG: An International Journal of Obstetrics and Gynaecology*, vol. 112, no. 5, pp. 678-679, 2005.

[11] A. Sebastian, M. Misterska-Skóra, M. Podolak-Dawidziak, M. Szmyrka-Kaczmarek, M. Sebastian, and P. Wiland, "Letter to the Editor Pregnancy exacerbates complications of acquired hemophilia in a patient with systemic lupus erythematosus," *Advances in Dermatology and Allergology*, vol. 3, no. 3, pp. 235–238, 2015.

[12] O. W. Rodrigues, I. de Oliveira Fernandes Junior, and A. Aparecida Ferreira, "Postpartum acquired hemophilia A: case report and literature review," *Journal of Blood Disorders and Medicine*, 2017.

[13] K. S. Lee, Y. J. Shim, K. M. Jang, and S. Y. Hyun, "Second case of postpartum acquired hemophilia A in a Korean female," *Blood research*, vol. 49, no. 3, pp. 205–207, 2014.

[14] K. Azam, Z. Batool, A. Malik, M. Chaudhry, and M. Abdullah, "Postpartum-acquired hemophilia presenting as hemoperitoneum: a case report," *Cureus*, vol. 12, no. 12, Article ID e11817, 2020.

[15] L. Qian, H. Ge, P. Hu et al., "Pregnancy-related acquired hemophilia A initially manifesting as pleural hemorrhage: a case report," *Medicine*, vol. 98, no. 3, Article ID e14119, 2019.

[16] J. A. Shavit and D. Ginsburg, "Hemophilias and other disorders of hemostasis," *Reference Module in Biomedical Sciences*, 2014.

[17] R. R. Lulla, G. A. Allen, A. Zakarija, and D. Green, "Transplacental transfer of postpartum inhibitors to factor VIII," *Haemophilia*, vol. 16, no. 1, pp. 14–17, 2010.

[18] M. P. Kosloski, D. S. Pisal, D. E. Mager, and S. V. Balu-Iyer, "Nonlinear pharmacokinetics of factor VIII and its phosphatidylinositol lipidic complex in hemophilia A mice," *Biopharmaceutics & Drug Disposition*, vol. 35, no. 3, pp. 154-163, 2014.

[19] M. Aringer, K. Costenbader, and D. Daikh, "European League against Rheumatism/American College of Rheumatology classification criteria for systemic lupus erythematosus," *Annals of the Rheumatic Diseases*, vol. 78, pp. 1151–1159, 2019.

[20] J. P. Buyon, "Clancy Neonatal lupus syndromes," *Current Opinion in Rheumatology*, vol. 15, no. 5, pp. 535–541, 2003.

[21] C. Gluhovschi, G. Gluhovschi, L. Petrica, S. Velciov, and A. Gluhovschi, "Pregnancy associated with systemic lupus erythematosus: immune tolerance in pregnancy and its deficiency in systemic lupus erythematosus--an immunological dilemma," *Journal of Immunology Research*, vol. 2015, Article ID 241547, 11 pages, 2015.

[22] K. S. Lee, Y. J. Shim, K. M. Jang, and S. Y. Hyun, "Second case of postpartum acquired hemophilia A in a Korean female," *Blood Research*, vol. 49, no. 3, pp. 205–207, 2014.

16

Utilization of Rituximab for Refractory Rowell Syndrome

Sukhraj Singh,[1] **Sandra Sheffield,**[2] **Nisha Chowdhury,**[2] **Swetha Nuthulaganti,**[2] **Zareen Vaghaiwalla,**[1] **and Karishma Ramsubeik**[1]

[1]*Division of Rheumatology, Department of Medicine, University of Florida Health Jacksonville, Jacksonville, FL, USA*
[2]*Division of Internal Medicine, Department of Medicine, University of Florida Health Jacksonville, Jacksonville, FL, USA*

Correspondence should be addressed to Sukhraj Singh; sukhraj.singh@jax.ufl.edu

Academic Editor: Gregory J. Tsay

Rowell syndrome describes the occurrence of erythema multiforme-like lesions in patients with cutaneous lesions of lupus erythematosus. The clinical picture of atypical erythema multiforme-like lesions, presence of chilblains, speckled ANA pattern, anti-Ro/SSA, or anti-La/SSB antibodies, and absence of infectious or pharmacologic triggers in a patient with systemic lupus erythematosus are some of the classic clinical and serologic features. Histopathologic and serologic findings can help differentiate this process from erythema multiforme. We present a case of young woman with systemic lupus erythematosus, end-stage renal disease due to lupus nephritis, and a remote history of Steven–Johnson syndrome due to sulfa allergy who presented to the hospital with a recurrent, progressive, targetoid erythematous rash involving more than 60% of her body surface area. Our patient had several hospitalizations in the recent past for this erythematous rash and had failed oral therapy with prednisone 1 mg/kg and hydroxychloroquine. In view of the minimal improvement and increasing severity and patient exhibiting early features of mast cell activation syndrome, the patient was treated with pulse intravenous glucocorticoids followed by rituximab with an excellent response. We highlight a unique case report of progressive Rowell syndrome refractory to standard of care with an excellent response to rituximab.

1. Background

Rowell syndrome (RS) is a rare clinical presentation first described in 1963 by Dr. Neville Rowell and colleagues as an association between systemic lupus erythematosus (SLE) and erythema multiforme (EM) [1]. The defining immunologic features include a speckled antinuclear antibody (ANA) pattern, anti-Ro/SSA or anti-La/SSB antibody, and positive rheumatoid factor (RF) [1]. Since its inception, less than 100 cases have been reported [2, 3]. Among these cases, a higher incidence of cases have been reported in women, with a ratio of women to men 8 : 1. Some cases have been linked to drug exposures, while others manifested with an initial presentation of SLE. Reported cases of RS often fluctuate in clinical and histological presentations and do not always meet the criteria, contributing to the debate on whether RS is its own distinct entity or simply the coexistence of two separate disease processes. Management of RS often overlaps with cutaneous lupus erythematosus and includes topical and oral steroids, antimalarials, immunosuppressive drugs, and pain management.

2. Case Presentation

A 26-year-old African American female with a medical history of SLE, ESRD due to LN, remote history of Steven–Johnson Syndrome due to sulfa allergy, and resistant hypertension presented to the emergency department with painful, peeling, blistering, rash and fever. She reported that the rash developed over a period of 3 months with an intermittent response to prednisone therapy. Three weeks prior to presentation, the rash became progressively worse. She developed fevers came on one week prior to presentation. The rash started on her arms and progressively spread. She admitted associated shortness of breath accompanied by a productive cough with green, bloody sputum, as well as nausea and vomiting. Patient reported compliance with her home dose of prednisone but may have not taken her mycophenolate mofetil regularly. She missed two sequential hemodialysis sessions due to pain with walking from the blistering rash on her soles of the feet.

Her physical exam was significant for fever of 100.6°F and tachycardia with heart rate of 130 beats per minute. Skin exam was evident for brown plaques on the forehead and bilateral cheeks with sparing of the nasolabial folds, with erosions and hemorrhagic crust involving the philtrum, ears, forehead, nose, chin, and lips. There were dark brown plaques with few erosions and atrophic scars on bilateral forearms and lower legs with deep red to violaceous painful targetoid lesions on the palms and plantar surfaces (Figures 1 and 2). The skin over the trunk had pink eroded macules, and there were pink patches on the back within a background of dusky necrotic plaques. There were multiple full-thickness epidermal necroses with large areas of bleeding with the denuded skin on the arms and chest in the sun exposed distribution (Figure 3). Oral mucosae were negative for any oral lesions.

Patient was found to be pancytopenic with white blood cell count (WBC) 2.03 (Ref: 3.4–10.8 × 10^3/UL), absolute neutrophil count (ANC) of 1.25 (Ref: 1.4–7.0 × 10^3/UL), hemoglobin (Hb) 8.8 g/dL (Ref: 11.1–15.9 g/dL), hematocrit (Hct) 28.9% (Ref: 34–46%), platelet 69 (150–450 × 10^3/UL), sodium 138 mmol/L, potassium 3.9 mmol/L, chloride 98 mmol/L, CO_2 21 mmol/L, BUN 41 mg/dL (Ref: 6–20 mg/dL), Cr 5.49 mg/dL (Ref: 0.57–1.0 mg/dL), calcium 7.2 mg/dL (8.7–10.2 mg/dL), albumin 3.2 g/dL, phosphorous 5.0 mg/dL (Ref: 1.2–2.2 mg/dL), AST 286 IU/L (Ref 0–40 IU/L), ALT 31 IU/L (0–32 IU/L), total bilirubin 0.5 mg/dL, alkaline phosphatase 136 IU/L, CK 91 U/L, serum lactate was 0.80 mmol/L, and ferritin was 5885 ng/mL (Ref: 15–50 ng/mL). Electrocardiogram was consistent with sinus tachycardia. Chest X-ray did not show any lung infiltrates or effusions. Ultrasound of the abdomen did not show an acute abdominal process, and the liver demonstrated normal echogenicity, echotexture, and size; the spleen was not enlarged. Sputum gram stain and cultures were unremarkable. Blood cultures were negative for bacteria and yeast. Patient was anuric due to chronic dialysis. Evaluation of lupus activity showed double-stranded DNA (dsDNA) antibody 42 IU/mL (Ref: 0–9 IU/L). Complement 3 (C3) was 43 mg/dL (Ref: 90–180 mg/dL) and complement 4 (C4) was 9 mg/dL (Ref: 10–40 mg/dL). Rheumatoid factor was negative. Sjogren's anti-SSA was >8.0 AI (Ref: 0–0.9 AI) and Sjogren's anti-SSB was <0.2 AI (Ref: 0–0.9 AI). HIV screen was negative, and viral hepatitis panels for hepatitis A, B, and C were negative. Skin biopsies showed focal interface changes, and periodic acid Schiff (PAS) stain was negative for fungal microorganisms. Gram stain highlighted surface cocci bacteria. VZV and herpes I/II immunostains were negative. The direct immunofluorescence revealed that finely granular deposition of C3, IgM, and fibrinogen is consistent with lupus.

Given her presentation of a fever, shortness of breath, and productive cough, there was a concern for postinfectious erythema multiforme. The nucleic acid amplification tests for multiple respiratory pathogens such as *Mycoplasma*, influenza A, influenza H1, influenza H3, influenza A virus H1 2009, influenza B, respiratory syncytial virus, parainfluenza virus type 1, 2, 3, 4, human metapneumovirus, rhinovirus/enterovirus, adenovirus, *Chlamydia pneumoniae*, and *Mycoplasma pneumoniae* were negative. Blood cultures did not grow any bacteria or fungal organisms. Skin wound cultures were also negative for any organisms except for skin flora. Historically, there were no preceding infections reported. Our presumptive primary diagnosis was acute on chronic cutaneous lupus with epidermal necrolysis due to noncompliance with medications; differentials included Rowell syndrome, bullous lupus, Steven–Johnsons syndrome, and toxic epidermal necrolysis (TEN). Hemophagocytic lymphohistiocytosis/mast cell activation syndrome (HLH/MAS) was also a concern given pancytopenia, fevers, elevated transaminases, and elevated ferritin. However, after further evaluation by hematology, HLH/MAS was less likely given halving of ferritin after first dose of intravenous steroids, lack of hepatosplenomegaly, lack of elevation in bilirubin and triglycerides, patient did not have persistent fevers, and soluble IL-2 receptor was 2021 pg/mL (Ref: 175.3–858.2 pg/mL), needed to be greater than 2400 pg/mL (greater than 2 standard deviations of reference range) to meet criteria, and clinical picture was also not as critical as usually seen. The clinical picture of atypical EM-like lesions, presence of chilblains, speckled ANA pattern, elevated anti-Ro/SSA, and absence of infectious or pharmacologic triggers in a patient with SLE confirmed our suspicion for Rowell syndrome.

Due to the extensive skin surface area involvement, the patient was treated with vancomycin intravenously for primary and secondary skin infection. Gram-negative coverage was held due to severe allergy to penicillin and cephalosporin antibiotics. The pancytopenia was suspected due to an acute flare of systemic lupus erythematosus, and the patient was initially started on methylprednisolone 1.5 mg/kg intravenously daily. Given more than 60% of body surface area (BSA) involvement, the patient was transferred to the burn unit for extensive debridement and multifaceted wound care. Mycophenolate mofetil was held given the elevated transaminases. Pulse doses of intravenous methylprednisolone were escalated to 1000 mg intravenous daily for three days given the concern for acute cutaneous lupus erythematosus with epidermal necrosis and concomitant MAS. After normalization of transaminases, negative testing for latent tuberculosis and hepatitis B and C, and negative blood cultures, the patient was given rituximab 375 mg/m^2 intravenously at day 0 and day 15 with excellent maintenance of remission of skin disease and cytopenias. This dose was chosen by the treating provider, given patient being dialysis dependent, thus more immunosuppressed state at baseline and recent elevation in transaminases.

It was reassuring that early suspicion for MAS appeared steroid-responsive to pulse intravenous methylprednisolone. The soluble IL-2 receptor alpha measurement was not elevated, and serum ferritin halved after the first dose of pulse steroids. Despite the improvements in serum and systemic symptoms, the skin manifestations were slow to respond. During 2-week and 12-week follow-up of the patient, there has been maintenance of clear skin without

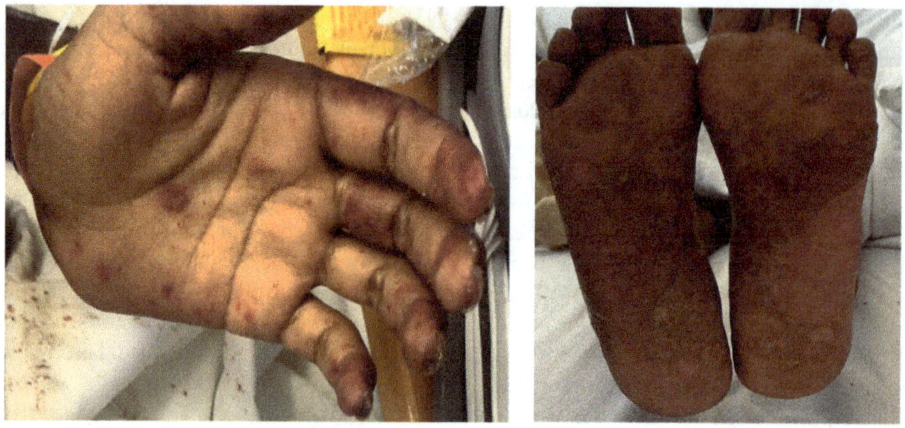

(a) (b)

Figure 1: Chilblain lupus erythematosus (LE), deep red to violaceous plaques on palms and soles. Some appear annular targetoid pain and pruritis.

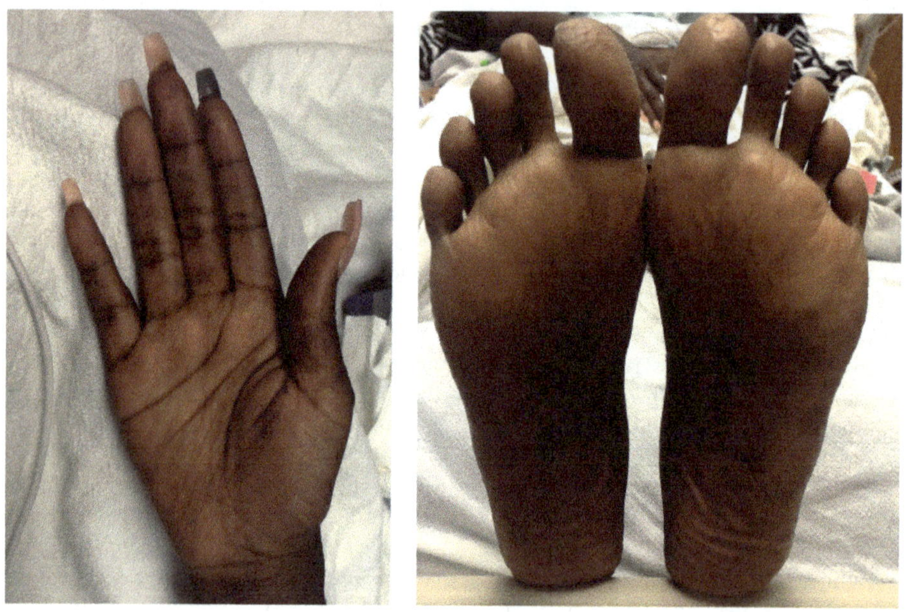

(a) (b)

Figure 2: Complete resolution of lesions seen in Figure 1 approximately 3 months after treatment.

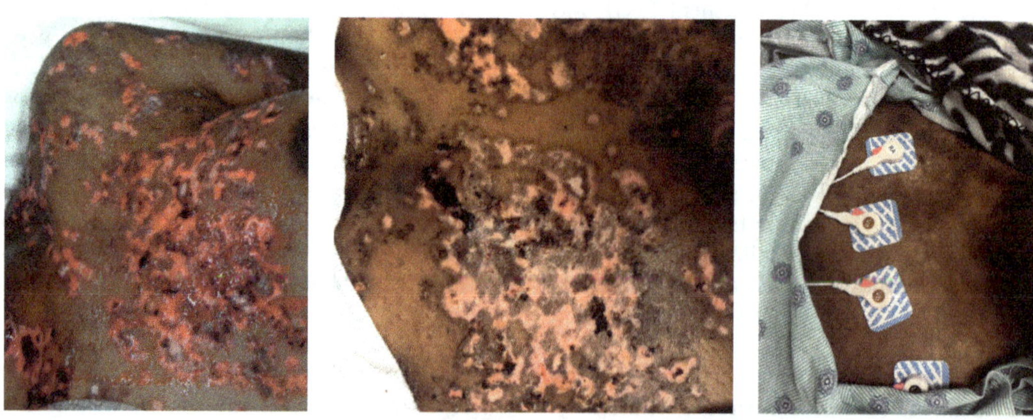

(a) (b) (c)

Figure 3: Left anterior chest wall demonstrating full-thickness epidermal necrosis with large areas of bleeding, denuded skin. Center image shows healing two weeks posttreatment and the image on the left shows complete resolution at 3 months since induction with rituximab.

Table 1: Summary of proposed diagnostic criteria for Rowell syndrome by different authors.

	Diagnosis
Rowell et al. [5] LE EM-like lesions (with the absence of any known precipitating factors) Speckled pattern of ANA Anti-SJT antibody (anti-La/SSB) Positive rheumatoid factor	All features required
Lee et al. [10] LE EM-like lesions (with the absence of any known precipitating factors) Chilblains Speckled pattern ANA Anti-La/SSB antibody Positive rheumatoid factor	All features required
Zeitouni et al. [1] Major criteria SLE, DLE, or SCLE EM-like lesions (with/without involvement of mucous membranes) Speckled pattern ANA Minor criteria Chilblains Anti-Ro/SSA or anti-La/SSB Positive rheumatoid factor	3 major + 1 minor criteria
Torchia et al. [8] Major criteria Presence of CCLE (DLE and/or chilblain) Presence of EM-like lesions (typical or atypical targets) At least one positivity among speckled ANA, anti-Ro/SSA, and anti-La/SSB antibodies Negative DIF on lesional EM-like lesions Minor criteria Absence of infectious or pharmacologic triggers Absence of typical EM location (acral and mucosal) Presence of at least one additional ARA criterion for diagnosis of SLE besides discoid rash and ANA and excluding photosensitivity, malar rash, and oral ulcers	Presence of all 4 major + 1 minor criteria

any active cutaneous lupus manifestations. Systemic Lupus Erythematosus Disease Activity Index 2000 (SLEDAI-2K) was 0 at 12-week follow-up.

3. Discussion and Conclusion

Erythema multiforme is an acute, immune-mediated condition characterized by the appearance of distinctive target-like lesions on the skin often accompanied by erosions or bullae involving the oral, genital, and/or ocular mucosae [4]. EM has very well-known causes in the literature including infections (herpes simplex virus or *Mycoplasma pneumoniae* infection), medications (nonsteroidal anti-inflammatory drugs (NSAIDs), antiepileptics, and antibiotics), malignancy, and autoimmune diseases [4]. Classical EM is precipitated by trigger factors such as infective agents or drugs and is not associated with any specific serological antibodies or with chilblains. The rare overlap of EM and SLE and the presence of serological criteria can help make the diagnosis of Rowell syndrome [1].

Rowell syndrome is a rare entity that has been described with all subtypes of systemic lupus erythematosus. Beck and Anderson first described unique and distinct features associated with Rowell syndrome [5]. These characteristics include coexistence of SLE, erythema multiforme-like lesions, and immunological changes. The first described unique characteristics include positive tests for rheumatoid factor, speckled pattern antinuclear antibody, and precipitating antibodies to saline extract of human tissue (anti-SjT) now known as La/SSB and Ro/SSA antibodies [6]. The erythema multiforme-like lesions are painful, pruritic, annular, erythematous, and red to violet plaques with blisters. The lesions are mainly seen in the arms and legs and less frequently on the face, neck, chest, and mouth. They could last from a few days to over a month [1]. Histopathologic findings of RS are controversial as well. The presence of necrotic keratinocytes is not specific to RS because it might be found in 54% of subacute cutaneous lupus erythematosus (SCLE) lesions [7]. The direct immunofluorescence of RS and EM exhibits similar findings to include deposits of C3 and immunoglobulin M in the dermal capillaries [6, 7]. Like SLE, Rowell syndrome is believed to be an autoimmune disease with an interplay of genetics, hormones, and environment factors. There are no specific autoantibodies associated with Rowell syndrome.

Since its first description in 1963, there has been controversy whether RS is a separate entity or a coincidental occurrence associated with cutaneous lupus erythematosus [1]. Approximately 95 cases have been described in the literature since it was first described [3]. We summarize the multiple different diagnostic criteria proposed over the last five decades (Table 1). Diagnostic criteria proposed by Torchia et al. seem to be the most comprehensive [8].

The response to treatment is variable, and frequent recurrences have been reported [7]. Different therapies studied for RS have produced variable results [7, 9, 10]. Various therapeutics options have been described for the management of RS including hydroxychloroquine, chloroquine, azathioprine, dapsone, thalidomide, and corticosteroid therapy [10]. Most RS patients respond well to the first-line therapies outlined above. Our patient continued to have breakthroughs of EM-like rash and progression despite the use of hydroxychloroquine and steroids. The development of early mast cell activation syndrome (MAS) in our patient with worsening cutaneous disease also warranted implementation of more powerful immunosuppression. We report the first case of persistent Rowell syndrome and LE nonspecific skin disease, which is treated with rituximab to maintain remission.

Rituximab is an anti-CD20 monoclonal antibody approved for the treatment of non-Hodgkin lymphoma, chronic lymphocytic leukemia, and rheumatoid arthritis, but it is used off-label for many other conditions [11]. Studies have shown its effectiveness in treating autoimmune skin disorders, such as pemphigus vulgaris, pemphigus foliaceus, vasculitis, SLE, and SCLE [12]. Currently, there are seventeen cases of cutaneous manifestation of SLE and eight cases with refractory SCLE treated with rituximab [12, 13]. Of the eight refractory SCLE cases, seven showed effective results except one. The dosing regimen was varied from 1 g every 2 weeks to 375 mg/m^2 weekly for 4 weeks [12]. Maintenance doses varied from every 2 months to 1 year. Although rituximab has shown effective results in treatment of SCLE, it has not been effective for chronic cutaneous lupus erythematosus. Rituximab therapy has been reported in treatment of five cases of erythema multiforme major [14]. However, these patients differed from the one presented in this case, as they did not have SLE and suffered from severe, chronic erythema multiforme major with positive antidesmoplakin antibodies in four of the five cases [14]. In other studies, 2 patients have been reported with LE nonspecific condition of vasculitis which had complete resolution of mucocutaneous disease after rituximab [15].

Rowell syndrome has a good prognosis with most cases reporting complete remission in one year; however, there are some cases citing recurrence of disease and up to two years until remission [16]. In the case presented, pulse intravenous glucocorticoids were used to induce remission, and two doses of rituximab 375 mg/m^2 two weeks apart were implemented to maintain remission. Although rituximab has been utilized as off-label treatment of SLE, this may be the first documented case of treatment of Rowell syndrome with rituximab.

Abbreviations

SLE: Systemic lupus erythematosus
ESRD: End-stage renal disease
SJS: Steven–Johnson syndrome
TEN: Toxic epidermal necrolysis
EM: Erythema multiforme
LE: Lupus erythematosus
ANA: Antinuclear antibody
SSA: Sjogren's syndrome-related antigen A
SSB: Sjogren's syndrome-related antigen B
RS: Rowell syndrome
MAS: Mast cell activation syndrome
LN: Lupus nephritis
VZV: Varicella zoster virus.

References

[1] N. C. Zeitouni, D. Funaro, R. A. Cloutier, E. Gagné, and J. Claveau, "Redefining Rowell's syndrome," *British Journal of Dermatology*, vol. 142, no. 2, pp. 343–346, 2000.

[2] E. Antiga, M. Caproni, D. Bonciani, V. Bonciolini, and P. Fabbri, "The last word on the so-called "Rowell's syndrome"?" *Lupus*, vol. 21, no. 6, pp. 577–585, 2012.

[3] L. Gallo, M. Megna, B. Festa et al., "Rowell syndrome: a diagnostic challenge," *The Journal of Clinical and Aesthetic Dermatology*, vol. 13, no. 4, pp. 40–42, 2020.

[4] D. A. Wetter, *Erythema Multiforme: Pathogenesis, Clinical Features, and Diagnosis*, UpToDate, Waltham, MA, USA, 2020.

[5] N. R. Rowell, J. S. Beck, and J. R. Anderson, "Lupus erythematosus and erythema multiforme-like lesions," *Archives of Dermatology*, vol. 88, no. 2, pp. 176–180, 1963.

[6] S. Khandpur, S. Das, and M. K. Singh, "Rowell's syndrome revisited: report of two cases from India," *International Journal of Dermatology*, vol. 44, no. 7, pp. 545–549, 2005.

[7] I. T. Andronache, C. Suta, C. Ionescu, A. Calistrat, and M. Suta, "Rowell syndrome-a controversial clinical entity," *Romanian Journal of Rhematology*, vol. 24, pp. 230–234, 2015.

[8] D. Torchia, P. Romanelli, and F. A. Kerdel, "Erythema multiforme and Stevens-Johnson syndrome/toxic epidermal necrolysis associated with lupus erythematosus," *Journal of the American Academy of Dermatology*, vol. 67, no. 3, pp. 417–421, 2012.

[9] R. Bhat, C. Varma, S. Bhatt, and C. Balachandran, "Rowell syndrome," *Indian Dermatology Online Journal*, vol. 5, no. Suppl 1, pp. S33–S35, 2014.

[10] A. Lee, P. Batra, V. Furer, W. Cheung, N. Wang Jr., and F. Andrew, "Rowell syndrome (systemic lupus erythematosus + erythema multiforme)," *Dermatology Online Journal*, vol. 15, no. 8, 2009.

[11] Lexicomp Rituximab, *Drug Information*, UpToDate, Waltham, MA, USA, 2020.

[12] M. Á. Penha, R. da Silva Libório, and H. A. Miot, "Rituximab in the treatment of extensive and refractory subacute cutaneous lupus erythematosus," *Anais Brasileiros de Dermatologia*, vol. 93, no. 3, pp. 467–469, 2018.

[13] S. Hofmann, M. Leandro, S. Morris, and D. Isenberg, "Effects of rituximab-based B-cell depletion therapy on skin manifestations of lupus erythematosus—report of 17 cases and review of the literature," *Lupus*, vol. 22, no. 9, pp. 932–939, 2013.

[14] G. Hirsch, S. Ingen-Housz-Oro, C. Fite et al., "Rituximab, a new treatment for difficult-to-treat chronic erythema multiforme major? five cases," *Journal of the European Academy of Dermatology and Venereology*, vol. 30, no. 7, pp. 1140–1143, 2016.

[15] E. M. Vital, M. Wittmann, S. Edward et al., "Brief report: responses to rituximab suggest B cell-independent inflammation in cutaneous systemic lupus erythematosus," *Arthritis & Rheumatology*, vol. 67, no. 6, pp. 1586–1591, 2015.

[16] D. Brănişteanu, S. Ianoşi, A. Dimitriu, G. Stoleriu, A. Oanţă, and D. Brănişteanu, "Drug-induced Rowell syndrome, a rare and difficult to manage disease: a case report," *Experimental and Therapeutic Medicine*, vol. 15, no. 1, pp. 785–788, 2018.

17

Cutaneous Polyarteritis Nodosa Presenting Atypically with Severe Pharyngeal Ulceration

Bayanne Olabi,[1,2] **Justin C. Mason,**[2] **and Ziad Farah**[2]

[1]*NHS Lothian, Department of Dermatology, Lauriston Building, Lauriston Place, Edinburgh EH3 9EN, UK*
[2]*Rheumatology Section, Imperial College Healthcare NHS Trust, Hammersmith Hospital, Du Cane Road, London W12 0HS, UK*

Correspondence should be addressed to Bayanne Olabi; bayanne@doctors.org.uk

Academic Editor: Jamal Mikdashi

Polyarteritis nodosa (PAN) is a multisystem, necrotising vasculitis of small- and medium-sized arteries with a predilection for the visceral vessels. Cutaneous PAN is a rare variant with symptomatic vasculitis limited to the skin, typically presenting as nodular lesions on the extremities with a propensity to ulcerate. We describe a rare case of histologically confirmed cutaneous PAN presenting in a 55-year-old Ghanaian woman with severe oropharyngeal ulceration. This was associated with dysphagia and significant weight loss. Oesophagoduodenoscopy showed that the ulceration extended throughout the oropharynx. Systemic polyarteritis nodosa was ruled out with magnetic resonance angiography. Our patient was treated successfully with corticosteroids and methotrexate. This case suggests that cutaneous PAN should be considered in the differential diagnosis of patients with oropharyngeal ulceration and that histological assessment is pivotal in establishing the diagnosis early in order to instigate appropriate therapy.

1. Introduction

Polyarteritis nodosa (PAN) is a multisystem, necrotising vasculitis of small- and medium-sized arteries with predilection for the visceral arteries. Cutaneous PAN is a rare variant with symptomatic vasculitis limited to skin, and at times, peripheral nerves [1]. The primary lesion is typically a subcutaneous nodule that affects the lower extremities, and these lesions often ulcerate [2]. Livedo reticularis has been reported in 50–80% of cases [3]. Commonly encountered symptoms include fever, malaise, myalgia, and arthralgia [4]. In this article, we present a rare case of histologically confirmed cutaneous PAN presenting with severe pharyngeal ulceration.

2. Case Presentation

A 55-year-old Ghanaian woman presented with a one-month history of mouth ulcers, painful swallowing, and fever. She had also developed cutaneous ulcers on the left lower leg, back, and scalp. She reported being nonspecifically unwell for 1 year, with fatigue, poor appetite, and 8 kg weight loss over three months. She was not taking any regular or new medications prior to this illness and had a background of asthma and asymptomatic mild-moderate mitral regurgitation. She did not consume alcohol or recreational drugs and smoked 10 cigarettes per day. She was born in Ghana and came to the UK aged 11. There was no travel history for 3 years prior to admission and no recent new sexual partners.

On admission, she was febrile at 38.2°C. Several painful mouth ulcers were seen, affecting the hard palate and the oropharynx (Figure 1(a)). No other mucous membrane involvement was present and specifically no genital ulcers. There was a 5 cm diameter circular pigmented nodule on the left calf, with central necrotic ulceration. She had a 10 cm diameter inflammatory well-demarcated plaque over the left central back (Figure 1(b)) and smaller ulcers over the scalp, all less than 1 cm diameter.

Laboratory tests revealed mild anaemia with a haemoglobin of 119 g/L, platelet count 227×10^9/L, white cell count 9.0×10^9/L, albumin 33 g/L (normal 35–55), an elevated

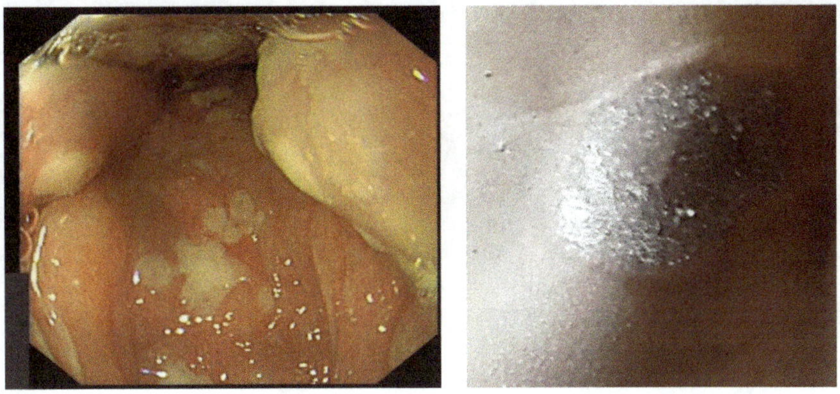

(a) (b)

FIGURE 1: (a) Oesophagogastroduodenoscopy demonstrating extensive pharyngeal ulceration. (b) Ulcerating plaque (10 cm diameter) over the left central back; photograph taken by the patient's family member prior to admission. Reproduced with patient consent.

erythrocyte sedimentation rate (ESR) of 69 mm/hr, and C-reactive protein (CRP) 73 mg/L (normal < 5). The ANCA test was negative, complement component C4 was elevated, and the rest of the autoimmune screen was negative. Blood and urine cultures and a scalp ulcer and throat swab revealed no bacterial growth. Viral throat swab was negative. Coeliac serology was also negative. Upper gastrointestinal endoscopy revealed marked oropharyngeal ulceration without contact bleeding (Figure 1(a)). A CT scan of the chest, abdomen, and pelvis revealed no evidence of malignancy, while an MR angiogram of the aorta revealed no evidence to suggest systemic PAN.

Two 4 mm punch biopsies were taken from the scalp lesions along with an 8 mm punch biopsy from the left lower leg nodule. These underwent haemotoxylin and eosin (H and E) and direct immunofluorescence staining. Immunohistochemistry from both locations revealed loss of epidermis with necrosis and a brisk inflammatory infiltrate in the dermis composed of neutrophils and histiocytes, the latter coalescing into poorly formed granulomas (Figures 2(a) and 2(b)). Abundant cytoclastic debris was present. In areas, the inflammatory cells were clearly centred around and obscuring blood vessels, which showed foci of fibrinoid necrosis (Figure 2(c)). The process involved small dermal blood vessels and larger muscular vessels deep in the biopsy. PAS (Periodic acid-Schiff) and ZN (Ziehl–Neelsen) stains were negative. Direct immunofluorescence was negative. The overall impression was of a necrotising vasculitis with granulomatous features, findings consistent with a diagnosis of cutaneous PAN.

Data are limited on the treatment used in cutaneous PAN. However, due to the severity of her presentation and oropharyngeal involvement precluding her from a safe swallow, systemic treatment was opted for in preference to topical therapy. The patient was initially prescribed intravenous hydrocortisone and subsequently oral prednisolone 40 mg and methotrexate 10 mg weekly. The latter was uptitrated to 15 mg weekly prior to discharge, and the prednisolone was slowly weaned. Once treatment was established, no further lesions developed and the existing oropharyngeal and cutaneous ulcers began to heal. After 23 days, when able to maintain good oral intake, the patient was discharged.

At clinic follow-up six weeks later, all the oral ulcers and the lesions on the leg, back, and scalp had healed, and no new lesions were seen. The patient reported persistent fatigue and muscle weakness, and there was evidence of mild proximal weakness in the hip flexors. Acute phase markers and serum albumin were within normal range. The methotrexate dose was increased from 15 mg to 17.5 mg weekly and the prednisolone dose was progressively weaned. At subsequent follow-up after 6 months, the patient was well with no active skin lesions. She continued methotrexate 20 mg weekly and prednisolone 5 mg daily. At 12-month follow-up, she remained in remission with CRP 2.0 g/L and ESR 24 mm/hr.

3. Discussion

The concept of a benign, limited cutaneous form of PAN has been debated since its first description in 1931 by Lindberg [5]. The precise pathogenesis of the condition is poorly understood. Cutaneous PAN presenting with typical nodular lesions on the extremities with a propensity to ulcerate is well recognised [2]. However, a presentation with severe mucocutaneous pharyngeal ulceration leading to significant weight loss has not been documented. Our case suggests that cutaneous PAN should be included in the differential diagnosis of oropharyngeal ulceration.

A diagnosis of cutaneous PAN requires exclusion of systemic PAN. This was confirmed in our patient by MR angiography. Although a diagnosis of systemic PAN can be supported by the aid of classification criteria, these do not include the cutaneous form of the disease [6]. In addition, whereas some have argued that cutaneous PAN can progress to the systemic form, Nakamura et al. concluded that although true cutaneous PAN may be associated with myalgia or neuropathy, this is limited to the same area as the skin lesions, and does not progress to the systemic form [7]. Moreland and Ball also discuss the differences between the two conditions, noting a 1 : 1 male to female ratio in cutaneous PAN and a significant male predominance in systemic PAN [8]. Unlike systemic PAN, the cutaneous form typically

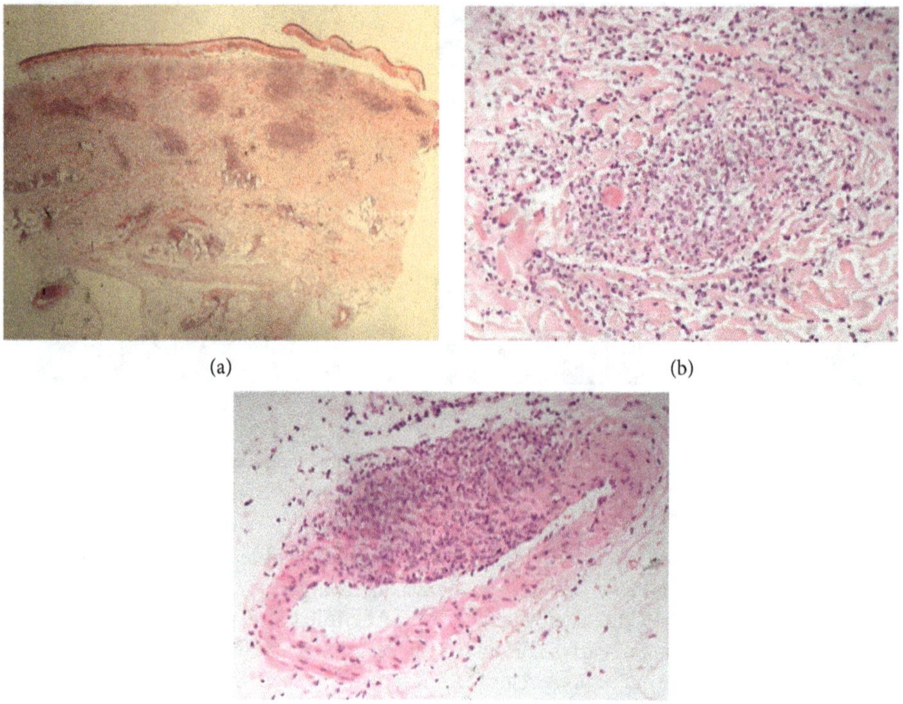

(a) (b) (c)

Figure 2: (a) H and E stained skin punch biopsy (x20 magnification) showing loss of the epidermis with an inflammatory infiltrate in the dermis composed of neutrophils and histiocytes, the latter coalescing into (b) poorly formed granulomas (x100 magnification). Abundant cytoclastic debris is present. (c) In areas the inflammation appears centred on blood vessels associated with fibrinoid necrosis (x200 magnification). The findings indicate a necrotising vasculitis with granulomatous features.

has a benign course with a good long-term prognosis and virtually no reports of mortality [2].

The subcutaneous tender, erythematous nodules (usually 0.5–3 cm in diameter) may disappear spontaneously or undergo ulceration. Other findings include petechiae, purpura, cutaneous necrosis, and autoamputations. Extracutaneous manifestations are not uncommon and include constitutional symptoms (commonly fever and malaise), arthralgia, myalgia, and peripheral neuropathy (mononeuropathy and mononeuritis multiplex) [1, 7].

Our case presented with pure cutaneous manifestations, and unusually oropharyngeal ulceration, without systemic involvement. Differential diagnoses for a blistering skin eruption and mucocutaneous ulceration were considered and excluded, including infection, underlying inflammatory bowel disease, dermatitis herpetiformis, Behçets syndrome, and drug reaction [9]. Oral ulceration is a very rare complication of polyarteritis nodosa and has been reported on occasion, including a study from the French vasculitis group [10]. There are no specific serological tests for cutaneous PAN, and diagnosis requires histopathologic confirmation [11]. Classically, skin biopsy reveals a necrotising vasculitis of the small arteries from the dermal-subcutaneous border to subcutaneous tissue, with infiltration of inflammatory cells into the media and intima together with fibrinoid degeneration [11]. Chen proposed a classification of cutaneous PAN into three stages: acute, repair, and scarring stages [12].

EULAR guidelines recommend the use of high-dose corticosteroids together with cyclophosphamide for remission induction in systemic PAN, followed by steroid-sparing agents including methotrexate, azathioprine, or leflunomide [13]. No specific guidelines for the management of cutaneous PAN have been developed. As cutaneous PAN is classically an ANCA-negative, nonorgan-threatening vasculitis, we adapted EULAR recommendations for the management of limited ANCA-associated vasculitis and prescribed corticosteroids and methotrexate [13]. This combination has proved effective for both cutaneous and oropharyngeal lesions to date, and use is supported by two previous reports of cutaneous PAN [14, 15].

Authors' Contributions

Justin C Mason and Ziad Farah contributed equally to this work.

Acknowledgments

This work received infrastructure report from the National Institute for Health Research Biomedical Research Centre at Imperial College.

References

[1] P. Borrie, "Cutaneous polyarteritis nodosa," *British Journal of Dermatology*, vol. 87, no. 2, pp. 87–95, 1972.

[2] J. L. Díaz-Pérez, Z. M. De Lagrán, J. Luis Díaz-Ramón, and R. K. Winkelmann, "Cutaneous polyarteritis nodosa," *Seminars in Cutaneous Medicine and Surgery*, vol. 26, no. 2, pp. 77–86, 2007.

[3] M. S. Daoud, K. P. Hutton, and L. E. Gibson, "Cutaneous periarteritis nodosa: a clinicopathological study of 79 cases," *British Journal of Dermatology*, vol. 136, no. 5, pp. 706–713, 1997.

[4] A. J. Morgan and R. A. Schwartz, "Cutaneous polyarteritis nodosa: a comprehensive review," *International Journal of Dermatology*, vol. 49, no. 7, pp. 750–756, 2010.

[5] K. Lindberg, "Ein beitrag zur kenntnis der periarteriitis nodosa," *Acta Medica Scandinavica*, vol. 76, no. 1-2, pp. 183–225, 1931.

[6] J. C. Jennette, R. J. Falk, P. A. Bacon et al., "2012 revised international chapel hill consensus conference nomenclature of vasculitides," *Arthritis & Rheumatism*, vol. 65, no. 1, pp. 1–11, 2013.

[7] T. Nakamura, N. Kanazawa, T. Ikeda et al., "Cutaneous polyarteritis nodosa: revisiting its definition and diagnostic criteria," *Archives of Dermatological Research*, vol. 301, no. 1, pp. 117–121, 2009.

[8] L. W. Moreland and G. V. Ball, "Cutaneous polyarteritis nodosa," *American Journal of Medicine*, vol. 88, no. 4, pp. 426–430, 1990.

[9] M. T. Keogan, "Clinical Immunology Review Series: an approach to the patient with recurrent orogenital ulceration, including Behçet's syndrome," *Clinical & Experimental Immunology*, vol. 156, no. 1, pp. 1–11, 2009.

[10] N. Kluger, C. Pagnoux, L. Guillevin, C. Francès, and French Vasculitis Study Group, "Comparison of cutaneous manifestations in systemic polyarteritis nodosa and microscopic polyangiitis," *British Journal of Dermatology*, vol. 159, no. 3, pp. 615–620, 2008 Sep.

[11] F. Furukawa, "Cutaneous polyarteritis nodosa: an update," *Annals of Vascular Diseases*, vol. 5, no. 3, pp. 282–288, 2012.

[12] K. R. Chen, *Polyarteritis Nodosa, Color Atlas Collagen Vascular Diseases Based on Skin Lesions*, Zennihon Byoin Shuppankai, Tokyo, Japan, 1st edition, 2006.

[13] C. Mukhtyar, L. Guillevin, M. C. Cid et al., "EULAR recommendations for the management of primary small and medium vessel vasculitis," *Annals of the Rheumatic Diseases*, vol. 68, no. 3, pp. 310–317, 2009.

[14] J. L. Jorizzo, W. L. White, C. M. Wise, M. D. Zanoffi, and E. F. Sherertz, "Low-dose weekly methotrexate for unusual neutrophilic vascular reactions: cutaneous polyarteritis nodosa and Behçet's disease," *Journal of the American Academy of Dermatology*, vol. 24, no. 6, pp. 973–978, 1991.

[15] N. E. C. Schartz, S. Alaoui, M. D. Vignon-Pennamen et al., "Successful treatment in two cases of steroid-dependent cutaneous polyarteritis nodosa with low-dose methotrexate," *Dermatology*, vol. 203, no. 4, pp. 336–338, 2001.

18

Trauma Induced Calcium Pyrophosphate Deposition Disease of the Lumbar Spine

Indrit Greca,[1] **Jihad Ben Gabr**,[1] **Andras Perl**,[1,2] **Stephanie Bryant**,[1] **and Dan Zaccarini**[1]

[1]*SUNY Upstate University Hospital, Syracuse, NY-13210, USA*
[2]*Departments of Medicine, Microbiology and Immunology, Biochemistry and Molecular Biology, State University of New York, UMU, College of Medicine, New York, USA*

Correspondence should be addressed to Indrit Greca; grecai@upstate.edu

Academic Editor: Mehmet Soy

Inflammatory arthritis, such as pseudogout or otherwise referred to as calcium pyrophosphate (CPP) crystal arthritis or calcium pyrophosphate deposition (CPPD) disease, is characterized by the deposition of crystal formation and deposition in large joints. CPPD is known to affect the elderly population and commonly manifests as inflammation of knees, hips, and shoulders. CPPD disease involving the spine has been infrequently encountered in practice and rarely described in the literature. Here, we describe a case of an 80-year-old female with no known history of inflammatory arthritis who presented with left lower extremity weakness and fall, initially thought to have discitis, later confirming CPPD of the spine through biopsy and ultimately resolution of symptoms with anti-inflammatory agents. Although consisting of different clinical presentations, two other case reports have described CPPD of the spine with similar radiographic findings, to this author's knowledge. With the radiologic similarities, this unique case serves to raise awareness in the medical community and possibly place pseudogout of the spine on the differential list when such cases are encountered. As a result, patients can be initiated on benign anti-inflammatory agents, avoiding invasive testing and unnecessary antibiotic exposure.

1. Introduction

Back pain is one of the most common symptoms experienced by an adult which oftentimes leads to medical evaluation. Approximately 84% of adults have experienced some degree of back pain in their lifetime [1]. Etiologies of back pain vary, but the majority of patients with these complaints will not have a definite known etiology [2]. Most common known etiologies appear to be muscular, whereas less than 1 percent of patients with back pain have nonbenign etiologies such as infection or malignancy [3]. Spinal inflammatory arthritis, such as acute CPP crystal arthritis, is not a typical etiology that would present as a differential of back pain and is not often thought of as a possible diagnosis. Acute CPP crystal arthritis is the deposition of calcium pyrophosphate dihydrate crystals in connective tissues, giving rise to inflammatory arthritis [4]. Etiology of acute CPP crystal arthritis is idiopathic, but joint trauma has been a linked factor [5]. The deposition of crystals most commonly affects the knees and the wrists. Here, we present an 80-year-old female with no past history of pseudogout who presented with back pain presumed to be of infectious origin but was ultimately found to have pseudogout of the lumbar spine. The purpose of this documentation is to bring awareness to pseudogout affecting the spine, which would otherwise be misdiagnosed as infection in patients with undistinguishable radiographic evidence, and expose these patients to unnecessary antibiotic treatment.

2. Case Presentation

80-year-old female with known medical history of hypothyroidism, gastroesophageal reflux disease, and hypertension presented to our hospital with left leg weakness with tingling prompting a fall, associated with progressive back pain. The patient started having back pain about one year prior to presentation after suffering a mechanical fall down a flight of stairs. At the time, she did not seek medical attention and pain improved with conservative treatment. However, six months ago the patient started having intermittent low back pain radiating to left buttock, for which she saw her primary care physician (PCP). Her PCP prescribed a short course of tramadol of unknown dosage and frequency. Approximately one month prior to presentation, the patient started experiencing exacerbations of her back pain associated with radiculopathy on bilateral lower extremities. She self-treated with aspirin 325 milligrams (mg) every 8 hours as needed along with Tylenol 650 mg every 6 hours as needed. On the day of hospitalization, the patient experienced severe left lower extremity numbness subsequently leading to her fall. She otherwise denied urinary or bowel incontinence, perineal paresthesia, fevers, chills, dizziness, palpitations, loss of consciousness, rashes, unintentional weight loss, and headaches.

On day 1 of examination, the patient was in no acute distress but appeared uncomfortable. The temperature was 36.4°C, the blood pressure was 104/65 mmHg, the pulse was 54 beats per minute, the respiratory rate was 16 breaths per minute, the oxygen saturation was 98% while she was breathing ambient air, and body mass index was 32.07 kilograms per meter squared (kg/m^2). Physical examination revealed pupils were equal, round, and reactive to light. Heart sounds were normal, with regular rate and rhythm. Lung sounds were clear bilaterally. The abdomen was soft and nontender. Musculoskeletal examination was remarkable for mild point tenderness of the lumbar spine. Rectal tone was intact. Strength and sensation were intact on bilateral upper and lower extremities. Patellar reflexes were plus one bilaterally. No clonus was noted, and Babinski sign was negative. There were no abrasions or discoloration of the skin noted on the paraspinal area. The paraspinal area was clean and nonerythematous. The patient was found to have abdominal fold and bilateral groin wounds that appeared moist and pale pink with some partial thickness and skin breakdown. There appeared to be some chronic skin changes with dark skin discoloration to the periphery as well.

Laboratory studies showed blood urea nitrogen of 32 mg/dL (reference range: 8–23 mg/dL; reference range is provided in the parentheses in the following laboratory studies), creatinine of 1.23 mg/dL (0.4–1.0 mg/dL), corrected calcium of 11.1 mg/dL (8.8–10.2 mg/dL), and a white blood cell count of 11.8 K/μL (4–10 K/μL). The rest of the basic laboratory studies were within normal range. The initial image of choice ordered was a computerized tomography (CT) scan, which showed advanced degenerative joint disease with severe spinal stenosis at the level of the lumbar 4-lumbar 5 (L4L5) spinal segment. Orthopedic spine specialty service was consulted and recommended to administer intravenous (IV) Decadron 6 milligrams every 6 hours and obtain a magnetic resonance imaging (MRI) for further evaluation of the abnormality noted on CT scan. MRI of the spine was completed on day 2, which depicted vertebral body edema and enhancement most evident at the L4L5 level and paravertebral soft tissue thickening seen at the L5-S1 level concerning of osteomyelitis/diskitis. (Figure 1). MRI also confirmed severe central canal stenosis at the L4L5 level with crowding of the cauda equina secondary to disk bulging and osteoarthropathy. Due to concerns of possible osteomyelitis of the spine, the patient was started empirically on vancomycin 2 grams every 12 hours and piperacillin/tazobactam 3.375 grams every 6 hours. A neurosurgery consult was requested.

Neurosurgery evaluated the patient and were concerned about the severe central canal and neuroforaminal stenosis as depicted by the imaging. They stated that the patient could have been a candidate for a L45 transforaminal lumbar interbody fusion (TLIF) as it appeared that there were significant sclerotic changes at this spinal level causing neurological deficits. However, further investigation needed to be done to determine the underlying etiology. Decadron was continued in the interim, and the patient's symptoms continued to improve. Due to stabilizing neurological physical examination, neurosurgery recommended biopsy of site to officially rule out osteomyelitis/discitis. In this setting, inflammatory markers were obtained. Erythrocyte sedimentation rate (ESR) was found to be 13 mm/hr (<30 mm/hr), and C-reactive protein was found to be 2.9 mg/L (<8.0 mg/dL). With normal inflammatory markers, antibiotics were discontinued on day 2 as likelihood of osteomyelitis was low.

On day 3, interventional radiology (IR) image-guided biopsy and aspiration of the L4L5 vertebral bone was done. Final pathology report showed fragments of cartilage with calcium pyrophosphate crystal deposition supporting a diagnosis of acute CPP crystal arthritis of the lumbar spine (Figures 2(a)–2(d)). Biopsy cultures for infection were negative. Blood cultures resulted as no growth. Given these findings, rheumatology service was consulted. The patient was started on colchicine 0.6 mg daily. Steroids were stopped on day 7 as initial symptoms improved. Rheumatology service also requested X-ray imaging of bilateral hands, wrists, and knees to assess for CPPD involvement. Imaging supported degenerative joint disease but did now show any signs of CPPD disease at these joints. The patient was eventually transferred to a rehabilitation center for the deconditioning. She was instructed to follow up with rheumatology services on an outpatient basis; however, the patient missed her appointment.

3. Discussion

Spinal pseudogout is a rare entity, with few case reports described in the literature, most of which depict pseudogout of the cervical region [6]. Based on literature review, the most commonly affected section of the spine has been reported to be the cervical spine [6, 7]. A study was conducted in the Rheumatology Department of Lariboisiere Hospital in Paris which attempted to find the prevalence of spinal involvement in patients with established diagnoses of widespread CPPD. It was noted that 24% of patients who were hospitalized with CPPD had spinal involvement, mostly affecting the cervical and lumbar spine; however, they had widespread CPPD disease [6]. In this case report, the patient had no previous history of pseudogout and had no other joint involvement after thorough investigation.

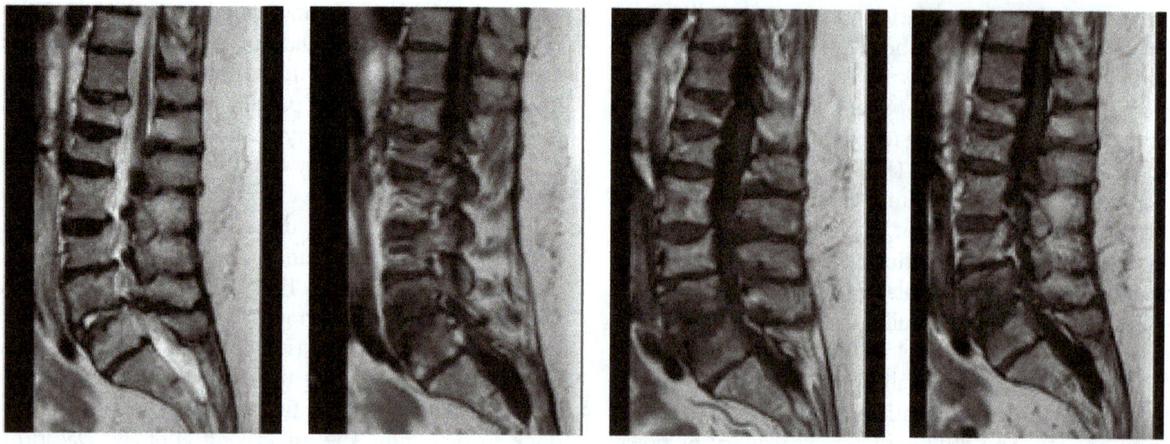

Figure 1: Axial and sagittal T1 and T2-weighted and coronal and sagittal short-TI inversion recovery (STIR) images of the lumbar spine without intravenous contrast administration. Axial and sagittal T1-weighted images were then acquired following intravenous administration of 80 mL of Gadavist. The image shows vertebral body edema and enhancement most evident at the L4L5 level. Paravertebral soft tissue thickening is seen at the L5-S1 level, with extension into the left neural foramina. Findings are suggestive of osteomyelitis/discitis.

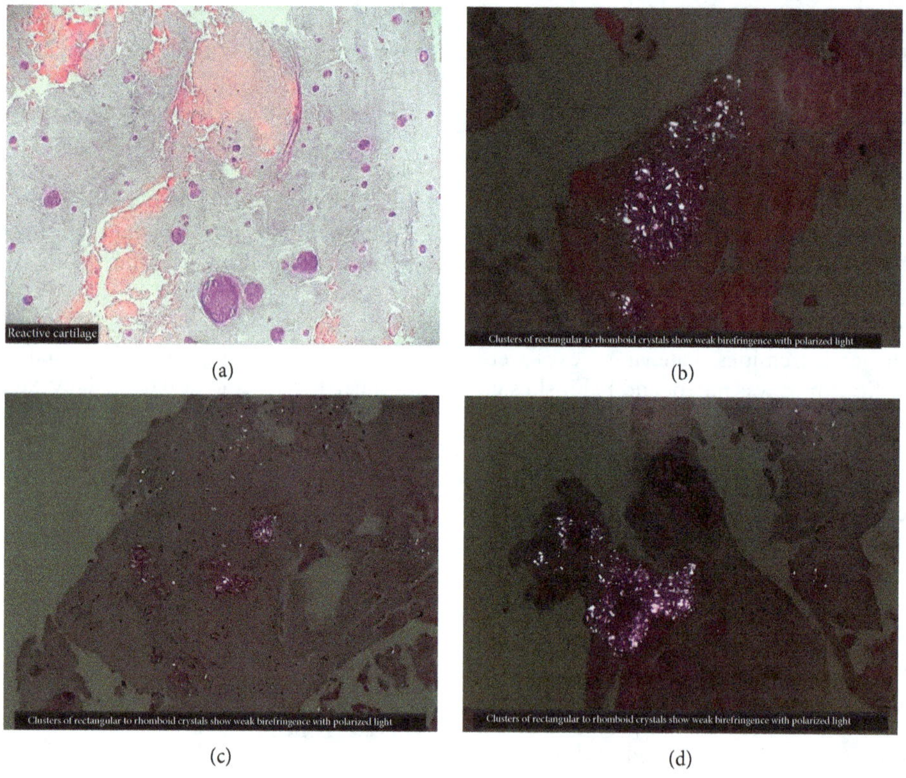

Figure 2: Fragments of cartilage with calcium pyrophosphate crystal deposition identified under microscopy. (a) H&E staining showing reactive cartilage. (b)–(d) Polarized light microscopy depicts clusters of rectangular to rhomboid crystals with weak birefringence.

The patient in this encounter obtained trauma at the site of crystal deposition prior to this hospitalization, which was rendered as the predisposition factor contributing to the formation of pseudogout. To the author's knowledge, there are no known case reports published which depict pseudogout formation of the spine after obtaining direct trauma. One case report by Bridges et al. described a 66-year-old female who underwent L2–5 laminectomies, bilateral foraminotomies, and L4–5 transforaminal lumbar interbody fusion with L4–5 posterior instrumented fusion for spinal stenosis and subsequently was found to have CPPD of the cervical and thoracic spine [8]. However, the patient had surgical intervention of the lumbar region, not involving the particular affected sites.

MRI is typically the method of choice when evaluating for pathologies of soft tissue, bone, and joints. MRI features of osteomyelitis or discitis commonly include descriptions of edema and disc degeneration of the affected site, according

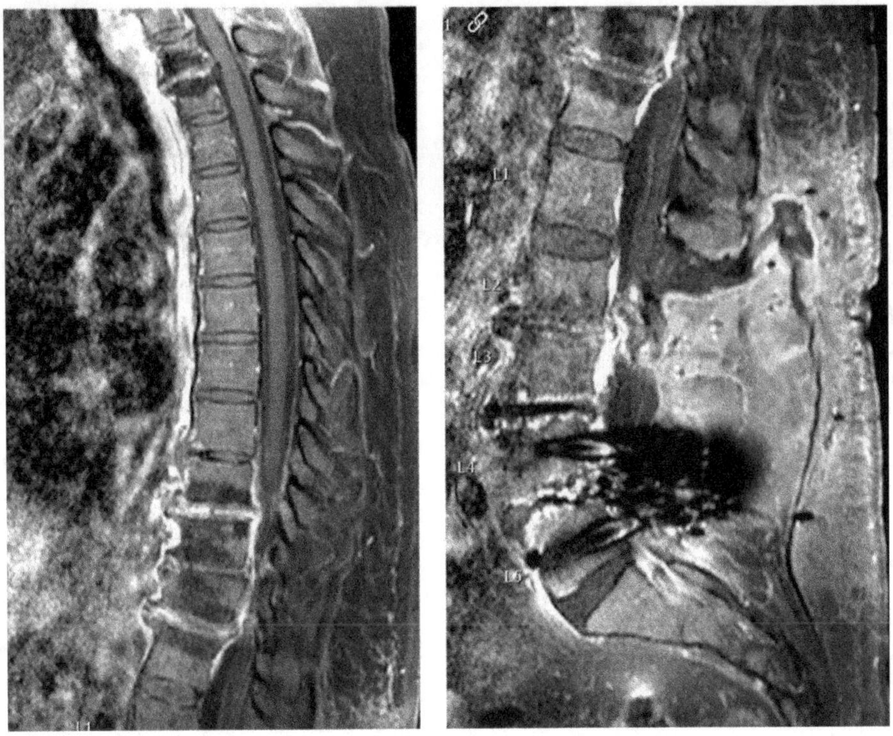

(a) (b)

FIGURE 3: Thoracic (a) and lumbar (b) spine MR images demonstrate some enhancement within the C7–T1 acet joints as well as the T1–2 and T9–12 intervertebral discs. There is also ventral epidural enhancement from T9 to T12 and some enhancement within the lumbar surgical site.

to a retrospective review of the database of spinal infections [9, 10]. An article written by Mechri et al. describes imaging features of malignant tumors of the spine [11]. According to this article, spinal tumors will be demonstrated typically as lytic lesions, well-formed tumors, or low to high signal intensity on T2-WI [11]. These findings are characteristic and are not to be confused with typical findings of pseudogout of the spine. Although there are limited data on the presentation of spinal pseudogout, a common theme of misdiagnosis of discitis or osteomyelitis has been reported due to common presenting symptoms of infection and image findings of edema, enhancement, and tissue thickening. Two case reports have been published which describe elderly patients presenting with fever, back pain, and subsequent elevated inflammatory markers [8, 12]. Moreover, the cases also describe similar findings on imaging, which further support including spinal pseudogout on the differential when such findings are recovered. In this case report, the MRI findings depicted vertebral body edema and enhancement, leading clinicians to the initial misdiagnosis of vertebral body osteomyelitis/discitis. The aim of this document along with the abovementioned articles is to establish radiological classification of pseudogout of the spine.

The case report by Bridges et al. depicts a case in which the clinical presentation and image findings were initially thought to be of infectious origin, as was the case in our patient. In this case report, the patient had surgical intervention of the spine and subsequently presented to the ED with complaints of fever, chills, and back spasms. The patient

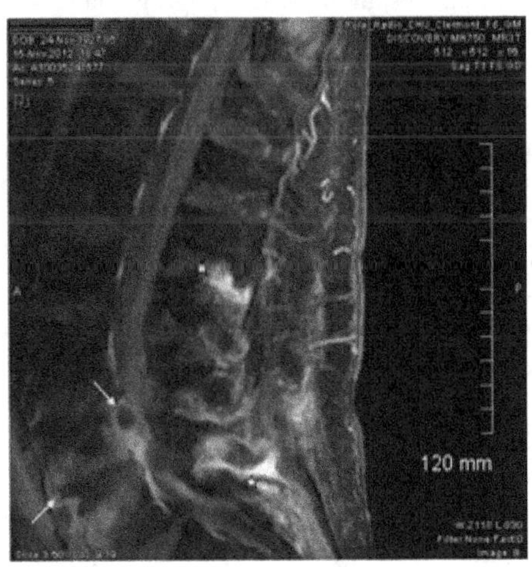

FIGURE 4: MRI of the lumbar spine (T1 fat sat + gadolinium): the gadolinium-enhanced sagittal T1-weighed MR image shows peripheral enhancement of L4-L5 disc and marrow edema extending from the L4 and L5 vertebrae with anterior epidural abscess-like spondylodiscitits (arrow). The MR image shows inflammation with enhancement of L1-L2 and L4-L5 zygapophysial joints (stars).

was found to have elevated inflammatory markers and had an MRI subsequently, which was concerning for infection.

Antibiotics were started empirically regardless of sterile biopsy results. As the patient's condition progressed on antibiotics, a full-spine MRI was done, which demonstrated "marked increase in the enhancement of the C (cervical)

7–T1 facet joints with extension into the paraspinal soft tissues and the posterior epidural space, resulting in spinal cord compression" (Figure 3). The patient underwent biopsy once again, which remained sterile; however, on further microscopic review, there was evidence of pseudogout. This patient shortly after developed widespread CPPD which further supported the diagnosis of spinal pseudogout. The patient's symptoms resolved after initiation of the interleukin-1 inhibitor [8].

Another case report documented by Grobost et al. illustrated a case of pseudogout of the lumbar spine presenting with clinical and image findings concerning for spondylodiscitis and epidural abscess with resultant lumbar percutaneous needle biopsy supporting pseudogout instead (Figure 4) [12]. The authors describe a case of an elderly male patient with recurrent back pain and history of CPPD. The patient was readmitted for back pain and obtained imaging prior to biopsy. MRI findings in this case depicted "peripheral enhancement of L4L5 disc and marrow edema extending from L4 and L5 vertebrae with anterior epidural abscess-like spondylodiscitis," as well as "inflammation with enhancement of L1L2 and L4L5 zygapophysial joints." The reading of this MRI shows similarities from the previous mentioned case by Bridges et al. as well as our case.

Both case reports demonstrated similar findings on imaging, depicting enhancement of the spinal region with extension into the paraspinal soft tissues. The MRI findings in our patient also showed enhancement at the affected spinal level with paravertebral soft tissue thickening. These depicted similarities, along with imaging analysis, can serve to establish guidelines in differentiating back pain. The manifestation of inflammatory joints in pseudogout originated from the deposition of calcium pyrophosphate dihydrate crystals in soft tissue. The approach to take in such scenarios, as depicted in the above cases, would be to try first-in-line treatments with anti-inflammatory agents, such as NSAIDs, Colchicine, and/or steroids. Although rare, it is crucial to suspect spinal pseudogout as its clinical manifestations can be debilitating, often leading to spinal cord compression, acute nerve compression, and spinal stenosis, amongst many other syndromes [13, 14]. Suspecting pseudogout in elderly patients with similar clinical presentation, and image findings can enable the medical community to initiate treatment promptly and avoid predisposing patients to unnecessary invasive procedures and exposure to antibiotics.

References

[1] R. A. Deyo and Y.-J. Tsui-Wu, "Descriptive epidemiology of low-back pain and its related medical care in the United States," *Spine*, vol. 12, no. 3, pp. 264–268, 1987.

[2] R. Chou, A. Qaseem, V. Snow et al., "Diagnosis and treatment of low back pain: a joint clinical practice guideline from the American College of Physicians and the American Pain Society," *Annals of Internal Medicine*, vol. 147, no. 7, p. 478, 2007.

[3] R. A. Deyo, J. Rainville, and Kent, "What can the history and physical examination tell us about low back pain?" *JAMA: The Journal of the American Medical Association*, vol. 268, no. 6, pp. 760–765, 1992.

[4] W. Zhang, M. Doherty, T. Bardin et al., "European League Against Rheumatism recommendations for calcium pyrophosphate deposition. Part I: terminology and diagnosis," *Annals of the Rheumatic Diseases*, vol. 70, no. 4, pp. 563–570, 2011.

[5] A. C. Jones, A. J. Chuck, E. A. Arie, D. J. Green, and M. Doherty, "Diseases associated with calcium pyrophosphate deposition disease," *Seminars in Arthritis and Rheumatism*, vol. 22, no. 3, pp. 188–202, 1992.

[6] A. Moshrif, J. D. Laredo, H. Bassiouni et al., "Spinal involvement with calcium pyrophosphate deposition disease in an academic rheumatology center: a series of 37 patients," *Seminars in Arthritis and Rheumatism*, vol. 48, no. 6, pp. 1113–1126, 2018.

[7] M. Salcman, A. Khan, and D. A. Symonds, "Calcium pyrophosphate arthropathy of the spine," *Neurosurgery*, vol. 34, no. 5, pp. 915–918, 1994.

[8] K. J. Bridges, C. L. Bullis, A. Wanchu, and K. D. Than, "Pseudogout of the cervical and thoracic spine mimicking infection after lumbar fusion: case report," *Journal of Neurosurgery: Spine*, vol. 27, no. 2, pp. 145–149, 2017.

[9] J. T. Bencardino and A. Hassankhani, "Calcium pyrophosphate dihydrate crystal deposition disease," *Seminars in Musculoskeletal Radiology*, vol. 7, no. 3, pp. 175–185, 2003.

[10] J. A. Dunbar, J. A. Sandoe, A. S. Rao, D. W. Crimmins, W. Baig, and J. J. Rankine, "The MRI appearance of early vertebral osteomyelitis and discitis," *Clinical Radiology*, vol. 65, no. 12, pp. 974–981, 2010.

[11] M. Mechri, H. Riahi, I. Sboui, M. Bouaziz, F. Vanhoenacker, and M. Ladeb, "Imaging of malignant primitive tumors of the spine," *Journal of the Belgian Society of Radiology*, vol. 102, no. 1, p. 56, 2018.

[12] V. Grobost, M. Vayssade, A. Roche, J. L. Kemeny, and M. Soubrier, "Axial calcium pyrophosphate dihydrate deposition disease revealed by recurrent sterile spondylodiscitis and epidural abscess," *Joint Bone Spine*, vol. 81, no. 2, pp. 180–182, 2014.

[13] N. Muthukumar and U. Karuppaswamy, "Tumoral calcium pyrophosphate dihydrate deposition disease of the ligamentum flavum," *Neurosurgery*, vol. 53, no. 1, pp. 103–109, 2003.

[14] P. Cabre, H. Pascal-Moussellard, S. Kaidomar et al., "Six cases of cervical ligamentum flavum calcification in Blacks in the French West Indies," *Joint Bone Spine*, vol. 68, no. 2, pp. 158–165, 2001.

19

Colchicine plus Dapsone in Colchicine-Resistant FMF Patients

Farhad Salehzadeh,[1] **A. Enteshary**,[2] **and M. Moshkbar**[3]

[1]*Professor in Pediatric Rheumatology, Pediatric Department, Bouali Children's Hospital, Ardabil University of Medical Sciences (ARUMS), Ardabil, Iran*
[2]*Assistant Professor of Rheumatology, Internal Medicine Department, Imam Khomeini Hospital, Ardabil University of Medical Sciences (ARUMS), Ardabil, Iran*
[3]*Pediatric Department, Bouali Children's Hospital, Ardabil University of Medical Sciences (ARUMS), Ardabil, Iran*

Correspondence should be addressed to A. Enteshary; afsanehenteshary@gmail.com

Academic Editor: Rustam Aminov

Five to ten percent of FMF patients have unfavorable response to the colchicine as a standard therapy. Biologic treatments have been shown to be highly effective, but there are often unavailable, because the price is unaffordably high. This study shows the striking effect of combined dapsone and colchicine therapy in such patients and recommends it as an alternative therapy in colchicine-resistant (CR) patients.

1. Introduction

Familial Mediterranean fever (FMF) is an auto-inflammatory monogenic disease that presents with recurrent painful attacks of fever, peritonitis, pleuritis and arthritis. In most patients, daily administration of colchicine can prevent a typical attack [1]. However, about five to ten percent of patients are completely resistant to colchicine or they have intolerable side effects due to this drug [2].

The therapeutic options for patients with colchicine-resistant FMF (CR-FMF) patients are biologic drugs; although recent studies have shown their efficacy and positive results, availability and the cost of this modality are the main limiting factors [3, 4].

A previous study about dapsone in children with CR-FMF suggests favorable results [5]; consequently, this study has been planned to evaluate dapsone plus colchicine as a combination therapy in adult and adolescent CR-FMF patients.

2. Case Reports

We tried this combination therapy in 6 patients; all of them have been checked for the G6PD enzyme before treatment and filled consent confirmation. The study has been confirmed by the local ethical committee of faculty of medicine.

Case 1 is a 26-year-old female with negative history of FMF in her family. The first presentation of this disease started at the age of 14 including: abdominal pain, fever, nausea, arthralgia in knee joints, and erythematous swelling of the limbs (erysipelas-like eruption). She usually had an attack every 2 weeks that would last for 1-2 days with a severity score of 10. Her *MEFV* gene mutation was: E148Q (heterozygous).

She started using colchicine 1 mg daily about 12 years ago but the results were not desirable enough, and she increased the dose to 2.5 mg daily, and then, the number of attacks was reduced to one attack every 20–30 days that would last 1 day with a severity of 5-6. We added dapsone 100 mg daily about 3.5 years ago, and since then, she did not have any similar attacks, except by discontinuation of the drug because of its unavailability in a short course period, her attacks recurred.

There have been no known side effects of colchicine or dapsone in this case.

Case 2 is a 40-year-old female with no history of FMF in her family. The onset of disease was from age 20 with abdominal pain, chills and fever, diarrhea, sweating, and

Table 1: Details of patients' data.

Patient no.	Age (years)	Sex	Duration (years)	Before colchicine	After colchicine		After dapsone plus colchicine	
				Attack interval	Dosage of colchicine	Attack interval	Number of attacks	Attack interval
1	26	F	12	14 days	2.5 mg daily	20–30 days	0	—
2	40	F	20	14 days	3 mg daily	2-3 months	0	—
3	38	M	24	1-2 weeks	1-2 mg daily	1 month	0	—
4	32	M	9	10 days	2 mg daily	30 days	0	—
5	12	F	9	3-4 days	1-2 mg daily	2 weeks	0	—
6	17	F	15	15–20 days	2.5 mg daily	1-2 months	1	5 months

arthralgia such as knee pain. She had an attack every 2 weeks that would last for 3-4 days with a high severity score near 10.

She started using colchicine 1 mg three times daily about 10 years ago, and then after the number of attacks was decreased to one episode every 2-3 months lasting for 1 day with a severity score of 7-8. Her MEFV gene mutations were M680I (G/C)/V726A (compound heterozygous).

From 9 months ago, we started using dapsone 50 mg daily, and since then, she was free of similar symptoms.

She suffers from occasional dizziness as known side effect of this drug.

Case 3 is a 38-year-old male with positive family history of FMF. He presented his first signs at the age of 14 but with delayed diagnosis until he was 30 years old. His symptoms were fever, arthralgia, body pain, and oral ulcer. The frequency of his attacks was variable, and each attack lasted for 3-4 days with a high severity score.

He started using colchicine 1 mg daily 8 years ago, and then after he suffered similar attacks with no response to colchicine although with high doses (2 mg). His *MEFV* gene mutations were C.1981G > T (D661Y), we submitted this as a new mutation in infevers.

From 9 months ago, we started dapsone 50 mg daily. Dapsone significantly controlled the attacks during this time. There have been no known side effects of this treatment in this case.

Case 4 is a 32-year-old male with negative family history of FMF. His first presentation was at the age of 23 years old with abdominal pain, vomiting, fever, chills, and limbs pain.

He was diagnosed with FMF at the age of 25, and his MEFV gene mutations were M680I (G/C) M680I (G/C) (homozygous). His attack intervals were almost 10 days, and it lasts for 3-4 days with a high severity score.

He started using colchicine 1 mg twice daily from 7 years ago, and since then, the number of attacks was decreased to one attack every month with similar pattern.

Seven months ago we added dapsone 50 mg daily, and since then, he was completely free of symptoms. There have been no known side effects of this therapy.

Case 5 is a 12-year-old female with negative family history. Her first signs presented at 3 years of age with: fever, abdominal pain, vomiting, chills, and sweating. She usually had an attack biweekly, lasting for 3-4 days with a high severity score. Her *MEFV* gene mutations were M694V/M680I (heterozygous).

She started using colchicine 1-2 mg daily from 6 years ago with unfavorable response. From 7 months ago, we added dapsone 50 mg daily, and since then, she has not have any attacks.

Case 6 is a 17-year-old female with negative family history. Her first sign was presented at one year of age with: fever and chills, nausea, and body pain with a high score. Her *MEFV* gene mutations were M694V (homozygous).

She started taking colchicine 0.25 mg daily 16 years ago then increased the dose to 2.5 mg daily; however, attacks persists to one episode every 1-2 months with similar severity.

From 7 months ago, we added dapsone 100 mg daily. Dapsone has reduced the frequency and severity of attacks (one attack in 5 months with a very low severity score). There have been no known side effects of this treatment in this case.

Table 1 shows these patients' data and summarized their findings.

3. Discussion

The exact mechanism of colchicine in controlling FMF attacks is not completely clear yet. Colchicine inhibits microtubule assembly in vitro conditions [6]. Microtubules are filamentous structures that help the maintenance of the structure of cells and are involved in cell movement for functions such as cytokine secretion, cell and nuclear divisions, and regulation of ion channels [7].

It is believed that the anti-inflammatory effect of colchicine in FMF is a result of microtubule disruption in neutrophils, which prevents their migration in response to chemotactic factors [8].

A new insight into colchicine efficacy is its effect in FMF through activation of the GTPase RhoA and subsequent phosphorylation of the 14-3-3 protein and inhibition of pyrin-induced inflammasome formation; Park et al. have found that colchicine resistance may also result when certain mutations in pyrin prevent binding to the 14-3-3 protein [9].

In review of the literature, there are some reports about alternative drugs especially biologics in CR-FMF patients. Intravenous colchicine 1 mg weekly in addition to the regular oral regime in patients suffering disabling attacks despite receiving maximal tolerated dose of oral colchicine may be beneficial [10].

In 2006, a young man with FMF and systemic amyloidosis who was not eligible for colchicine treatment because of gastrointestinal toxicity and ongoing dialysis was successfully treated with anakinra [11], and there is a report about a child who had frequent severe FMF attacks despite colchicine therapy was treated with this drug [12]. A small randomized placebo-controlled trial showed that Rilonacept, an IL-1 inhibitor, significantly reduced the frequency of FMF attacks [13].

Canakinumab, a high-affinity human anti-IL1b monoclonal antibody [14], was used for treating two children with colchicine-resistant FMF [15]. Recently, the efficacy of biologic drugs has been shown it has been shown an effective biologic drug in different auto-inflammatory diseases.

Two months of canakinumab therapy in another case, a 14-year-old female patient nonresponsive to colchicine and anakinra, resulted in remission of FMF attacks and improvement in inflammatory markers [17]. Several case reports have showed that TNF inhibitors such as etanercept and infliximab can be effective in controlling and improvement of FMF attacks [18–20].

The anti-inflammatory effect of dapsone is believed to be related to stabilization of neutrophil lysosomes [21]. Different studies showed that dapsone may impair neutrophil chemotaxis [22]. Dapsone could suppress integrin-mediated neutrophil adherence function. It also inhibits chemo attractant-induced signal transduction and thus suppresses neutrophil recruitment and local production of toxic products in the affected skin of neutrophilic dermatoses [23]. It can also suppress human neutrophil superoxide production and elastase release [24].

Therefore, it can be concluded that neutrophils and neutrophil products are the main targets of dapsone. patients' complete clinical response, lack of attacks by using a combination of two anti-inflammatory drugs was significant.

It seems that the synergetic effect of colchicine and dapsone in disturbing the neutrophils function as a combination therapy in controlling of FMF attacks in CR-FMF patients' emphasis this positive clinical response.

4. Conclusion and Recommendations

The combination of colchicine plus dapsone appears remarkably effective in controlling the attacks in CR-FMF patients, and our suggestion of a prospective controlled trial of this promising drug is warranted.

References

[1] M. Tunca, S. Akar, F Onen et al., "Familial Mediterranean fever (FMF) in Turkey: results of a nationwide multicenter study," *Medicine (Baltimore)*, vol. 84, no. 1, pp. 1–11, 2005.

[2] M. Lidar and A. Livneh, "Familial Mediterranean fever: clinical, molecular and management advancements," *Netherlands Journal of Medicine*, vol. 65, no. 9, pp. 318–324, 2007.

[3] P. Portincasa, "Colchicine, biologic agents and more for the treatment of familial Mediterranean fever. The old, the new, and the rare," *Current Medicinal Chemistry*, vol. 23, no. 1, pp. 60–86, 2016.

[4] T. Koga, K. Migita, and A. Kawakami, "Biologic therapy in familial Mediterranean fever," *Modern Rheumatology*, vol. 26, no. 5, pp. 637–641, 2016.

[5] F. Salehzadeh, S. Jahangiri, and E. Mohammadi, "Dapsone as an alternative therapy in children with familial Mediterranean fever," *Iranian Journal of Pediatrics*, vol. 22, no. 1, pp. 23–27, 2012.

[6] J. M. Andreu and S. N. Timasheff, "Interaction of tubulin with single ring analogs of colchicine," *Biochemistry*, vol. 21, no. 3, pp. 534–543, 2002.

[7] J. P. Caviston and E. L. F. Holzbaur, "Microtubule motors at the intersection of trafficking and transport," *Trends in Cell Biology*, vol. 16, no. 10, pp. 530–537, 2006.

[8] E. Ben-Chetrit, S. Bergmann, and R. Sood, "Mechanism of the anti-inflammatory effect of colchicine in rheumatic diseases: a possible new outlook through microarray analysis," *Rheumatology*, vol. 45, no. 3, pp. 274–282, 2005.

[9] Y. H. Park, G. Wood, D. L. Kastner, and J. J. Chae, "Pyrin inflammasome activation and RhoA signaling in the autoinflammatory diseases FMF and HIDS," *Nature Immunology*, vol. 17, no. 8, pp. 914–921, 2016.

[10] M. Lidar, R. Kedem, P. Langevitz, M. Pras, and A. Livneh, "Intravenous colchicine for treatment of patients with familial Mediterranean fever unresponsive to oral colchicine," *Journal of Rheumatology*, vol. 30, no. 12, pp. 2620–2623, 2003.

[11] J. J. Chae, G. Wood, S. L. Masters et al., "The B30.2 domain of pyrin, the familial Mediterranean fever protein, interacts directly with caspase-1 to modulate IL-1beta production," *Proceedings of the National Academy of Sciences*, vol. 103, no. 26, pp. 9982–9987, 2006.

[12] L. M. Kuijk, A. M. A. P. Govers, W. J. D. Hofhuis, and J. Frenkel, "Effective treatment of a colchicine-resistant familial Mediterranean fever patient with anakinra," *Annals of the Rheumatic Diseases*, vol. 66, no. 11, pp. 1545-1546, 2007.

[13] P. J. Hashkes, S. J. Spalding, E. H. Giannini et al., "Rilonacept for colchicine resistant or -intolerant familial Mediterranean fever," *Annals of Internal Medicine*, vol. 157, no. 8, pp. 533–541, 2012.

[14] R. Alten, H. Gram, L. A. Joosten et al., "The human anti-IL-1β monoclonal antibody ACZ885 is effective in joint inflammation models in mice and in a proof-of-concept study in patients with rheumatoid arthritis," *Arthritis Research & Therapy*, vol. 10, no. 3, p. R67, 2008.

[15] I. Mitroulis, P. Skendros, A. Oikonomou, A. G. Tzioufas, and K. Ritis, "The efficacy of canakinumab in the treatment of a patient with familial Mediterranean fever and longstanding destructive arthritis," *Annals of the Rheumatic Diseases*, vol. 70, no. 7, pp. 1347-1348, 2011.

[16] F. De Benedetti, M. Gattorno, J. Anton et al., "Canakinumab for the treatment of autoinflammatory recurrent fever syndromes," *New England Journal of Medicine*, vol. 378, no. 20, pp. 1908–1919, 2018.

[17] D. O. Hacihamdioglu and S. Ozen, "Canakinumab induces remission in a patient with resistant familial Mediterranean fever," *Rheumatology*, vol. 51, no. 6, p. 1041, 2012.

[18] A. Mor, M. H. Pillinger, M. Kishimoto, A. M. Abeles, and A. Livneh, "Familial Mediterranean fever successfully treated with etanercept," *JCR: Journal of Clinical Rheumatology*, vol. 13, no. 1, pp. 38–40, 2007.

[19] S. Ozgocmen, L. Özçakar, O. Ardicoglu, E. Kocakoc, A. Kaya, and A. Kiris, "Familial Mediterranean fever responds well to infliximab: single case experience," *Clinical Rheumatology*, vol. 25, no. 1, pp. 83–87, 2005.

[20] O. Sakallioglu, A. Duzova, and S. Ozen, "Etanercept in the treatment of arthritis in a patient with familial Mediterranean fever," *Clinical and Experimental Rheumatology*, vol. 24, no. 4, pp. 435–437, 2006.

[21] K. Williams, R. B. Capstick, D. A. Lewis, and R. Best, "Anti-

inflammatory actions of dapsone and its related biochemistry," *Journal of Pharmacy and Pharmacology*, vol. 28, no. 7, pp. 555–558, 2011.

[22] S. A. Booth, C. E. Moody, M. V. Dahl, M. J. Herron, and R. D. Nelson, "Dapsone suppresses integrin-mediated neutrophil adherence function," *Journal of Investigative Dermatology*, vol. 98, no. 2, pp. 135–140, 1992.

[23] S. M. Debol, M. J. Herron, and R. D. Nelson, "Anti-inflammatory action of dapsone: inhibition of neutrophil adherence is associated with inhibition of chemoattractant-induced signal transduction," *Journal of Leukocyte Biology*, vol. 62, no. 6, pp. 827–836, 1997.

[24] T. Suda, Y. Suzuki, T. Matsui et al., "Dapsone suppresses human neutrophil superoxide production and elastase release in a calcium-dependent manner," *British Journal of Dermatology*, vol. 152, no. 5, pp. 887–895, 2005.

20

Genital Ulcer of Behçet Disease Localized in the Vagina may Lack Pain, Making it Difficult to Assess

Soichiro Obata[1], **Koji Kobayashi**[2], **Misaki Toda**[1], **Etsuko Miyagi**[3] **and Shigeru Aoki**[1]

[1]*Perinatal Center for Maternity and Neonates, Yokohama City University Medical Center, Yokohama, Japan*
[2]*Center for Rheumatic Disease, Yokohama City University Medical Center, Yokohama, Japan*
[3]*Department of Obstetrics and Gynecology, Yokohama City University Hospital, Yokohama, Japan*

Correspondence should be addressed to Soichiro Obata; soobata@yokohama-cu.ac.jp

Academic Editor: Suleyman Serdar Koca

Genital ulcer is one of the main clinical symptoms of Behçet disease; ulcers mostly occur in the vulva and are usually quite painful. We present an unusual case of Behçet disease wherein a painless genital ulcer was localized in the vagina. Our case is of a 43-year-old woman diagnosed with Behçet disease that was controlled with prednisolone. She became pregnant and developed fever, oral ulcers, and arthralgia at 16 weeks of gestation. Although a relapse of Behçet disease was suspected, ulceration and pain of the vulva were not observed. At 18 and 28 weeks of gestation, a vaginal ulcer was observed during regular prenatal examination, but the patient had no pain or other symptoms in the vulva. The vaginal ulcer healed at 29 weeks of gestation. No recurrence of the vaginal ulcer and other symptoms of Behçet disease were seen on subsequent follow-up examination at 1 month after delivery. Although genital ulcers of Behçet disease are common in the vulva and are generally painful, if they are located in the vagina, they can be painless. If Behçet disease is suspected based on other symptoms, a vaginal examination should be conducted as necessary for accurate evaluation of Behçet disease.

1. Introduction

Behçet disease presents with systemic symptoms triggered by vasculitis [1–3]. Genital ulcer is one of the main clinical symptoms; ulcers mostly occur in the vulva and are usually quite painful [1–3]. We present an unusual case of Behçet disease wherein a painless genital ulcer was localized in the vagina.

2. Case Presentation

Our case is that of a 43-year-old primiparous woman. She was diagnosed with Behçet disease at the age of 34 years; she presented with recurrent oral ulceration, recurrent genital ulceration, and pseudofolliculitis with characteristic acneiform nodules. She had no eye lesions. Her condition was well controlled with prednisolone (PSL) 8 mg/day oral dose. She fell pregnant spontaneously and visited our perinatal center for her prenatal care. As she was detected with hypertension at her first visit, we recommended that she check her blood pressure regularly at home. She developed fever, oral ulcers, and arthralgia at 16 weeks of gestation, due to which a relapse of Behçet disease was suspected. Because her condition was controlled well with PSL, the daily oral dose of PSL was increased from 8 mg to 10 mg. At this time, ulceration and pain of the vulva were not observed. She visited our outpatient clinic for a regular prenatal examination at 18 weeks and 4 days of gestation, which was when an ulcer localized in the vagina was incidentally observed (Figure 1). The ulcer was painless and the patient had no symptoms in the vulva either (Figure 2). Chlamydial and gonococcal infection were not detected, and cytology of the vaginal wall showed no findings suggesting malignancy. As the other symptoms of Behçet disease were resolved after the dose of PSL had been increased, the same dose was maintained. At the next prenatal care visit, at 22 weeks and 4 days of gestation, the vaginal ulcer had disappeared and other symptoms of Behçet disease were not seen. At 28 weeks and

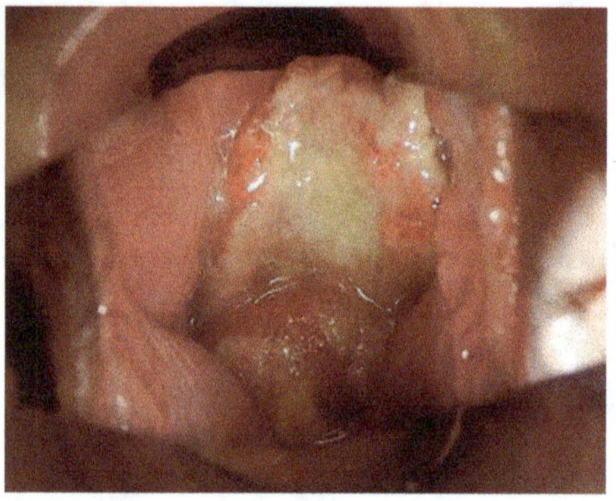

FIGURE 1: Genital ulcer localized in the vagina at 18 weeks of gestation.

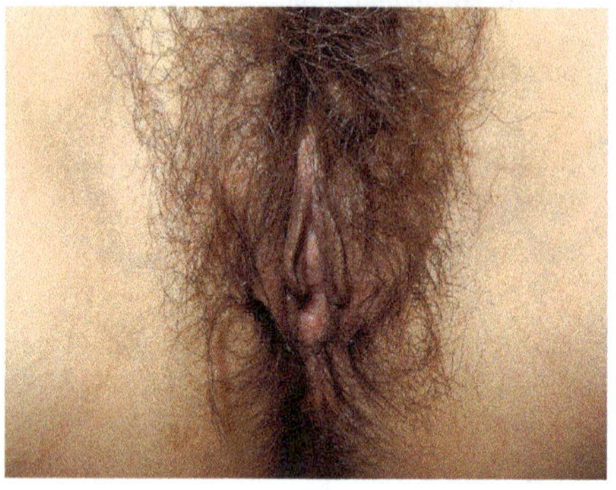

FIGURE 2: There were no symptoms in the vulva at 18 weeks of gestation.

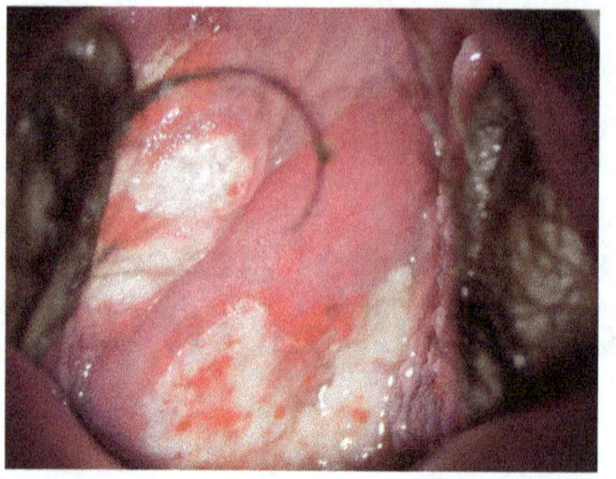

FIGURE 3: Relapse of vaginal ulcer at 28 weeks of gestation.

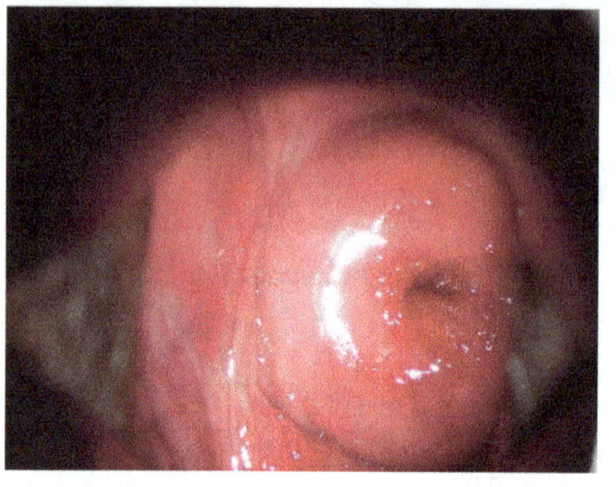

FIGURE 4: Vaginal ulcer was healed in the postpartum period.

0 days of gestation, atypical genital bleeding and vaginal ulcer recurrence were observed (Figure 3). At the same time, recurrence of the oral ulcer and arthralgia as well as a mild increase in the fever were observed; based on these symptoms, she was diagnosed with a relapse of Behçet disease and the daily dose of PSL was increased from 10 mg to 15 mg. The vaginal ulcer disappeared at 29 weeks and 2 days of gestation (Figure 4). Thereafter, there was no relapse of the symptoms of Behçet disease.

At 33 weeks and 0 days of gestation, her blood pressure had increased, due to which she was admitted to the hospital. She was diagnosed with severe preeclampsia superimposed. Induction of labor was conducted but it was not effective, and we performed cesarean section at 37 weeks and 6 days of gestation. She delivered a male infant weighing 2002 g. There were no complications in the postoperative course, and she was discharged with her baby at 7 days after cesarean section. No recurrence of the vaginal ulcer and other symptoms of Behçet disease were seen on subsequent follow-up examination at 1 month after delivery.

The patient was explained about the possibility of publishing this case as a case report and the accompanying images. She provided consent.

3. Discussion

In Behçet disease, genital ulcers are a common symptom. However, they primarily occur in the vulva and are often painful [1–3]. However, in rare cases, ulcers can be localized in the vagina; in such cases, the ulcers may be painless. Intravaginal examination is usually not performed during regular medical check-ups; in cases with painless vaginal ulcer, there is a possibility of missing the ulcer, resulting in insufficient evaluation of Behçet disease.

In this case, although there were no vulval symptoms, she was diagnosed with a relapse of Behçet disease based on the presence of oral ulcers, arthralgia, and mild increase in fever. In our patient, the painless vaginal ulcer was incidentally noticed during a regular prenatal examination. Senusi et al. examined 137 cases of Behçet disease with primary genital lesions and reported that only 9% patients had ulcers in the vagina; the remaining ulcers were located in the labia or vulva [4]. When a vaginal ulcer is detected, it is necessary to rule out infectious diseases, malignant tumors, and Crohn's disease [5–7]. As the case patient was pregnant, HIV, syphilis, chlamydia, and gonococcal infections had been ruled out due to the regular prenatal examinations. Moreover, cytology of the ulcer yielded no findings indicating malignancy. The patient had no gastrointestinal symptoms that would suggest Crohn's disease. The vaginal ulcer was healed after the PSL dose was increased for relieving the other symptoms of Behçet disease, mainly the intraoral ulcers and arthralgia. Therefore, we diagnosed the vaginal ulcer as one of the symptoms of relapse of Behçet disease.

When ulcers occur in the vulva, such as in Behçet disease or vulvar herpes, it generally causes severe pain [8]. However, most vaginal lesions are painless because there is no nerve ending in the upper part of the vaginal wall. For example, in cases of vaginal wall erosion occurring after pessary use for uterine prolapse, patients report no pain [9]. Similarly, in cases of lacerations limited to the superficial vaginal wall after normal delivery, very few complaints of pain are noted. Moreover, unless there is sexual intercourse, pain may not manifest due to the absence of physical contact. Our patient had not had sexual intercourse as she was pregnant; therefore, pain and bleeding were not observed.

If the genital ulcer is localized in the vagina, the clinical symptoms may be poor and there is a possibility that the evaluation of Behçet disease will be insufficient. Although the other symptoms of Behçet disease were observed in our case, it was initially judged that there was no genital ulcer because there was no ulcer or pain in the vulva. The ulcer was an incidental finding during a regular prenatal examination. In general medical examination, if there is no pain or other symptoms, detailed genital examination is usually not performed, possibly causing insufficient assessment of Behçet disease. In recent years, there is a recommendation for checking the symptoms of intestinal Behçet disease for sufficient evaluation [10]. In a similar vein, accurate genital assessment is also needed. If there is a vaginal ulcer, it is often accompanied by vaginal bleeding. Thus, if relapse of Behçet disease is suspected based on other symptoms, the presence or absence of vaginal bleeding should be confirmed. Especially, in a patient with vaginal bleeding without a vulval ulcer, a vaginal examination should be conducted by a gynecologist for a more accurate evaluation of Behçet disease. Vaginal examination is also needed for ruling out other diseases, such as cervical or endometrial cancer.

To conclude, although genital ulcers of Behçet disease are common in the vulva and are generally painful, if they are located in the vagina, they can be painless. If Behçet disease is suspected based on other symptoms, a vaginal examination should be conducted as it is necessary for an accurate evaluation of Behçet disease, especially in patients with vaginal bleeding without vulval ulcers.

References

[1] International Study Group for Behçet's Disease, "Criteria for diagnosis of Behçet's disease," *Lancet*, vol. 335, no. 8697, pp. 1078–1080, 1990.

[2] I. Bulur and M. Onder, "Behçet disease: new aspects," *Clinics in Dermatology*, vol. 35, no. 5, pp. 421–434, 2017.

[3] J. R. Nair and R. J. Moots, "Behçet's disease," *Clinical Medicine: Journal of the Royal College of Physicians of London*, vol. 17, no. 1, pp. 71–77, 2017.

[4] A. Senusi, N. Seoudi, L. A. Bergmeier et al., "Genital ulcer severity score and genital health quality of life in Behçet's disease," *Orphanet Journal of Rare Diseases*, vol. 10, no. 1, p. 117, 2015.

[5] N. M. Zetola and C. D. Pilcher, "Diagnosis and management of acute HIV infection," *Infectious Disease Clinics of North America*, vol. 21, no. 1, pp. 19–48, 2007.

[6] V. N. Sehgal, D. Pandhi, and A. Khurana, "Nonspecific genital ulcers," *Clinics in Dermatology*, vol. 32, no. 2, pp. 259–274, 2014.

[7] S. M. Bruisten, "Genital ulcers in women," *Current Women's Health Reports*, vol. 3, no. 4, pp. 288–298, 2003.

[8] S. M. Garland and M. Steben, "Genital herpes," *Best Practice & Research Clinical Obstetrics & Gynaecology*, vol. 28, no. 7, pp. 1098–1110, 2014.

[9] T. Manchana, "Ring pessary for all pelvic organ prolapse," *Archives of Gynecology and Obstetrics*, vol. 284, no. 2, pp. 391–395, 2011.

[10] J. H. Cheon and W. H. Kim, "An update on the diagnosis, treatment, and prognosis of intestinal Behçet's disease," *Current Opinion in Rheumatology*, vol. 27, no. 1, pp. 24–31, 2015.

21

Tophaceous Gout in the Pancreas: Case Reports and Review of the Literature

Soo Choi,[1] Natalie Voskanian,[1] Jeffrey Ramos,[2] and Katherine H.Y. Nguyen[1]

[1]*University of California, San Diego, CA, USA*
[2]*Scripps Memorial Hospital, San Diego, CA, USA*

Correspondence should be addressed to Katherine H.Y. Nguyen; khn022@health.ucsd.edu

Academic Editor: Mario Salazar-Paramo

We report 3 patients who presented with abnormal pancreatic contents that were initially nondiagnostic but were eventually found to have urate crystal deposition consistent with pancreatic tophaceous gout. Our first case involved an ICU patient who had fever of unknown origin and refractory pancreatic pseudocyst. The other 2 patients presented with abdominal pain associated with a pancreatic mass which mimicked malignancy. After further investigation, we were able to identify pancreatic tophaceous gout as the diagnosis. Initiation of therapy led to resolution of pancreatitis in the first patient and resolution of abdominal pain and decrease in size of a pancreatic mass in the other 2 patients. The recognition of clinical gout involving the pancreas has important implications in the evaluation and care of these patients who are at high risk for tophaceous gout. In addition, the importance of specimen preparation that preserves crystals for viewing is discussed.

1. Introduction/Background

Gout is an inflammatory process initiated by macrophage ingestion of monosodium urate crystals that are needle-shaped and negatively birefringent under polarized microscopy. Tophaceous gout typically favors peripheral sites such as fingers, hands, knees, feet, toes, forearms, olecranon bursa, ears, or Achilles' tendons. Rare cases have been reported in the colon, pelvic muscles, kidneys, and spine [1–5]. However, there are very few case reports in the literature documenting tophaceous gout in the pancreas to our knowledge.

1.1. Case #1. A 71-year-old man with hypertension, hyperlipidemia, myocardial infarction, and distant history of gout not on treatment was brought to the hospital for slurred speech and confusion preceded by three weeks of nausea, vomiting, decreased food intake, and progressive malaise and four days of abdominal pain following escalated consumption of a bottle of vodka daily. Medications on admission were HCTZ, lisinopril, and lovastatin.

Laboratory studies revealed a significantly elevated lipase level of 6797 U/L and amylase level of 550 U/L. Other notable labs included the following: WBC 14.7 thousands/μL, 80 segs and 5 bands, alkaline phosphatase 52 U/L, AST 169 U/L, ALT 71 U/L, MCV 106 fl, BUN 16 mg/dL, creatinine 12.5 mg/dL, glucose 833 mg/dL, hemoglobin A1c 5.5, creatine kinase 1986 U/L, and troponin I 0.24 ng/ml. ABG showed oxygen saturation of 89% on FiO_2 of 60%. Blood cultures were negative throughout his hospitalization. Chest X-ray showed atelectasis and left greater than right consolidation, consistent with pneumonia. Admission CT of the abdomen and pelvis showed diffuse enlargement and edema of the pancreas and inflammatory changes of peripancreatic fat. No fluid collections, gallstones, or ductal dilatation were noted. Of interest, his lipase fell precipitously to 921 on day 2 and normalized on day 4 of hospitalization without ever being elevated again during his stay.

Despite successful treatment and resolution of his pneumonia, pleural effusions, and *C. difficile* colitis, the patient developed new onset of leukocytosis and fever up to 102 Fahrenheit. Repeat abdominal CT showed hypoperfusion of the pancreas and new development of a large fluid collection along the upper pancreatic body and tail consistent with a pseudocyst measuring 15 × 9 cm. On hospital day 22, the patient was taken to the OR for exploration and was found to have a "fully necrotic gland" and peripancreatic fluid collection. The pancreas was surgically debrided and drained, and three surgical drains were placed. Culture of the fluid contents grew out *Pseudomonas*. Another course of antibiotics was completed. The patient's surgical wound site underwent dehiscence and evisceration so he was taken back to the OR on hospital day 30 and again on day 37 for further debridement. The output from his abdominal drains was consistently greater than 100 mL daily.

On hospital day 29, the patient developed pain, swelling, and erythema of his right olecranon bursa. Bursal fluid WBC was 16,875/μL with 98% neutrophils. Gram stain and culture were negative. Rheumatology was consulted on hospital day 56 for recurrent pain and swelling in the right 2nd and 3rd metacarpal joints and olecranon bursa. The serum uric acid level was 2.5 mg/dL. Aspiration of bursa fluid revealed chalky material positive for negatively birefringent crystals. Careful review of the surgically obtained pancreatic tissue and drain fluid confirmed the presence of birefringent monosodium crystals consistent with pancreatic tophaceous gout.

The patient's fever of 101.2 F resolved six hours after he received 20 mg Kenalog injection into the olecranon bursa. Two days later, he was placed on IV solu-medrol 40 mg, and within a day, his abdominal drain output decreased by 30% and within a week, it decreased by 90%. Patient was transferred out of ICU on day 59 and discharged after 63 days of hospitalization.

1.2. Case #2. A 74-year-old Asian woman with a history of CVA, hypertension, hyperlipidemia, CKD, and diuretic therapy was admitted to the hospital with two days of abdominal pain radiating to the back with normal lipase. The pain was nonpositional and not associated with eating, nausea, vomiting, or dysuria. She denied diarrhea, constipation, appetite or weight changes, fevers, chills, or night sweats.

Abdominal CT with IV contrast showed a hypoattenuating superior pancreatic mass, measuring 2.4 × 4.7 cm, and a second mass in the pancreatic head, measuring 2.2 × 1.8 cm. There was no pancreatic or biliary ductal dilatation or liver abnormality.

Her hospital course was notable for new onset polyarthritis affecting both ankles, new development of subcutaneous mass on her right ankle, fevers to 100–101 F, and an elevated white count of 12,000/μL. The soft tissue mass on her ankle was aspirated, yielding 20 cc of chalky white substance that was positive for negatively birefringent crystals. The uric acid level was 10 mg/dL.

A diagnostic CT-guided FNA biopsy of the pancreatic mass revealed a necrotic and crystalline material with chronic inflammatory cells. There was no evidence of malignancy or infection. Subsequent transfer to a tertiary care hospital and endoscopic biopsy confirmed numerous needle-shaped negatively birefringent urate crystals consistent with tophaceous gout, with no evidence of malignancy or infection.

We started the patient on prednisone taper and colchicine prophylaxis with improvement of her gouty arthritis. Lasix was discontinued and allopurinol was initiated. Six months later, the pancreatic mass was unchanged on repeat CT and the patient was asymptomatic.

1.3. Case #3. A 71-year-old woman with JRA, type 2 DM, hypertension, and CKD stage 4 presented with 6 weeks of acute onset abdominal pain. CT abdomen and pelvis showed masslike area in the pancreas, measuring 4.1 × 2.7 cm (Figure 1). Endoscopic ultrasound showed 6 masses in peripancreatic, perihilar, and periportal regions. Fine-needle aspiration of the peripancreatic mass near the tail showed necrotic material with acute and chronic inflammation and rare clusters of histiocytes suggestive of granulomas. GMS and AFB stains are negative.

Rheumatology was consulted. Having previous experience with pancreatic tophaceous gout, we performed a retroactive analysis of the FNA material and confirmed the presence of needle-shaped negative birefringent crystals. The patient was started on steroid therapy and experienced significant improvement of her abdominal pain. Her uric acid was 9.0 g/dL prior to initiation of allopurinol.

Subsequent CT abdomen performed 10 months later showed decrease in the size of the lesion, measuring 1.8 × 1.7 cm, and repeat scan in 22 months showed complete resolution of the lesion (Figure 2).

2. Discussion

There have only been 4 cases of pancreatic gout reported in the literature according to our search in the PubMed database for articles published in English language [6–9]. We report 3 additional cases which highlight the importance of recognizing uric acid deposition in the differential diagnosis of pancreatic lesions.

In 2002, Khanna et al. presented the first case of gouty tophi in pancreatic pseudocyst mimicking infection. In 2009, a second case of pancreatic gout was reported masquerading as neoplasm. Two additional cases of pancreatic gout mimicking neoplasm were reported in 2016 and 2019. In this case series, we report one additional case mimicking infection and two more cases mimicking malignancy. In all cases presenting as pancreatic masses, imaging findings were highly suggestive of malignancy. Biopsy of the pancreatic lesions in all of the reported cases demonstrated necrotic material and/or debris. There have been several prior case reports documenting tophaceous gout mimicking infections and malignancy in various other sites/organs [1–3]. We suggest that tophaceous gout be considered in the differential diagnosis of any soft tissue mass or fluid collection including pancreatic pseudocysts and masses.

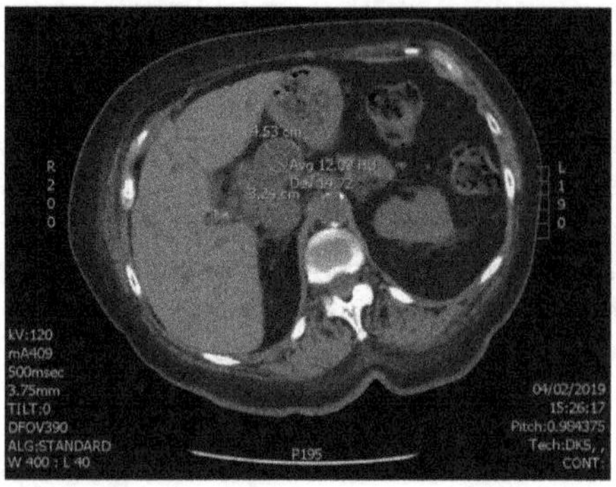

FIGURE 1: CT scan image of the abdomen without contrast showing the pancreatic mass before treatment.

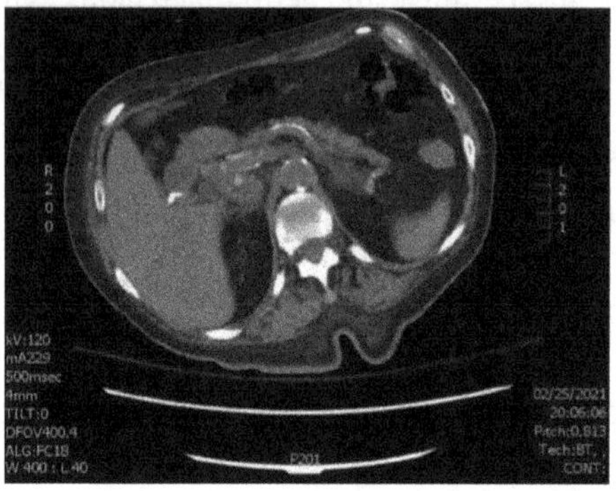

FIGURE 2: CT scan image of the abdomen without contrast showing resolution of the pancreatic mass after allopurinol therapy.

It is important to note that 4 cases of total 7 (2 of the 4 previously reported cases and 2 of our current 3 cases) occurred in patients without a prior known history of gout. Three of the cases also had normal uric acid level at the time of diagnosis. These features may explain the paucity of pancreatic gout diagnosed reported in the literature and underscore the importance of considering pancreatic gout even in patients without a prior history of gout and with normal uric acid level. We hypothesize that pancreatic gout may explain cases of pancreatitis previously labeled idiopathic. It should be noted that the usual method by which surgical tissue is prepped using aqueous fixations, especially with use of formalin, often results in dissolution of the urate crystals. We suspect that the diagnosis of pancreatic gout may have been missed due to the fixation and preservation process dissolving the crystals. We suggest that any patient with a history of gout who is undergoing surgery or biopsy of the pancreas in the setting of pancreatitis have additional specimens sent to look for urate crystals in a nonaqueous solution [10].

All of the previously reported cases of pancreatic gout were either asymptomatic or only associated with mild nonspecific abdominal pain. Our case #1 is the first case documenting pancreatic gout associated with fever and leukocytosis. Our case demonstrates that pancreatic gout can explain fever of unknown origin in a patient with pancreatic fluid collection. In this case, refractory fever after >50 days of ICU admission and several courses of antibiotics and surgeries resolved within six hours of initiation of steroid therapy and his pancreatic drain output decreased by 30% within 1 day and by 90% within 1 week of starting solumedrol. In all of the reported cases, urate-lowering therapy was associated with clinical improvement. In cases associated with pancreatic lesions, the lesions remained stable at 6 months in 2 cases and improved or resolved at 8–18 months in 3 cases. These cases highlight the importance of exploring the possibility of pancreatic gout and considering steroid and urate-lowering therapy in patients with pancreatic fluid collections/lesions.

We have shown that tophaceous gout in the pancreas can mimic pseudocyst, pancreatic abscess, or malignancy. We hope that this case series expands awareness of pancreatic gout and encourages additional evaluation in future patients who present with pancreatic abnormalities and gout risk factors. Making the appropriate diagnosis is crucial in preventing unnecessary studies, interventions (i.e., antibiotics, chemotherapy), surgeries, and prolonged hospitalization and results in overall improved patient care.

References

[1] W. Huiqing, M. J. Klein, R. E. Stahl, and M. A. Sanchez, "Intestinal pseudotumorous gouty nodulosis: a colonic tophus without manifestation of gouty arthritis," *Human Pathology*, vol. 35, no. 7, pp. 897–899, 2004.

[2] L. McLean, "Tophaceous pseudotumors in Polynesian patients with gout," *Journal of Rheumatology*, vol. 31, no. 9, pp. 1866–1868, 2004.

[3] C. H. Chen, C. K. H. Chen, L. R. Yeh, H. B. Pan, and C. F. Yang, "Intra-abdominal gout mimicking pelvic abscess," *Skeletal Radiology*, vol. 34, no. 4, pp. 229–233, 2005.

[4] C. P. Beier, A. Hartmann, C. Woertgen, A. Brawanski, and R. D. Rothoerl, "A large, erosive intraspinal and paravertebral gout tophus," *Journal of Neurosurgery: Spine*, vol. 3, no. 6, pp. 485–487, 2005.

[5] R. Wernick, C. Winkler, and S. Campbell, "Tophi as the initial manifestation of gout. Report of six cases and review of the literature," *Archives of Internal Medicine*, vol. 152, no. 4, pp. 873–876, 1992.

[6] D. Khanna, S.-J. Tang, W. D. Wallace, B. E. Roth, and B. H. Hahn, "Gouty tophi in a pancreatic pseudocyst," *Arthritis & Rheumatism*, vol. 46, no. 2, pp. 565-566, 2002.

[7] S. Gupta, Z. McMahan, P. C. Patel, D. W. Markham, M. H. Drazner, and P. P. A. Mammen, "Pancreatic gout masquerading as pancreatic cancer in a heart transplant candidate," *Journal of Heart and Lung Transplantation*, vol. 28, no. 10, pp. 1112-1113, 2009.

[8] S. Shrestha, F. Kamal, M. Ali Khan, and C. R. Tombazzi, "Gouty tophi manifesting as a pancreatic foci," *American Journal of the Medical Sciences*, vol. 358, no. 4, pp. 294–298, 2019.

[9] T. M. Nenasheva, "Gouty Visceropathies," *Voen Med Zh*, no. 2, pp. 30–32, 1995.

[10] V. Shidham, M. Chivukula, Z. Basir, and G. Shidham, "Evaluation of crystals in formalin-fixed, paraffin-embedded tissue sections for the differential diagnosis of pseudogout, gout, and tumoral calcinosis," *Modern Pathology*, vol. 14, no. 8, pp. 806–810, 2001.

22

Chronic Myeloid Leukemia in a Patient Receiving Tofacitinib: A Case Report and Literature Review

Georgio Medawar,[1] Joseph Chahrouri,[1,2] and Rabih Said[1,3]

[1]*Internal Medicine Department, St George Hospital University Medical Center and the University of Balamand, Beirut, Lebanon*
[2]*Rheumatology Division, St George Hospital University Medical Center and the University of Balamand, Beirut, Lebanon*
[3]*Hematology/Oncology Division, St George Hospital University Medical Center and the University of Balamand, Beirut, Lebanon*

Correspondence should be addressed to Georgio Medawar; georgiomed@gmail.com

Academic Editor: George S. Habib

Background. Tofacitinib is a new oral Janus kinase inhibitor that has shown promising clinical benefit in various rheumatologic diseases. However, many concerns related to the development of malignancies have been reported with its use. *Case Presentation.* A 43-year-old female patient received tofacitinib for refractory rheumatoid arthritis (RA). Two years after 5 mg bid daily dosing, the patient developed chronic myelogenous leukemia (CML), for which she received imatinib and tofacitinib was discontinued. She then remained in remission for rheumatoid arthritis and within the expected milestone outcome for her CML. *Conclusion.* This is the first reported case of CML after the use of tofacitinib. This event is of particular interest knowing the possible benefits tofacitinib carries in the treatment of CML demonstrated in a few studies.

1. Introduction

Tofacitinib is an oral Janus kinase (JAK) inhibitor that was approved in 2012 for moderate to severe active rheumatoid arthritis (RA), in 2017 for active psoriatic arthritis, and recently in 2018 for induction and maintenance of moderate to severe ulcerative colitis [1]. It primarily acts by inhibiting JAK3 and/or JAK1; subsequently, it leads to the inhibition of IL-15-induced phosphorylation of STAT5 and IL-6-induced phosphorylation of STAT1 and STAT3 [2].

The immune-modulator effect of tofacitinib in such a relatively new mechanism of action has raised a concern about adverse events, particularly malignancies [1, 3].

Herein, we report a case of a patient who developed CML after receiving tofacitinib for rheumatoid arthritis.

2. Case Presentation

A 43-year-old female patient with Hashimoto's thyroiditis was diagnosed with seropositive RA (anti-CCP 140, ref <20) in April 2013 when she presented with bilateral wrist, PIP, elbow, shoulder, knee, and ankle synovitis. She was started on prednisone taper at 20 mg/day and methotrexate 10 mg once a week optimized in increments up to 25 mg/week, with calcium, vitamin D, and folic acid supplements. Despite this therapy and despite significant improvement, there was recurrent, intermittent low-grade synovitis in both wrists. In mid-2016, X-rays revealed early erosions in the left ulnar styloid and capitate as well as the bases of the left second and third metacarpal bones. It was then decided, in January 2016, to start her on targeted therapy with tofacitinib 5 mg bid. The patient had rapid favorable response, and within 3 months, she was in clinical remission. The dose of methotrexate was progressively tapered down and stopped by the end of December 2016. The patient then remained in remission. Unfortunately, a routine laboratory test on June 23, 2016, showed leukocytosis of 27,500. The hemoglobin count was 11.3, and the platelet count was 610,000. A repeat CBC 5 days later confirmed leukocytosis with a WBC of 32,300 (7% metamyelocytes, 3% myelocytes, and 2% promyelocytes), hemoglobin count of 10.6, and platelet count of 703,000. Tofacitinib was discontinued, and the patient was referred to hematology/oncology.

Initial blood work was positive for t(9; 22) BCR-ABL (p210 b3a2) on FISH analysis. Bone marrow aspirate and biopsy showed myeloid and megakaryocytic hyperplasia with 2% blasts and a myeloid-to-erythroid ratio of 10 : 1. The karyotype showed t(9; 22) detected in all the examined cells. The flow cytometry showed that 5-6% of flow events express early myeloid markers.

The patient was diagnosed with chronic myelogenous leukemia (CML), and she was started on imatinib 400 mg. Two weeks later, blood tests showed a WBC of 18,200, platelet count of 514,000 and hemoglobin count of 9.9 that later further dropped to 6.5 with significant fatigue. Therefore, imatinib was decreased to 300 mg/day. Three months later, the patient remained in clinical remission for rheumatoid arthritis with hematological remission with WBC 4,700, Hg 12.5, and platelets 291,000. Her repeat quantitative PCR for BCR-ABL was 0.86%.

3. Discussion

Various malignancies have been reported after the use of tofacitinib in previous case reports and meta-analyses (Table 1). However, ongoing debate about the higher incidence rate of cancer after tofacitinib is not confirmed in the real-world, postmarketing treated population [12].

For instance, in the rheumatoid arthritis clinical development program, the incidence rate of malignancies in patients treated with tofacitinib, excluding nonmelanoma skin cancer (NMSC), was reported to be 0.85/100 patient-year (py) (107 out of 5671 patients) in a total tofacitinib exposure of 12,644 py. These include both solid cancers (lung, breast, and gastric cancer) and hematologic malignancies (lymphoma and T-cell CLL) [3]. Cohen et al. present a more extended analysis with 6,194 patients included and a total exposure of 19,406 py (over 8.5 years). The incidence rate of malignancies was 0.89/100 py, and they included lung disorders, breast disorders, and lymphoma/lymphoproliferative disorders [4]. In both analyses, there was no association between the dose of tofacitinib and the risk of malignancy (except for NMSC), and the malignancy rate remained relatively stable by 6-month intervals. Similarly, a Japanese long-term extension (LTE) study reported an incidence rate of 1.2/100 py of malignancies (19 out of 486 patients) that include gastric, breast, ovarian, colon, lung, fallopian tube, thyroid, and esophageal cancer, in addition to acute myeloid leukemia (AML), lymphoproliferative disorders, liposarcoma, and transitional cell carcinoma [5]. However, a large meta-analysis showed that there is no statistically significant increase in any type of malignancies with the use of tofacitinib in patients with RA [12]. Furthermore, the risk of NMSC, lung cancer, and lymphoma/lymphoproliferative disorders was previously reported to be increased in patients with rheumatoid arthritis [13, 14]; therefore, the analysis of cancer development in this patient population would be challenging.

On the contrary, the data on cancer development in psoriatic arthritis patients treated with tofacitinib are more unclear. For instance, two out of three phase 3 clinical trials reported malignancies as adverse events. In OPAL Broaden, 3 patients developed solid tumors (excluding NMSC) out of 107 patients (2.8%) taking continuous 5 mg bid tofacitinib for up to 12 months [6]. In the ongoing OPAL Balance trial, after 24 months of follow-up, 2 cases of malignancies were reported among the 680 enrolled patients (0.3%) [7], whereas in OPAL Beyond, no malignancies were reported [8].

Likewise, in ulcerative colitis, three phase 3 clinical trials (OCTAVE Induction 1, OCTAVE Induction 2, and OCTAVE Sustain) evaluated the safety and efficacy of tofacitinib in induction and maintenance. No malignancies (excluding NMSC) were reported in any of these trials, but an ongoing LTE study revealed 8 cases giving an overall incidence rate of 0.48/100 py (combining OCTAVE trials with the LTE study) [9, 10].

In addition, Xie and Ma reported a case of AML 2 years after the use of tofacitinib for refractory ulcerative colitis [11], despite a possible increased risk of AML with ulcerative colitis [15].

Natural killer (NK) cells, in addition to other cytokine transduction signaling (such as interferon types I and II), have been shown to have a major inhibitory role in tumorigenesis [16]. Tofacitinib has been shown to decrease the number of NK cells as well as the signaling transduction of various cytokines [2, 17]. This might hypothetically be a mechanism by which tofacitinib can increase the risk of some malignancies.

From another perspective, various studies have investigated the role of the JAK/STAT pathway in the pathophysiology of CML [18, 19]; BCR-ABL activates several signaling pathways such as PI3K, RAF, ERK, MEK, and JAK. The latter transduces signals via STAT and plays essential roles in cell proliferation and differentiation in leukemia [18]. In addition, few in vitro studies have shown that the use of JAK inhibitors with or without imatinib on CML cell lines had a modest positive outcome with JAK2/JAK3 inhibitors alone and a marked effect when combined (synergic effect). This suggests that targeting JAK may carry a potential therapeutic option for CML [18–21]. These findings led to the integration of JAK inhibitors in recent recruiting/ongoing clinical trials for treatment of CML (see Web References [22] and [23]).

To our knowledge, this is the first reported case of CML that occurred 2 years after tofacitinib use at 5 mg bid in a patient with rheumatoid arthritis. It is difficult to tell whether our patient developed a de novo CML or she already had acquired the BCR-ABL translocation during her treatment for rheumatoid arthritis which was possibly "silenced" by inhibiting the JAK3 pathway with tofacitinib. Moreover, a solid cause-effect relationship between the use of tofacitinib and the development of CML cannot be established. However, by discontinuing tofacitinib and treating her with imatinib, the patient has been so far in remission for her rheumatoid arthritis and within the expected milestone outcome for her CML.

Whether imatinib contributed to the maintenance of her rheumatoid arthritis in remission or not is not known. An extensive mutational workup and studying the effect of reintroduction of tofacitinib in case of relapse of either

Table 1: Reported cases of malignancies with the use of tofacitinib.

	Reported malignancies (excluding NMSC)	Malignancy crude IR	Malignancy IR/100 py
Rheumatoid arthritis			
Curtis et al. [3]	Lung, breast, and gastric lymphoma and T-cell CLL	1.88	0.85
Cohen et al. [4]	Lung disorders, breast disorders, and lymphoma/ lymphoproliferative disorders	2.79	0.89
Yamanaka et al. [5]	Gastric, breast, ovarian, colon, lung, fallopian tube, thyroid, esophageal, and lymphoproliferative disorders, acute myeloid leukemia, liposarcoma, and transitional cell carcinoma	3.9	1.2
Psoriatic arthritis			
OPAL trials [6–8]*	Breast carcinoma, transitional cell carcinoma, and vulvar squamous cell carcinoma	2.8 (OPAL Broaden)	2.8 (OPAL Broaden)
		0.3 (OPAL Balance)	— (OPAL Balance)
Ulcerative colitis			
OCTAVE trials + LTE [9, 10]**	—	0.48	—
Xie and Ma [11]	Acute myeloid leukemia	—	—

*The cancer types mentioned were only reported in OPAL Broaden. In the ongoing OPAL Balance, there was no specification of the cancer types. **In the ongoing LTE study (NCT014770612), there was no specification of the cancer types.

rheumatoid arthritis or CML would be interesting to perform in this case.

4. Conclusion

Despite the potential benefits of tofacitinib in the treatment of CML, we illustrated a unique case of CML that developed after its use for RA. It may represent a potential side effect that may be added to the list of malignancies associated with this drug. In contrast, the response of both RA and CML to imatinib shed the light on the interrelation of pathways between RA and CML and may be the subject of many interesting studies.

Abbreviations

JAK: Janus kinase
RA: Rheumatoid arthritis
CML: Chronic myelogenous leukemia
AML: Acute myelogenous leukemia
NMSC: Nonmelanoma skin cancer
LTE: Long-term extension.

Additional Points

Clinical Practice. Many solid and hematologic malignancies have been reported after the use of tofacitinib. Our first-time reported case of CML is of special interest: (i) It is the first malignancy type that has a direct pathway relation with the drug's targets. (ii) The drug itself has potential benefits in treatment of CML. (iii) We are not sure if the drug delayed or potentiated the development of CML. (iv) Treatment of CML with imatinib led to good response to both RA and CML. These observations raise many questions that can be addressed in the future: (i) What is the mutational status of patients receiving JAK3 inhibitors who develop CML? (ii) Do JAK inhibitors really work in CML? (iii) What is the effect of reintroducing JAK3 inhibitors in patients with relapsed CML who previously received JAK inhibitors? (iv) Does imatinib play a role in rheumatoid arthritis?

Acknowledgments

We are grateful to the medical record team at Saint George Hospital University Medical Center, Beirut, Lebanon, who provided us with all the necessary documents to complete the case. We also appreciate Dr. Omar Zmerli for medical writing assistance.

References

[1] XELJANZ (tofacitinib) [package insert on the internet] Pfizer Inc., New York, NY, USA, November 2018, https://www.accessdata.fda.gov/drugsatfda_docs/label/2018/203214s018lbl.pdf.

[2] J. A. Hodge, T. T. Kawabata, S. Krishnaswami et al., "The mechanism of action of tofacitinib—an oral Janus kinase inhibitor for the treatment of rheumatoid arthritis," *Clinical and Experimental Rheumatology*, vol. 34, no. 2, pp. 318–328, 2016.

[3] J. R. Curtis, E. B. Lee, I. V. Kaplan et al., "Tofacitinib, an oral Janus kinase inhibitor: analysis of malignancies across the rheumatoid arthritis clinical development programme," *Annals of the Rheumatic Diseases*, vol. 75, no. 5, pp. 831–841, 2016.

[4] S. B. Cohen, Y. Tanaka, X. Mariette et al., "Long-term safety of tofacitinib for the treatment of rheumatoid arthritis up to 8.5 years: integrated analysis of data from the global clinical trials," *Annals of the Rheumatic Diseases*, vol. 76, no. 7, pp. 1253–1262, 2017.

[5] H. Yamanaka, Y. Tanaka, T. Takeuchi et al., "Tofacitinib, an oral Janus kinase inhibitor, as monotherapy or with background methotrexate, in Japanese patients with rheumatoid arthritis: an open-label, long-term extension study," *Arthritis Research & Therapy*, vol. 18, no. 1, pp. 1–12, 2016.

[6] P. Mease, S. Hall, O. FitzGerald et al., "Tofacitinib or adalimumab versus placebo for psoriatic arthritis," *New England Journal of Medicine*, vol. 377, no. 16, pp. 1537–1550, 2017.

[7] T.-S. Wang and T.-F. Tsai, "Tofacitinib in psoriatic arthritis," *Immunotherapy*, vol. 9, no. 14, pp. 1153–1163, 2017.

[8] D. Gladman, W. Rigby, V. F. Azevedo et al., "Tofacitinib for psoriatic arthritis in patients with an inadequate response to

TNF inhibitors," *New England Journal of Medicine*, vol. 377, no. 16, pp. 1525–1536, 2017.

[9] W. J. Sandborn, C. Su, B. E. Sands et al., "Tofacitinib as induction and maintenance therapy for ulcerative colitis," *New England Journal of Medicine*, vol. 376, no. 18, pp. 1723–1736, 2017.

[10] G. R. Lichtenstein, M. A. Ciorba, G. Rogler et al., "Sa1763—tofacitinib for the treatment of ulcerative colitis: analysis of malignancy rates from the octave clinical program," *Gastroenterology*, vol. 154, no. 6, pp. S-385-386, 2018.

[11] M. Xie and H. Ma, "Acute myeloid leukemia in a patient receiving phase iii clinical trial of tofacitinib (xeljanz) therapy for ulcerative colitis: a case study with literature review," *International Journal of Current Medical Sciences*, vol. 6, no. 11, pp. 185–187, 2016.

[12] J. R. Maneiro, A. Souto, and J. J. Gomez-Reino, "Risks of malignancies related to tofacitinib and biological drugs in rheumatoid arthritis: systematic review, meta-analysis, and network meta-analysis," *Seminars in Arthritis and Rheumatism*, vol. 47, no. 2, pp. 149–156, 2017.

[13] K. M. Wilton and E. L. Matteson, "Malignancy incidence, management, and prevention in patients with rheumatoid arthritis," *Rheumatology and Therapy*, vol. 4, no. 2, pp. 333–347, 2017.

[14] L. Mellemkjær, M. S. Linet, G. Gridley, M. Frisch, H. Møller, and J. H. Olsen, "Rheumatoid arthritis and cancer risk," *European Journal of Cancer*, vol. 32, no. 10, pp. 1753–1757, 1996.

[15] J. Askling, L. Brandt, A. Lapidus et al., "Risk of haematopoietic cancer in patients with inflammatory bowel disease," *Gut*, vol. 54, no. 5, pp. 617–622, 2005.

[16] R. D. Schreiber, L. J. Old, and M. J. Smyth, "Cancer Immunoediting: integrating suppression and promotion," *Science*, vol. 331, no. 6024, pp. 1565–1571, 2011.

[17] M. Harigai, "Growing evidence of the safety of JAK inhibitors in patients with rheumatoid arthritis," *Rheumatology*, vol. 58, no. 1, pp. 34–42, 2019.

[18] K. Yagi, A. Shimada, and T. Sendo, "Pharmacological inhibition of JAK3 enhances the antitumor activity of imatinib in human chronic myeloid leukemia," *European Journal of Pharmacology*, vol. 825, pp. 28–33, 2018.

[19] A. Samanta, B. Perazzona, S. Chakraborty et al., "Janus kinase 2 regulates Bcr-Abl signaling in chronic myeloid leukemia," *Leukemia*, vol. 25, no. 3, pp. 463–472, 2011.

[20] P. Valent, "Targeting the JAK2-STAT5 pathway in CML," *Blood*, vol. 124, no. 9, pp. 1386–1388, 2014.

[21] M. Massimino, S. Stella, E. Tirrò et al., "Non ABL-directed inhibitors as alternative treatment strategies for chronic myeloid leukemia," *Molecular Cancer*, vol. 17, no. 1, pp. 1–15, 2018.

[22] https://clinicaltrials.gov/ct2/show/NCT01702064, November 2018.

[23] https://clinicaltrials.gov/ct2/show/NCT01751425, October 2018.

23

Antiphospholipid Syndrome Associated with Nonradiographic Axial Spondyloarthritis

Jozélio Freire De Carvalho[1] **and Antoniella Fernanda Mendanha Sousa**[2]

[1]*Institute for Health Sciences from Federal University of Bahia, Salvador, Bahia, Brazil*
[2]*INPOS, Goiania-GO, Brazil*

Correspondence should be addressed to Jozélio Freire De Carvalho; jotafc@gmail.com

Academic Editor: Ljudmila Stojanovich

Herein, we describe a patient with antiphospholipid syndrome (APS) associated with nonradiographic axial spondyloarthritis (NRAS). A 31-year-old woman with a past medical history of uveitis experienced a pulmonary thromboembolism in March 2014 and was treated with rivaroxaban (20 mg/day). Five months later, she started complaining of low back pain. The results on contrast-enhanced sacroiliac magnetic resonance imaging were normal. Laboratory tests revealed positive HLA-B27 and the presence of lupus anticoagulant and IgM anticardiolipin. The diagnoses of APS and NRAS were made. The patient was treated with rivaroxaban for APS and sulfasalazine (2 g/day), respectively. As she showed the presence of lupus anticoagulant antibodies in blood, she did not receive nonsteroidal anti-inflammatory drugs. After 6 months, the patient was asymptomatic, without lumbar pain; she also showed normalization of the erythrocyte sedimentation rate and the C-reactive protein and vitamin D levels, good control of lumbar pain, and no new uveitis episodes. The APS was also stable. To the best of our knowledge, this is the first reported case of NRAS associated with APS.

1. Introduction

Antiphospholipid syndrome (APS) is a systemic autoimmune disease characterized by recurrent thrombosis associated with obstetric complications and/or thrombocytopenia in the presence of persistent antiphospholipid antibodies [1]. This coagulopathy, when isolated, is called primary APS, or it may be associated with other autoimmune conditions (i.e., secondary APS), commonly with systemic lupus erythematosus [1].

In an extensive study with 1,000 patients with APS, the diseases associated with APS, apart from primary APS in 53.1% of the cases, were lupus in 36.2% of the cases, lupus-like syndrome in 5%, Sjögren syndrome in 2.2%, rheumatoid arthritis in 1.8%, systemic sclerosis in 0.7%, systemic vasculitis in 0.7%, and dermatomyositis in 0.7% [2].

APS with spondyloarthritis is quite rare; only five cases have been previously reported [3–7]. To the best of our knowledge, no case of nonradiographic axial spondyloarthritis (NRAS) associated with APS has been reported. Therefore, herein, we report the first case of APS associated with NRAS.

2. Case Report

A 31-year-old woman had a past medical history of obesity, dyslipidemia, and breast nodules, as well as a family history for vitiligo in her sister, multiple sclerosis in her cousin, and pulmonary thromboembolism in an aunt who died of it. She also had a childhood history of transient polyarthralgia and had received glucocorticoids. When she was 23 years of age, she was diagnosed with uveitis in her left eye. In March 2014, she started complaining of radiating pain in her left flank and left shoulder while breathing, and a diagnosis of pulmonary thromboembolism was confirmed on the basis of the results of perfusion scintigraphy and pulmonary angiotomography. The patient was hospitalized and treated in an intensive care unit, receiving intravenous heparin. She was discharged after being prescribed rivaroxaban (20 mg/day). In September 2014, the patient started complaining of inflammatory low back pain that had persisted for more than 3 months. Physical examination demonstrated a blood pressure of 140/80 mmHg, weight of 95.15 kg, height of 1.64 m, and body mass index of 35.38 kg/m^2. The sacroiliac joints were normal on the physical examination. The results on contrast-enhanced sacroiliac magnetic resonance imaging were normal. Laboratory tests revealed the presence of HLA-B27, as well as positive results for lupus anticoagulant antibodies (in February and June 2014) and low titer IgM anticardiolipin antibodies (15.7 MPL; positive value > 10 MPL); the results for IgG anticardiolipin antibodies were negative. The patient was heterozygous for the presence of both mutant prothrombin and methylenetetrahydrofolate reductase. All other thrombophilia factors were within the normal ranges, including antithrombin III (128%), protein C (170%), protein S (130%), and homocysteine (9.4 μmol/L); factor V Leiden was absent. The patient was negative for antinuclear antibodies, anti-Sm, anti-dsDNA, anti-RNP, anti-Ro/SS-A, anti-La/SS-B, anti-CCP, rheumatoid factor, and ANCA; complement levels were within the normal ranges. The 25-OH-vitamin D level was 20.4 ng/mL (normal >30 ng/mL), the erythrocyte sedimentation rate (ESR) was 30 mm/h, and the C-reactive protein (CRP) level was 30.4 mg/L. A diagnosis of APS was made on the basis of the occurrence of pulmonary thromboembolism and the results of at least two tests that showed positive lupus anticoagulant antibodies over 12 weeks, and a diagnosis of NRAS was made on the basis of the observation of inflammatory low back pain for more than 3 months in a patient aged <45 years, as well as the positive result for HLA-B27, the presence of uveitis, and high levels of CRP. The patient was treated with rivaroxaban for APS and sulfasalazine (2 g/day); a single subcutaneous injection of vitamin D3 (600,000 IU) was also added as part of her treatment. As the patient showed the presence of lupus anticoagulants in blood, she did not receive nonsteroidal anti-inflammatory drugs. After 6 months, she was asymptomatic, with good control of lumbar pain, as well as normalized ESR and CRP and vitamin D levels; she also did not show any new episodes of uveitis. The APS was also stable without any new clinical or laboratory features.

3. Discussion

To the best of our knowledge, herein, we describe the first patient with APS and NRAS.

Antiphospholipid antibodies have been observed in patients with spondyloarthritis. In a study of 84 patients with axial spondyloarthritis and 40 healthy controls, antiphospholipid antibodies were more frequently observed in patients with axial spondyloarthritis (29% vs. 5% in the controls, $p < 0.002$). Importantly, no patient had thrombosis or other clinical manifestations of APS [8]. However, antiphospholipid antibodies have not been detected in patients with axial spondyloarthritis in other studies [9].

NRAS is more frequently observed in women than in men. Although patients with NRAS have a shorter disease duration and do not show radiological alterations, they experience a substantial illness burden, with self-reported disease activity and functional impairments comparable to those of patients with radiographic disease. Interestingly, radiographic progression was observed in approximately 10% of these patients over 2 years [10].

The first description of APS in a patient with axial spondyloarthritis was reported in 1991 by Blanchard et al. in a 60-year-old man with leg ulcers and persistent lupus anticoagulants [5]. Two other cases of APS associated with axial spondyloarthritis have been described in the medical literature by Mateo et al. in 1992 [3, 4]; the first patient with axial spondyloarthritis developed a pons infarction associated with high titers of anticardiolipin antibodies, and the second patient had deep vein thrombosis with the presence of lupus anticoagulant antibodies [3, 4]. The fourth case of APS in a patient with axial spondyloarthritis was described in 1993; the patient had axial spondyloarthritis with deep venous thrombosis and positive lupus anticoagulant antibodies [6]. The fifth case of APS in a patient with axial spondyloarthritis was reported in a 67-year-old woman with spondyloarthritis who was treated with adalimumab. After the 3rd dose of this biological drug, she experienced ischemic changes in her distal fingers and toes, showed positivity for IgM anticardiolipin antibodies, and showed the appearance of antinuclear antibodies and ANCA anti-dsDNA. The authors linked the autoimmunity and thrombosis to a drug-induced manifestation secondary to adalimumab use [7].

In conclusion, herein, we describe a rare case of APS with NRAS. The patient was treated with anticoagulants and sulfasalazine and had good outcomes for both diseases.

Additional Points

Highlights. Antiphospholipid syndrome (APS) is characterized by recurrent thrombosis and/or obstetric events.Nonradiographic axial spondyloarthritis (NRAS) is a type of spondyloarthritis characterized by the clinical features of spondyloarthritis but no imaging evidence of sacroiliitis or spine involvement. No case of APS associated with NRAS has been previously described.We describe the first case of APS with NRAS.

Authors' Contributions

JFC carried out conception, analysis, writing, interpretation, revision, and submission. AFMS performed analysis, interpretation, and revision.

Acknowledgments

The authors would like to thank Sergio Ribeiro for the English revision of the manuscript.

References

[1] G. R. Hughes, "Thrombosis, abortion, cerebral disease, and the

lupus anticoagulant," *BMJ*, vol. 287, no. 6399, pp. 1088-1089, 1983.

[2] R. Cervera, J.-C. Piette, J. Font et al., "Antiphospholipid syndrome: clinical and immunologic manifestations and patterns of disease expression in a cohort of 1,000 patients," *Arthritis & Rheumatism*, vol. 46, no. 4, pp. 1019–1027, 2002.

[3] L. Mateo, X. Juanola, J. M. Nolla, J. del Blanco, F. Rubio, and D. Roig Escofet, "Antiphospholipid syndrome in patients with ankylosing spondylitis. Presentation of 2 cases," *Medical Clinics of North America*, vol. 98, no. 10, pp. 381–383, 1992.

[4] L. Mateo, X. Juanola, J. M. Nolla, and J. del Blanco, "Antiphospholipid syndrome in patients with ankylosing spondylitis," *Journal of Rheumatology*, vol. 20, no. 8, pp. 1451-1452, 1993.

[5] B. Blanchard, I. Lazareth, C. Brossel, L. Saporta, M. Letanoux, and P. Priollet, "Lupus anticoagulant and leg ulcers associated with ankylosing spondylitis," *Journal of Rheumatology*, vol. 18, no. 12, pp. 1922-1923, 1991.

[6] P. R. Ames, E. Lubrano, R. Scarpa, L. Iannaccone, and V. Brancaccio, "Lupus anticoagulant, ankylosing spondylitis, and thrombosis," *Journal of Rheumatology*, vol. 20, no. 9, pp. 1626–1628, 1993.

[7] I. Hemmati and J. Kur, "Adalimumab-associated antiphospholipid syndrome: a case report and review of the literature," *Clinical Rheumatology*, vol. 32, no. 7, pp. 1095–1098, 2013.

[8] X. Juanola, L. Mateo, P. Domenech et al., "Prevalence of antiphospholipid antibodies in patients with ankylosing spondylitis," *Journal of Rheumatology*, vol. 22, no. 10, pp. 1891–1893, 1995.

[9] R. R. Buchanan, J. R. Wardlaw, A. G. Riglar, G. O. Littlejohn, and M. II. Miller, "Antiphospholipid antibodics in thc connective tissue diseases: their relation to the antiphospholipid syndrome and forme fruste disease," *Journal of Rheumatology*, vol. 16, no. 6, pp. 757–761, 1989.

[10] A. Boonen, J. Sieper, D. van der Heijde et al., "The burden of non-radiographic axial spondyloarthritis," *Seminars in Arthritis and Rheumatism*, vol. 44, no. 5, pp. 556–562, 2015.

24

Hydroxychloroquine and Fabry Disease: Three Case Reports Examining an Unexpected Pathologic Link and a Review of the Literature

Rouhin Sen,[1] **Kathleen Borghoff,**[2] **Kirk W. Foster,**[3] **Stanley J. Radio,**[3] **Alan Erickson,**[4] **and Michelene Hearth-Holmes**[4]

[1]*University of Colorado Denver, Division of Rheumatology, Barbara Davis Center, Mail Stop B115, 1775 Aurora Court, Aurora 80045, Colorado, USA*
[2]*University of Nebraska Medical Center, Division of Diabetes, Endocrinology, and Metabolism, 984130 Nebraska Medical Center, Omaha 68198, NE, USA*
[3]*University of Nebraska Medical Center, Department of Pathology and Microbiology, 985900 Nebraska Medical Center, Omaha 68198, NE, USA*
[4]*University of Nebraska Medical Center, Division of Rheumatology, 986270 Nebraska Medical Center, Omaha 68198, NE, USA*

Correspondence should be addressed to Rouhin Sen; rouhin.sen@cuanschutz.edu

Academic Editor: Gregory J. Tsay

Background. Hydroxychloroquine is an effective and widely used treatment in multiple autoimmune connective tissue diseases that gained a lot of publicity in the coronavirus disease 2019 (COVID-19) pandemic. Our case reports are unique in that they explore the rare and sometimes overlooked effects of this drug on multiple organ systems, specifically the kidney, cardiac muscle, and skeletal muscle. We include key histologic features in images which aid in identifying and distinguishing hydroxychloroquine toxicity from mimickers. Lastly, we report the very interesting similarity in the intracellular action of hydroxychloroquine to the pathology of Fabry disease (and its associated lysosomal enzyme, α-galactosidase A). *Case Presentation.* We will examine the case presentations of three female Caucasian patients: a 22-year-old with lupus nephritis class V, a 72-year-old with long-standing systemic lupus erythematosus, and a 74-year-old with undifferentiated connective tissue disease. All three patients were on hydroxychloroquine therapy for varying amounts of time with histologic evidence of hydroxychloroquine toxicity that is three is present in histological samples of the kidney, the heart, and the skeletal muscle. *Conclusions.* Hydroxychloroquine is a very important and beneficial medication used for various autoimmune connective tissue diseases. Clinicians should be aware of the rare but sometimes serious side effects that can result from the medication, which at times can mimic manifestations of the connective tissue disease itself or Fabry disease. A thorough investigation should be performed in these cases to properly elucidate the cause followed by the appropriate targeted therapy.

1. Introduction

Hydroxychloroquine (HCQ) was thrust into the public spotlight due to the pandemic caused by the severe acute respiratory syndrome coronavirus 2 (SARS-CoV-2). Though its efficacy against SARS-CoV-2 is questionable, the drug certainly has gained tremendous popularity leading to subsequent demand and worldwide shortages.

HCQ is an old drug that is quite well-known to rheumatologists. The drug traces its ancestry to quinine, a compound present in the bark of the cinchona, "the fever tree." Quinine was first isolated in the 1800s, but cinchona bark extracts were in use for at least two centuries prior in Peru and Europe for the treatment of "ague" (malaria). Quinine supplies were reduced during the ravage of World War II leading to the development of synthetic substitutes—chloroquine and quinacrine [1].

Because of perceived toxicity, chloroquine and quinacrine were largely ignored for years until postwar studies in the United States showed their tremendous value in treating malaria [1]. Chloroquine emerged as one of the principal weapons in the World Health Organization's fight against the disease. Around the same time, anecdotal reports from veterans described improvement in symptoms from systemic lupus erythematosus (SLE) and rheumatoid arthritis (RA) leading up to a 1951 study in Lancet describing the benefits of quinacrine on several patients with lupus [2].

Within the next few years, quinacrine, chloroquine, and the newer HCQ (differing from chloroquine by one hydroxyl group) were used to treat SLE and RA [1]. For various reasons including side effects and efficacy, chloroquine and quinacrine fell out of favor and were not widely prescribed. HCQ, an oral cost-effective medication with excellent bioavailability, became a cornerstone drug and ubiquitous in the treatment of several connective tissue diseases and eventually approved by the US Food and Drug Administration for discoid lupus, SLE, and RA [3]. For many of these conditions including SLE, HCQ reduced clinical flare while improving survival, undoubtedly earning its place on the World Health Organization's "List of Essential Medicines" as a disease-modifying agent used in rheumatic disorders.

In its more than half-century of use, HCQ has been generally considered safe, well-tolerated, and with minimal interactions; it notably requires regular eye exams for retinopathy screening and commonly causes nausea and mild diarrhea. Only isolated cases of nephropathy, cardiomyopathy, and skeletal myopathy have been reported. This case series examines some of these lesser-known but serious side effects of HCQ, related histology and pathology, and most interestingly, similarity to the lysosomal storage disorder, Fabry disease.

2. Case Reports

2.1. Case One. A 22-year-old Caucasian female 10 weeks pregnant was admitted with complaints of nausea, vomiting, diarrhea, and fevers. She has a known history of systemic lupus erythematosus and Sjogren syndrome diagnosed at the age of 17; treatment has been primarily with HCQ since the time of diagnosis. At the time of admission, she was on HCQ 400 mg daily. Previously, she had tried azathioprine which was not tolerated due to vomiting and mycophenolate mofetil which was stopped prior to conception. In the past, she has also required treatment with both high- and low-dose oral and intravenous steroids for flares and inflammatory joint pains. She was on prednisone 15 mg daily at the time of admission.

Admission serology was as follows: anti-nuclear-antibody (ANA) positive (1 : 640, homogenous pattern), anti-SSA 201 AU/mL, anti-SSB 664 AU/mL, anti-Smith 411 AU/mL, anti-RNP 306 AU/mL, anti-dsDNA 290 AU/mL, and anti-histones 276 AU/mL. Complete blood count showed stable normocytic normochromic anemia and complete metabolic panel was significant only for a potassium level of 3 mg/dL which was replaced. Complement levels were within normal limits. Her urine analysis showed increased proteins at greater than 300 mg/dL. Subsequent urine protein to creatinine ratio was 5.1 which was a significant change from outpatient labs obtained approximately 3 months prior to admission.

During her hospital course, her symptoms showed improvement with symptomatic treatment and fluids. Due to the increased proteinuria and to assess renal involvement of lupus, she agreed to undergo a kidney biopsy. Pathology showed Class V membranous lupus nephritis. In addition to these findings, electron microscopy showed that intracellular inclusions were found within many podocytes and some tubular epithelial cells (Figure 1). The inclusions were composed of lamellated electron-dense material with the appearance of myelin bodies. The findings were consistent with what had been described in patients receiving HCQ therapy. HCQ was stopped and she was put on increased doses of oral prednisone; her proteinuria resolved two months later. She was restarted on mycophenolate mofetil alone after her pregnancy came to term.

2.2. Case Two. A 72-year-old Caucasian female was transferred from an outside hospital for progressively worsening heart failure (New York Health Association Class IV) and evaluation of cardiac replacement therapy and ventricular assistive device. Her past medical history was significant for SLE diagnosed 50 years prior to our initial encounter. Her disease was controlled well with HCQ 200 mg daily for more than 20 years. For flares, she reported taking low-dose oral prednisone as needed.

Her initial admission vitals were stable. Physical exam showed a cachectic appearing elderly female with ulnar drift across her metacarpal joints which were completely reducible. The exam also revealed lower extremity bunions bilaterally with cock-up deformities. No joint effusions were noted. She had 2+ pedal edema bilaterally and hyper- and hypopigmentation on her lower extremities.

Her initial labs were significant for pancytopenia which from outside records seemed chronic. A complete metabolic panel was significant for an elevated creatinine of 1.9 mg/dL but otherwise, normal electrolytes.

Transthoracic echocardiogram reported dilated left ventricle with a globally depressed ejection fraction of 15%, grade III diastolic dysfunction, severe mitral regurgitation, severe tricuspid regurgitation, and elevated right ventricular systolic pressure (RVSP). Previous but recent cardiac catheterization findings were consistent with a nonischemic cause for her cardiomyopathy. Right heart catheterization was performed to evaluate for pulmonary artery hypertension and showed a pulmonary artery wedge pressure of 47 mmHg.

An endomyocardial biopsy was performed to evaluate the cause of her cardiomyopathy and showed mild ventricular myocyte hypertrophy and focal mild interstitial fibrosis. Myeloid bodies and curvilinear bodies were present on ultrastructural examination (Figure 2). The finding of curvilinear bodies was known to be highly specific for HCQ toxicity, and the drug was discontinued. The patient was deemed a poor candidate for a ventricular assistive device

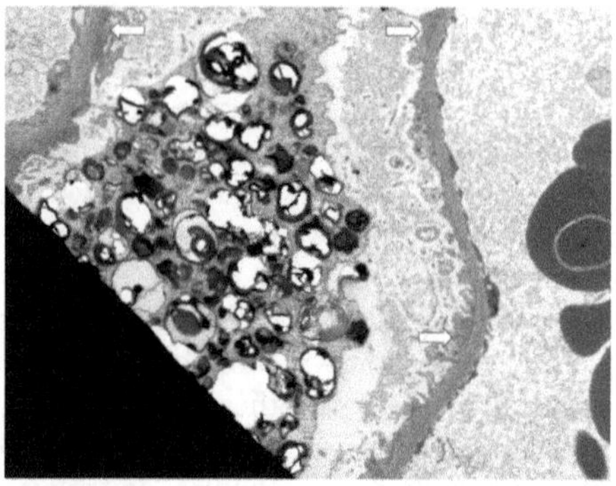

Figure 1: Electron micrograph showing subepithelial electron-dense deposits consistent with class 5 lupus nephritis and intracytoplasmic lamellated bodies (also known as curvilinear bodies-white arrows) within the overlying podocyte. Original magnification 1000×.

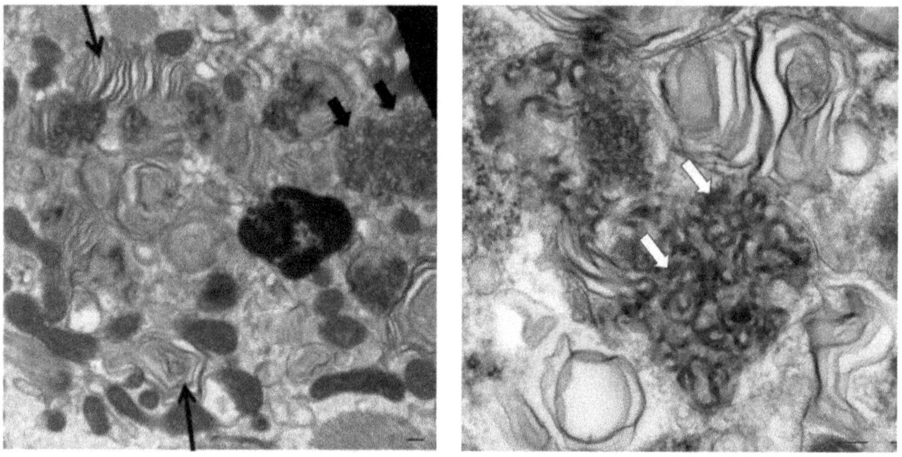

(a) (b)

Figure 2: On the left (a), an electron micrograph of endomyocardial biopsy with myeloid bodies (single black arrows) is present including a "zebra" type in the upper part of the figure. Curvilinear bodies (white double arrows) are also present. On the right (b), higher magnification of curvilinear bodies.

due to poor nutritional status and thrombocytopenia. She was discharged home on milrinone infusion and life-vest but passed away shortly after discharge.

2.3. Case Three. A 76-year-old Caucasian female was seen in the clinic for progressive weakness in her upper and lower extremities. She was known to have a history of an undifferentiated connective tissue disorder manifested by inflammatory arthritis, Raynaud phenomenon, high ANA titer (1 : 640, homogenous pattern), dsDNA of 70 AU/mL, anti-RNP IgG >8 AU/mL, and anti-Smith antibodies 2.3 AU/mL. She also had a history of Sjogren syndrome confirmed via lip biopsy and positive Schirmer test but with negative anti-SSA/SSB.

She was taking HCQ 200 mg twice daily, methotrexate 7.5 mg weekly, and prednisone 5 mg daily for her rheumatic diseases. She was on HCQ for approximately 4 years. She was recently admitted inpatient for muscle weakness but continued to have trouble with activities of daily living following discharge despite physical therapy.

Her initial vital signs in the clinic were stable. Her physical exam revealed 4/5 strength in bilateral deltoids, biceps, triceps, and iliopsoas and 5/5 strength elsewhere. Her creatine kinase was normal at 109 U/L, and aldolase was slightly elevated at 8.6 U/L (the normal range is 1.5–8.1 U/L) in a hemolyzed sample. Repeat aldolase was normal at 7.5 U/L.

She had electromyography (EMG) which showed chronic, primarily axonal, sensory motor peripheral neuropathy of an estimated moderate degree. Of note, the EMG was limited in quality due to a recent history of cellulitis in her lower extremities. A muscle biopsy (Figure 3) showed more than 50% lobulated myofibers, some with excessive mitochondrial activity, small numbers of myofibers with nemaline rods, lysosomal curvilinear bodies, and fiber type grouping, all consistent with chronic denervation and reinnervation. The lysosomal curvilinear bodies were known to be consistent with HCQ therapy. Her HCQ was stopped, and she began following up with neurology for nemaline myopathy.

3. Discussion

The immunomodulatory properties of HCQ are likely due to its effects on the innate immune system and acidic cellular compartments [4]. HCQ is a weak amphiphilic base that can

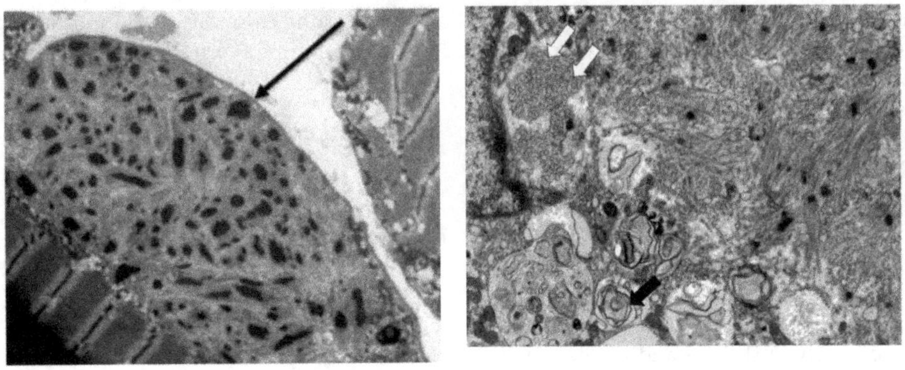

(a) (b)

FIGURE 3: On the left (a), an electron micrograph of skeletal muscle biopsy with Nemaline rod (black arrow). On the right (b), an electron micrograph of the myeloid body, black arrow and curvilinear bodies (white double arrows).

easily cross the plasma membrane into acidic cytoplasmic vesicles, such as lysosomes, where it is protonated and trapped. The accumulation of HCQ raises the pH in vesicles interfering with functions that are dependent upon acidic environments. This interferes with the action of Toll-like receptors and their ligands which plays an important role in receptor recycling, intracellular processing, and the secretion of proteins [3]. This interference leads to decreased production of cytokines and other inflammatory mediators, decreased lymphocytic proliferation and natural killer cell activity, altered antibody production, and interference with antigen processing [5]. Thus, through various actions, HCQ decreases the activity of the innate immune system in autoimmune diseases [3].

3.1. Relation of HCQ to Fabry Disease. The increased intravacuolar pH inhibits the action of lysosomal enzymes, one of which is α-galactosidase A [6]. This very same enzyme is deficient in the rare X-linked recessive lysosomal disorder, Fabry disease. The absence of the enzyme in Fabry disease causes an accumulation of intracellular glycolipid globotriaosylceramide in cells of the kidney, vascular endothelium, cardiac, skeletal, and smooth muscles [7]. Accumulation of this globotriaosylceramide causes impairment in the function of these tissues. The rare side effects seen in our cases could result from a similar pathology as Fabry disease due to inhibition of α-galactosidase A and subsequent aggregation of globotriaosylceramide.

Renal manifestations of Fabry disease include proteinuria and unexplained renal insufficiency similar to case one. Our patient had no family history of lysosomal storage disorders making it an unlikely cause of the renal pathology. Ultrastructural kidney biopsy findings in Fabry disease include lamellated myeloid bodies and zebra bodies found in both podocytes and endothelial cells. This was once thought to be exclusive to the disease but now, has also been described in other conditions that cause renal phospholipidosis including the use of drugs such as HCQ [8]. Ultrastructural analyses have also shown a feature unique to HCQ use and never reported in Fabry disease-curvilinear inclusion bodies [9].

3.2. Curvilinear Inclusion Bodies. Curvilinear inclusion bodies were first described by Muller-Hocker et al. in 2003 [10]. Inclusion bodies are nuclear or cytoplasmic aggregates of proteins. A curvilinear inclusion body is this protein aggregate in a lamellated and twisted structure surrounded by a membrane. Cases by Ferluga [11] and Costa et al. [8] reported that patients on HCQ therapy had histopathological and ultrastructural findings similar to Fabry disease. In these case series, the majority of patients had curvilinear inclusion bodies. Though not considered a uniform finding, this is specific to HCQ toxicity not only in the kidney but also in the cardiac and skeletal muscles.

HCQ-induced damage to cardiac and skeletal muscle is rare and hard to quantify. One study identified nearly 10% prevalence and 1.2% annual incidence of just skeletal myopathy with HCQ use [12]. Another case series reported 1 case of skeletal myopathy in 100 patient-years of therapy [13]. Risk factors for developing cardiac or skeletal myopathy include female gender, Caucasian race, older age, and renal dysfunction. Long-standing treatment with HCQ is also thought to increase the risk of myopathies with effects usually seen after 10 years of use [14]. Discontinuation of therapy is thought to improve skeletal myopathy but this process can take months given the long half-life of HCQ [3].

Cardiac and skeletal myopathy related to HCQ use and Fabry disease clinically present similarly, which is not surprising given their pathologic similarity. HCQ cardiomyopathy can manifest as systolic or diastolic heart failure, conduction anomalies, left or right ventricular hypertrophy, valvular disease, coronary artery disease, or hypertension [14]. The most common presentation for HCQ cardiomyopathy is typically heart failure. A recent case series by Tselios et al. demonstrated 8 out of 8 patients with abnormal cardiac biomarkers and left ventricular hypertrophy in patients with HCQ cardiomyopathy [15]. The question as to why HCQ causes cardiac issues may be explained by its affinity to melanocytes which have been shown to exist in the human heart [16].

HCQ skeletal myopathy and Fabry disease typically present with proximal lower extremity weakness or atrophy [17]. Serum creatine kinase and lactate dehydrogenase can be mildly elevated, which may be overlooked in the context of rheumatic diseases. Due to the higher-than-expected prevalence of HCQ skeletal myopathy, some experts have recommended monitoring for myopathies using a physical exam, serologic tests, and electromyography [18]. Biopsy of the cardiac or skeletal muscle provides a definitive diagnosis, as is the case for HCQ nephropathy.

Typical histopathologic findings in HCQ skeletal and cardiac myopathy are similar to and consistent with what is seen in Fabry disease [18]. Vacuolar myopathy is a finding in nearly all reported cases [19]. Like HCQ nephropathy, the electron microscopic finding of curvilinear inclusion bodies is considered specific for HCQ skeletal and cardiac myopathy and present in over 90% of biopsies [17, 18].

Mortality for anti-malarial induced cardiomyopathy is high; a review of cases by Tselios et al. showed mortality of 45% within 3-4 months after diagnosis [17]; in keeping with this observation, our patient did expire within months of diagnosis. Interestingly, there have been reports suggesting possible reversibility of skeletal and cardiac myopathy with cessation of the drug [19]. In some case reports, patients had improved subjective complaints such as shortness of breath or skeletal muscle weakness. There have also been reports of improved systolic function, evidence of regression of ventricular hypertrophy, and even complete resolution of pathologic changes [17] within 6 months to 2 years of drug cessation. Earlier diagnosis of HCQ cardiomyopathy may lead to better survival. Cardiac magnetic resonance imaging (MRI) using T1 mapping has been used to detect subclinical heart damage in Fabry disease, and there is some hope it can be used for early detection in those with suspected HCQ cardiomyopathy [20]. However, there are also several case reports showing no improvement of either cardiac or skeletal myopathy despite stopping HCQ due to the reservoir of the drug in deposited tissue.

It is unclear how to predict the patients who may develop HCQ nephropathy or myopathy. The development of retinopathy, which is very closely monitored in those on HCQ therapy, has not been consistently found in patients with myopathy; only about 13% of patients with myopathy had preceding or concurrent ocular disease [14, 17]. Another study has suggested that skin hyperpigmentation could be a marker for those who are at higher risk of HCQ toxicities [21] since the skin is a reservoir for the drug but this association has also not been proven.

4. Conclusion

There are only a few case reports of HCQ-induced nephropathy, skeletal myopathy, and cardiac myopathy in the literature. Given the use of HCQ for the past 60–70 years, the prevalence of nephropathy or myopathy related to the drug's use seems negligible. This may be because many cases are subclinical, under-recognized, or attributed to another cause such as the connective tissue disease itself. In the future, it would be interesting to investigate a correlation between partial or reduced α-galactosidase A activity and the higher risk of developing HCQ toxicity and if the activity level correlated inversely to the degree of toxicity. The high mortality and potential reversibility of HCQ nephropathy and myopathy emphasize the importance of recognition and consideration of alternative therapy in these patients.

References

[1] C. Radis, *Plaquenil: From Malaria Treatment to Managing Lupus, RA*, The Rheumatologist, Atlanta, GA, USA, 2015.

[2] F. Page, "Treatment of lupus erythematosus with mepacrine," *The Lancet*, vol. 258, no. 6687, pp. 755–758, 1951.

[3] E. A. Shippey, V. D. Wagler, and A. N. Collamer, "Hydroxychloroquine: an old drug with new relevance," *Cleveland Clinic Journal of Medicine*, vol. 85, no. 6, pp. 459–467, 2018.

[4] D. J. Wallace, V. S. Gudsoorkar, M. H. Weisman, and S. R. Venuturupalli, "New insights into mechanisms of therapeutic effects of antimalarial agents in SLE," *Nature Reviews Rheumatology*, vol. 8, no. 9, pp. 522–533, 2012.

[5] R. I. Rynes, "Antimalarial drugs in the treatment of rheumatological diseases," *British Journal of Rheumatology*, vol. 36, 1997.

[6] P. Fredman, G. W. Klinghardt, and L. Svennerholm, "Effect of chloroquine on the activity of some lysosomal enzymes involved in ganglioside degradation," *Biochimca Biophysica Acta*, vol. 917, 1987.

[7] J. Alroy, S. Sabnis, and J. B. Kopp, "Renal pathology in Fabry disease," *Journal of the American Society of Nephrology*, vol. 13, 2002.

[8] R. M. Costa, E. V. Martul, J. M. Reboredo, and S. Cigarrán, "Curvilinear bodies in hydroxychloroquine-induced renal phospholipidosis resembling Fabry disease," *Clinical Kidney Journal*, vol. 6, no. 5, pp. 533–536, Oct. 2013.

[9] H. Yogasundaram, B. N. Putko, J. Tien et al., "Hydroxychloroquine-induced cardiomyopathy: case report, pathophysiology, diagnosis, and treatment," *Canadian Journal of Cardiology*, vol. 30, no. 12, 2014.

[10] J. Müller-Höcker, H. Schmid, M. Weiss, U. Dendorfer, and G. S. Braun, "Chloroquine-induced phospholipidosis of the kidney mimicking fabry's disease: case report and review of the literature," *Human Pathology*, vol. 34, no. 3, pp. 285–289, 2003.

[11] D. Ferluga, "Nephropathy in Fabry Disease and Iatrogenic Phospholipidosis Mimicking Fabry Disease," in *Proceedings of the Presented at the First International Renal Pathology Conference (Coruna) in La Coruna*, Coruna, Spain, 2010.

[12] E. Casado, J. Gratacós, C. Tolosa et al., "Antimalarial myopathy: an underdiagnosed complication? Prospective longitudinal study of 119 patients," *Annals of the Rheumatic Diseases*, vol. 65, no. 3, pp. 385–390, Mar. 2006.

[13] J. A. Avtna-Zubieta, E. S. Johnson, M. E. Suarez-Almazor, and A. S. Russell, "Incidence of myopathy in patients treated with antimalarials. A report of three cases and a review of the literature," *Rheumatology*, vol. 34, no. 2, pp. 166–170, 1995.

[14] J. E. Nord, P. K. Shah, R. Z. Rinaldi, and M. H. Weisman, "Hydroxychloroquine cardiotoxicity in systemic lupus erythematosus: a report of 2 cases and review of the literature," *Seminars in Arthritis and Rheumatism*, vol. 33, no. 5, pp. 336–351, 2004.

[15] K. Tselios, M. Deeb, D. D. Gladman et al., "Antimalarial-induced cardiomyopathy in systemic lupus erythematosus: as rare as considered?" *Journal of Rheumatology*, vol. 46, no. 4, pp. 391–396, 2019.

[16] I. Yajima and L. Larue, "The location of heart melanocytes is specified and the level of pigmentation in the heart may

correlate with coat color," *Pigment Cell & Melanoma Research*, vol. 21, no. 4, pp. 471–476, 2008.
[17] K. Tselios, M. Deeb, D. D. Gladman, P. Harvey, and M. B. Urowitz, "Antimalarial-induced cardiomyopathy: a systematic review of the literature," *Lupus*, vol. 27, no. 4, pp. 591–599, 2018.
[18] M. Azimian, S. H. Gultekin, J. L. Hata et al., "Fatal antimalarial-induced cardiomyopathy: report of 2 cases," *Journal of Clinical Rheumatology*, vol. 18, no. 7, pp. 363–366, 2012.
[19] J. B. Kwon, A. Kleiner, K. Ishida, J. Godown, E. Ciafaloni, and R. J. Looney, "Hydroxychloroquine-induced myopathy," *Journal of Clinical Rheumatology*, vol. 16, no. 1, pp. 28–31, 2010.
[20] S. Pica, D. M. Sado, V. Maestrini et al., "Reproducibility of native myocardial T1 mapping in the assessment of Fabry disease and its role in early detection of cardiac involvement by cardiovascular magnetic resonance," *Journal of Cardiovascular Magnetic Resonance*, vol. 16, no. 1, p. 99, 2014.
[21] T. P. Millard, A. Kirk, and R. Ratnavel, "Cutaneous hyperpigmentation during therapy with hydroxychloroquine," *Clinical and Experimental Dermatology*, vol. 29, no. 1, pp. 92-93, 2004.

25

Three's Company: Coexistence of Silicosis, Scleroderma and Sjogren Syndrome in a Single Patient

Alexis Ziebelman,[1,2] **Shir Raibman-Spector**,[2,3] **and Omer Gendelman**[1,2,4]

[1]*Department of Medicine "B", Sheba Medical Center, Tel-Hashomer, Ramat Gan, Israel*
[2]*Sackler Faculty of Medicine, Tel Aviv University, Tel-Aviv, Israel*
[3]*Department of Medicine "E", Sheba Medical Center, Tel-Hashomer, Ramat Gan, Israel*
[4]*Rheumatology Unit, Sheba Medical Center, Tel-Hashomer, Ramat Gan, Israel*

Correspondence should be addressed to Alexis Ziebelman; aziebelman@gmail.com

Academic Editor: Mario Salazar-Paramo

We describe a patient who presented with silicosis, scleroderma, and Sjogren syndrome all at the same time. The diagnoses in this case are all associated with continuous exposure to crystalline silica at the patient's workplace. The following report discusses this unique presentation.

1. Introduction

The etiology of autoimmune diseases is complex and multifactorial [1]. Genetics has been proven to play a role in the development of autoimmune diseases; however, it is not the sole contributing risk factor. Over the past few years, environmental factors have been found to play a complementary and significant role in the initiation and propagation of different autoimmune diseases and can be linked to up to 70% of all autoimmune diseases [2].

Environmental exposure to crystalline silica is a well-known occupational hazard among those involved in stone quarrying, mining, and sand blasting, and continuous exposure is associated with an increased risk for a variety of silica-related diseases [1, 3]. Silicosis is an inflammatory lung disease that results from inhalation and retention of crystalline silica in the lung [4]. Several forms of clinical silicosis have been reported:

(1) Acute silicosis occurring after relatively short (a few months to as long as 2 years) but intense exposure to high concentrations of silica. Clinical symptoms include fatigue, cough, dyspnea, pleuritic pain, and uncommonly, rapid progression occurs, resulting in respiratory failure [5].

(2) Accelerated silicosis occurs within 10 years from the initial exposure to a large amount of respirable crystalline. Clinical manifestations are variable, ranging from individuals with only abnormal chest imaging without symptoms to those presenting with cough and dyspnea [6].

(3) Chronic silicosis, subdivided into simple (nodular) silicosis and progressive massive fibrosis, occurs after 15–20 years of moderate to low exposure. Clinical symptoms may not appear until years after exposure, ranging from mild cough to severe dyspnea and respiratory failure [7].

In addition, exposure to inhaled silica possesses risks for other pulmonary diseases including lung cancer and tuberculosis [8].

Exposure to crystalline silica has also been found to be associated with the development of various autoimmune diseases including systemic lupus erythematosus (SLE), rheumatoid arthritis, systemic sclerosis, and antineutrophil cytoplasmic antibody (ANCA)-related vasculitis [9].

Autoimmune/inflammatory syndrome induced by adjuvants (ASIA) encompasses diverse inflammatory phenomena that occur due to exposure to an adjuvant. The disease spectrum can vary widely in clinical presentation and extent of severity of the manifestations. It has been reported that some individuals develop constitutional symptoms, antibody production, or worsening of current inflammatory conditions in response to exposure to and adjuvant. Watad et al. first introduced this syndrome in 2011 and considered silica to be an adjuvant [10]. There are also several case reports of women presenting with autoimmune symptoms after silicone breast implantation. De Carvalho and Shoenfeld described a case report of the first patient with silicone breast implantation to develop systemic sclerosis sine scleroderma (ssSSc), an atypical form of systemic sclerosis that lacks skin involvement [11]. Yet, in case-control studies, there is no association seen between the presence of connective tissue disorders and silica exposure [12].

In the current case report, we describe a patient who simultaneously developed three different inflammatory and autoimmune diseases after prolonged exposure to crystalline silica.

The patient is a 52-year-old male, who worked as a marble mason for over 20 years. His medical history is significant for type II diabetes mellitus and smoking. He presented with a 7-month history of polyarthralgia and numbness, mainly involving the palms and feet and accompanied by morning stiffness lasting for one hour. He also suffered from episodic bluish discoloration of fingers and toes upon exposure to cold, which was suggestive of Raynaud's phenomenon. In addition, he noticed recurrent small sores on the tip of his fingers. Finally, he also complained of dry mouth and mild dyspnea over the last year. The patient was then hospitalized for further work-up.

Upon admission, examination of the head and neck revealed an enlarged, smooth, nontender left parotid gland. Physical examination of the hand joints revealed puffy fingers and arthralgia without signs of arthritis over the MCP and PIP joints. Sclerodactyly distal to the MCPs was noted bilaterally, accompanied by pitting scars at the tip of the digits. Pigmentary changes with areas of hypopigmentation were observed over the MCP and PIP joints (Figures 1 and 2). Additionally, the perioral skin was tight with reduced oral aperture.

Laboratory investigations including complete blood count, urinalysis, liver, and renal function tests were within normal limits. The erythrocyte sedimentation rate (ESR) was elevated: 85 mm/h. Rheumatoid factor (RF) and anticyclic citrullinated peptide (CCP) were negative. Antinuclear antibodies (ANA), homogeneous and speckled, were positive with the titer of 1 : 1280 together with high titers of both anti-Ro/SSA and anti-La/SSB (>8, normal 0–0.99) and Scl-70 (>8, normal 0–0.99). HCV Ab and HBV surface Ag and core-Ab were negative.

Chest X-ray demonstrated a bulla and small rounded consolidation in the right upper lobe, while high resolution computed tomography (HRCT) of the chest revealed bilateral apical fibrosis, upwards hilar traction, mediastinal and hilar adenopathy with coarse eggshell calcification, and esophageal dilation (Figure 3).

Spirometry and lung function were as follows: FEV1 77%, FVC 70%, DLCO 84%, TLC 93%, FRC 100%, RV 131%, and SaO_2 98% on room air reflecting a restrictive lung disease pattern.

Accordingly, the patient was diagnosed with pulmonary silicosis, scleroderma, and Sjogren syndrome.

The patient was prescribed methotrexate (10 mg/week), prednisone (5 mg/day), and amlodipine (10 mg/day) and discharged for ambulatory follow-up in the rheumatology and pulmonology outpatient clinics.

2. Discussion

The diagnoses of pulmonary silicosis, scleroderma, and Sjogren syndrome observed in this case are all associated with continuous exposure to crystalline silica at the patient's workplace.

The connection between silicosis and inhalation of crystalline silica is well established [3]. The silica particles are phagocyted by macrophages, which in turn stimulates the production of proinflammatory cytokines such as IL-1 and TNF. In addition, activation of the NALP3 protein inflammasome induces regulatory T cells to express cytotoxic T-lymphocyte antigen 4, IL-10, and transforming growth factor-beta (TGF-β). This process results in lung tissue inflammation and fibrosis [13].

The development of systemic sclerosis after silica exposure is a newer concept, initially described by Erasmus et al. in 1957 based on Witwatersrand gold miners who developed scleroderma [14]. Today, silica exposure is considered a major environmental risk factor for scleroderma [15,16]. A case–control study including 80 cases and 160 matched controls investigating the relation between systemic sclerosis and occupational exposure found a significantly increased OR (odds ratio) for systemic sclerosis following exposure to crystalline silica (OR 5.57, 95% CI 1.69–18.37) [17]. In a meta-analysis by Memuric et al. encompassing 16 series (1101 cases in 3 cohorts and 9 case–control series), assessing the association between silica exposure and scleroderma, only three studies reported lower risk or no association between silica exposure and scleroderma. The combined estimator of relative risk (CERR) for scleroderma was 3.20 (95% CI 1.89–5.43), reaching 15.49 (95% CI 4.54–52.87) for the cohort studies included in the analysis [16]. Finally, a prospective study evaluating the association between systemic sclerosis and occupational exposure to various chemicals and pollutants found an increased risk (OR 5.32, $p < 0.0001$) for systemic sclerosis following exposure to crystalline silica [18].

The direct mechanism of how crystalline silica induces scleroderma is unclear. However, there is a theory that silica particles stimulate and induce responder T cells, but not T regulatory cells, to avoid apoptosis. This imbalance shifts the immune system towards autoimmunity, contributing to the development of scleroderma [19]. Interestingly, scleroderma associated with silica exposure differs clinically from "idiopathic" scleroderma. According to a systematic review by Freire et al., scleroderma associated with silica exhibits a male predominance, is more of the diffuse subtype, and shows lower survival [20]. In a retrospective study of clinical and laboratory features of patients with scleroderma associated with silica ("Erasmus syndrome"), the majority of patients were male (78%), smokers (68%), and presented

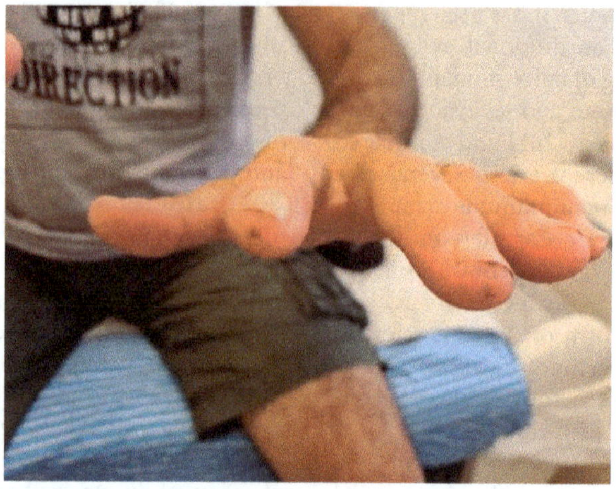

FIGURE 1: Pitting scars at the tip of the digits.

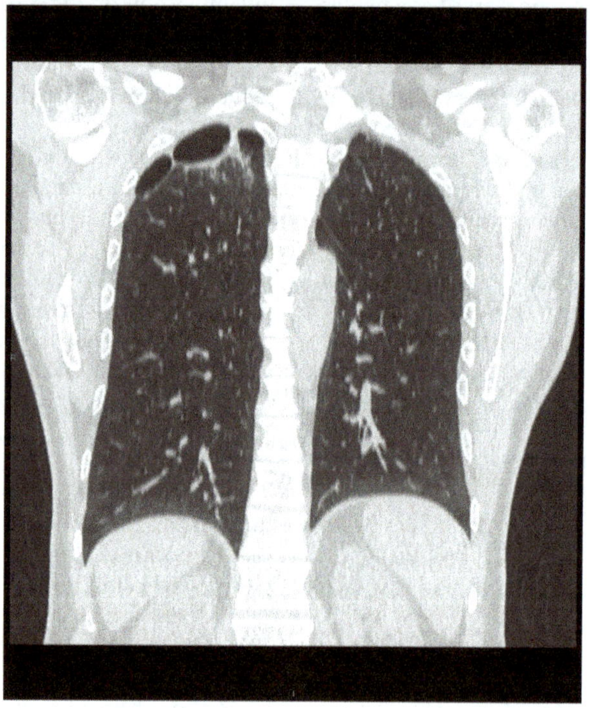

FIGURE 2: Chest CT demonstrating apical fibrosis.

with diffuse scleroderma (67%). Antinuclear antibodies were positive in all patients, while antitopoisomerase I was positive in 44% [21]. It is critical to mention that the observed male predominance might be a reflection of the higher rate of man workers in the mining and dusty industries [22].

Compared with scleroderma, the causality between Sjogren syndrome and silicone exposure is less well understood. There are a few case reports that reported an association, yet the underlying mechanism remains unclear [23, 24]. Colafrancesco et al. considered silicone as an adjuvant, a substance that acts to accelerate, prolong, or enhance antigen-specific immune responses and capable to induce the ASIA syndrome (an autoimmune/inflammatory syndrome induced by adjuvants). The ability of adjuvants to initiate an immune response in the glandular epithelium and the shared symptoms in both Sjogren's and ASIA syndromes may explain the impact of silicone on the pathogenesis of Sjogren syndrome [25].

It is also critical to note that in patients with scleroderma, an association exists with Sjogren syndrome that can reach up to 10%, irrespective of occupational exposure [26]. Furthermore, anti-Ro antibody positive disease, such as in this patient, has been noted to account for 20% of scleroderma cases [27]. Anti-Ro positivity is itself a worse prognostic factor and can be viewed independently of the silica stimulation pathway and must be considered in this patient [28].

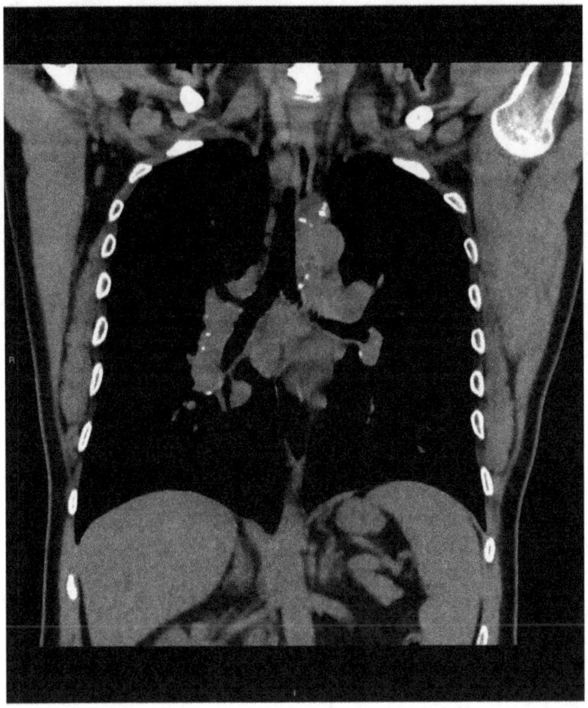

FIGURE 3: Chest CT: mediastinal and hilar adenopathy with coarse eggshell classification.

Exposure to crystalline silica is a significant occupational hazard for a variety of immune-mediated diseases. Scleroderma and Sjogren syndrome, appearing simultaneously in our patient after continuous exposure to silica, are both noncurable autoimmune diseases, associated with significant morbidity and increased mortality. As modifiable risk factors for autoimmune diseases are scarce, active surveillance, screening, and protective measures must be initiated in those with hazardous exposure to crystalline silica. Hopefully, this will decrease the prevalence of the diseases associated with such exposure in the future.

References

[1] M. F. Khan and H. Wang, "Environmental exposures and autoimmune diseases: contribution of gut microbiome," *Frontiers in Immunology*, vol. 10, p. 3094, 2020.

[2] A. Vojdani, K. M. Pollard, and A. W. Campbell, "Environmental triggers and autoimmunity," *Autoimmune Diseases*, vol. 2014, Article ID 798029, 2 pages, 2014.

[3] R. F. Hoy and D. C. Chambers, "Silica-related diseases in the modern world," *Allergy*, vol. 75, no. 11, pp. 2805–2817, 2020.

[4] R. K. Sharma, A. K. Sharma, and A. Sharma, "Erasmus syndrome: association of silicosis and systemic sclerosis," *Indian Dermatol Online J*, vol. 9, no. 3, pp. 185–187, 2018.

[5] M. I. Greenberg, J. Waksman, and J. Curtis, *Disease-a-Month*, vol. 53, no. 8, pp. 394–416, 2007.

[6] V. Leso, L. Fontana, R. Romano, P. Gervetti, and I. Iavicoli, "Artificial stone associated silicosis: a systematic Review," *International Journal of Environmental Research and Public Health*, vol. 16, no. 4, p. 568, 2019.

[7] R. A. Cohen, A. Patel, and F. H. Green, "Lung disease caused by exposure to coal mine and silica dust," *Seminars in Respiratory and Critical Care Medicine*, vol. 29, no. 06, pp. 651-661, 2008.

[8] T. Sato, T. Shimosato, and D. M. Klinman, "Silicosis and lung cancer: current perspectives," *Lung Cancer: Targets and Therapy*, vol. 9, pp. 91-101, 2018.

[9] J. M. Mayeux, G. M. Escalante, J. M. Christy, R. D. Pawar, D. H. Kono, and K. M. Pollard, "Silicosis and Silica-induced autoimmunity in the diversity outbred mouse," *Frontiers in Immunology*, vol. 9, p. 874, 2018.

[10] A. Watad, K. Sharif, and Y. Shoenfeld, "The ASIA syndrome: basic concepts," *Mediterranean Journal of Rheumatology*, vol. 28, no. 2, pp. 64-69, 2017.

[11] J. F. de Carvalho and Y. Shoenfeld, "Systemic sclerosis sine scleroderma after silicone breast implants," *Journal of Clinical Rheumatology*, vol. 39, 2020.

[12] J. G. Hortolam, J. F. Carvalho, and S. Appenzeller, "Connective tissue diseases following silicone breast implantation: where do we stand?" *Clinics*, vol. 68, no. 3, p. 281, 2013.

[13] H. Barnes, N. S. L. Goh, T. L. Leong, and R. Hoy, "Silica-associated lung disease: an old-world exposure in modern industries," *Respirology*, vol. 24, no. 12, pp. 1165–1175, 2019.

[14] L. D. Erasmus, "Scleroderma in goldminers on the Witwatersrand with particular reference to pulmonary manifestations," *South African Journal of Laboratory and Clinical Medicine*, vol. 3, no. 3, pp. 209–231, 1957.

[15] U. F. Haustein, V. Ziegler, K. Herrmann, J. Mehlhorn, and C. Schmidt, "Silica-induced scleroderma," *Journal of the American Academy of Dermatology*, vol. 22, no. 3, pp. 444–448, 1990.

[16] Z. D. Mc Cormic, S. S. Khuder, B. K. Aryal, A. L. Ames, and S. A. Khuder, "Occupational silica exposure as a risk factor for scleroderma: a meta-analysis," *International Archives of Occupational and Environmental Health*, vol. 83, no. 7, pp. 763–769, 2010.

[17] E. Diot, V. Lesire, J. L. Guilmot et al., *Occupational and Environmental Medicine*, vol. 59, no. 8, pp. 545–549, 2002.

[18] I. Marie, J.-F. Gehanno, M. Bubenheim et al., "Prospective study to evaluate the association between systemic sclerosis and occupational exposure and review of the literature," *Autoimmunity Reviews*, vol. 13, no. 2, pp. 151–156, 2014.

[19] S. Lee, H. Hayashi, H. Mastuzaki, N. Kumagai-Takei, and T. Otsuki, "Silicosis and autoimmunity," *Current Opinion in Allergy and Clinical Immunology*, vol. 17, no. 2, pp. 78–84, 2017.

[20] M. Freire, M. Alonso, A. Rivera et al., "Clinical peculiarities of patients with scleroderma exposed to silica: a systematic review of the literature," *Seminars in Arthritis and Rheumatism*, vol. 45, no. 3, pp. 294–300, 2015.

[21] L. F. Rocha, A. P. Luppino Assad, R. G. Marangoni, A. P. T. Del Rio, J. F. Marques-Neto, and P. D. Sampaio-Barros, "Systemic sclerosis and silica exposure: a rare association in a large Brazilian cohort," *Rheumatology International*, vol. 36, no. 5, pp. 697–702, 2016.

[22] M. T. Turner, S. R. Samuel, E. J. Silverstone, and D. H. Yates, "Silica exposure and connective tissue disease: an under-recognized association in three Australian artificial stone workers," *American Journal of Respiratory and Critical Care Medicine*, vol. 201, no. 3, pp. 378–380, 2020.

[23] L. Astudillo, L. Sailler, M. Ecoiffier, J. Giron, B. Couret, and E. Arlet-Suau, "Exposure to silica and primary Sjögren's syndrome in a dental technician," *Rheumatology*, vol. 42, no. 10, pp. 1268-1269, 2003.

[24] F. Puisieux, E. Hachulla, M. Brouillard, P. Hatron, and

B. Devulder, "Silicosis and primary Sjögren's syndrome," *La Revue de Medecine Interne*, vol. 15, no. 9, pp. 575–579, 1994.

[25] S. Colafrancesco, C. Perricone, R. Priori, G. Valesini, and Y. Shoenfeld, "Sjögren's syndrome: another facet of the autoimmune/inflammatory syndrome induced by adjuvants (ASIA)," *Journal of Autoimmunity*, vol. 51, pp. 10–16, 2014.

[26] A. Balbir-Gurman and Y. Braun-Moscovici, "Scleroderma overlap syndrome," *The Israel Medical Association Journal*, vol. 13, no. 1, pp. 14–20, 2011.

[27] M. Hudson, J. Pope, M. Mahler, S. Tatibouet, R. Steele, and M. Baron, "clinical significance of antibodies to ro52/TRIM21 in systemic sclerosis," *Arthritis Research and Therapy*, vol. 14, no. 2, p. R50, 2012.

[28] A. A. Drosos, A. P. Andonopoulos, J. S. Costopoulos, E. D. Stavropoulos, C. S. Papadimitriou, and H. M. Moutsopoulos, "Sjögren's syndrome in progressive systemic sclerosis," *Journal of Rheumatology*, vol. 15, no. 6, pp. 965–968, 1988.

26

Pneumomediastinum as a Manifestation of Granulomatosis with Polyangiitis

Ahmed Alhazmi,[1] Mohamed Moulaye Cheikh,[2] and Rola Yousef Hassan[1]

[1]*Department of Medicine, Division of Rheumatology, King Fahad Armed Forces Hospital, Jeddah, Saudi Arabia*
[2]*Doctor Soliman Fakeeh Hospital, Jeddah, Saudi Arabia*

Correspondence should be addressed to Rola Yousef Hassan; r.toufiq@hotmail.com

Academic Editor: Mehmet Soy

A 38-year-old hypertensive male with a smoking history presented to the emergency room with significant hemoptysis, arthritis, and a purpuric rash. Other findings included a dropping hemoglobin and acute kidney injury with microscopic hematuria. The pulmonary computed tomography was significant for alveolar hemorrhage and a rarely reported pneumomediastinum. Along with this constellation of findings, a positive antiproteinase 3 helped to confirm this patient's diagnosis of granulomatosis with polyangiitis. Treatment commenced with sessions of plasma exchange and pulse steroids along with cyclophosphamide infusions. The patient had since improved and made a full recovery. This case report highlights the rarely described pneumomediastinum in association with vasculitides.

1. Introduction

Vasculitides are a group of uncommonly seen and diverse inflammatory diseases that affect blood vessels. These conditions may arise unprompted or may be precipitated by an underlying disease. It was first classified by the American College of Rheumatology in 1990 [1], with the Chapel Hill Consensus Conference providing a nomenclature system that more comprehensively covers all types of vasculitides, last updated in 2012 [2]. The most widely known branch of vasculitides is the antineutrophil cytoplasmic antibody-positive vasculitis (ANCA) which encompasses microscopic polyangiitis (MPA), granulomatosis with polyangiitis (GPA), and eosinophilic granulomatosis with polyangiitis (EGPA) [2].

GPA is a necrotizing, granulomatous vasculitis which affects multiple organs including the upper and lower respiratory tract and the kidneys [3]. Common pulmonary radiographic features include nodules, reticulations, segmental atelectasis, widespread opacities associated with air bronchograms, pleural lesions, and rarely hilar lymphadenopathy [4]. The most serious respiratory complication of this disease is alveolar hemorrhage, necessitating aggressive therapy with plasma-pharesis and immunosuppressive drugs [5].

Pneumomediastinum is the existence of air in the mediastinal cavity. This condition can either present spontaneously or secondary to manipulation of the patient's respiratory and digestive systems by trauma, infections, a perforated viscus, or via medical interventions [6]. Data reporting associations between pneumonediastinum and rheumatological diseases are limited, and this association, however, was more commonly pronounced in patients with concomitant interstitial lung disease, as with inflammatory myopathies, systemic lupus erythematosus and systemic sclerosis [7]. There was a case report published in 2014 documenting a presentation of pneumomediastinum in a patient with microscopic polyangitis that was preceded by interstitial pneumonia [8].

2. The Case Report

We are presenting the case of a 38-year-old male who was previously known to be hypertensive and a heavy smoker. He had presented to the emergency room with a 10-day history of productive cough which was associated initially with blood-tinged sputum but had escalated to massive hemoptysis. Further examination revealed the presence of arthritis and a purpuric rash scattered over his lower limbs (Figures 1 and 2). His arthritis was polyarticular, affecting mainly the small joints of the hands (the right first, second, and third proximal interphalangeal joints and the left second proximal interphalangeal joint were tender), and an ultrasound also confirmed grade 1 synovitis in both wrists.

The laboratory investigations were significant for a dropping hemoglobin, acute kidney injury, and microscopic hematuria (Table 1). On admission, his chest x-ray showed extensive bilateral ground glass opacities (Figure 3). A pulmonary high-resolution computed tomography (HRCT) was ordered for further assessment and demonstrated evidence of alveolar hemorrhage in the form of diffuse scattered patchy areas of ground glass opacities in both lungs involving all lobes except the apical segments of the upper lung lobes and the subpleuretic areas (Figure 4). There was also a linear lucency noted in the left mediastinum representing pneumomediastinum (Figure 4). A preliminary diagnosis of pulmonary renal vasculitis was made, and a full autoimmune panel was sent.

A few hours after admission, the patient had developed significant hypoxia mandating transfer to the intensive care unit where he was stabilized and promptly started on pulse steroids (methylprednisone 1 gram intravenous daily) and plasma exchange sessions. He required intubation and mechanical ventilation two days after his admission due to deteriorating pulmonary functions and the development of acute respiratory distress syndrome. The patient was started urgently on cyclophosphamide 750 mg intravascular infusion according to the National Institute of Health protocol. He underwent a skin biopsy which gave no evidence of vasculitis. A bronchoalveolar lavage was also performed and grew *Pseudomonas* and *Alicyclobacillus* for which he received colistin and tigecycline for a probable health-care-associated pneumonia (HCAP). After bronchoscopy, the patient had developed right pneumothorax which required the insertion of a chest tube.

The patient's overall condition gradually improved after receiving five sessions of plasma exchange and 5 days of pulse steroids. He was extubated and transferred to the medical ward. His test results came back positive for C antineutrophil cytoplasmic antibodies (cANCA) with a titer of 1 : 20 and anti-proteinase 3 (PR3), whilst P antineutrophil cytoplasmic antibodies (pANCA), myeloperoxidase (MPO), and the antiglomerular basement membrane (anti GBM) were negative (Table 1). A final diagnosis of granulomatosis with polyangitis was made after the exclusion of other causes. The differential included systemic lupus erythematosus which was ruled out based on the absence of supportive clinical features and autoantibodies (Table 1). Other differentials included Goodpasture's syndrome which was deemed less likely with negative anti-GBM and as this condition is not associated with arthritis or purpura. Other small vessel vasculitides such as eosinophilic granulomatosis with polyangitis and microscopic polyangitis were also less likely given that the patient gave no prior history of bronchial asthma, his investigation showed no eosinophilia, and a negative P ANCA/MPO (Table 1).

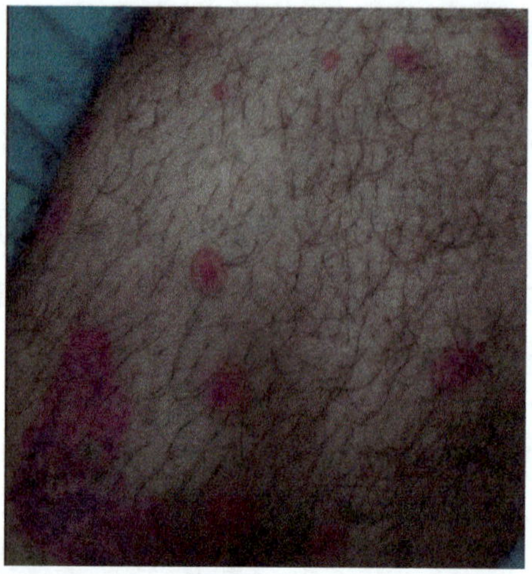

FIGURE 1: Purpuric rash scattered over the patient's lower limbs.

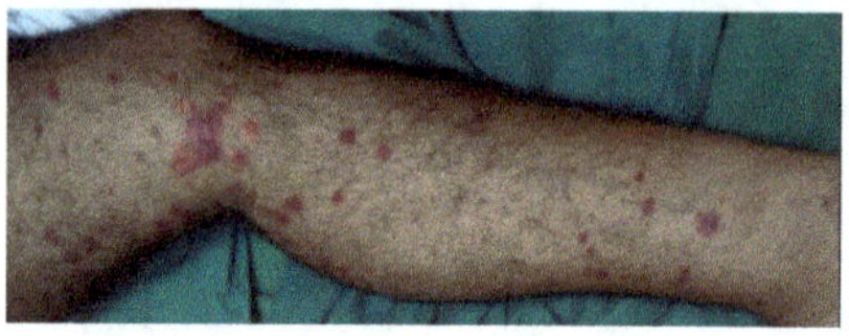

FIGURE 2: Purpuric rash scattered over the patient's lower limbs.

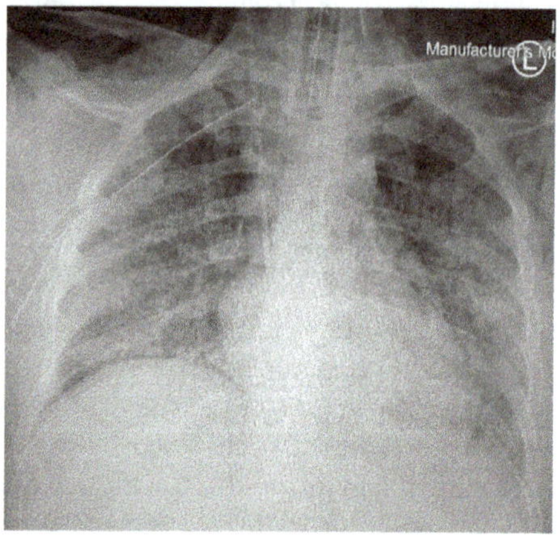

FIGURE 3: Admission chest X-ray showing bilateral extensive ground glass opacities.

The patient had received a second dose of cyclophosphamide during his stay. After a month spent in the hospital, the patient was discharged in a stable condition and given follow-up doses of cyclophosphamide along with tapering steroids in the outpatient setting. A repeated HRCT conducted 12 months after his initial presentation showed complete resolution of his ground glass opacities and pneumomediastinum (Figure 5).

3. Discussion

GPA is a multisystemic disease with involvement mainly affecting the respiratory and renal systems [3]. One of the earliest and most impactful papers that closely studied the

TABLE 1: Laboratory investigations.

	Pretreatment	3 months after treatment
White blood cells	10.9 × 109	8.67 × 109
Absolute neutrophil count	5.6 × 109	8.1 × 109
Absolute lymphocyte count	1.9 × 109/L	3.9 × 109/L
Absolute eosinophil count	0.2 × 109/L	0.108 × 109/L
Hemoglobin	8.68 g/dL	12.9 g/dL
Platelet	265 × 109	334 × 109
Creatinine	120 umol/L	114 umol/L
Urea	14 nmol/L	14 umol/L
C-reactive protein	6.5 mg/L	5.5 mg/L
Erythrocyte sedimentation rate	110 MM/HR	17 MM/HR
Urine analysis		
Blood	+3	+1
Red blood cells	+2 (10–34 cells)	Negative
Protein	Negative	Negative
White blood cells	Negative	Negative
Casts	No casts seen	No casts seen
Antinuclear Ab	<1 : 40	
P ANCA	<1 : 20	<1 : 20
C ANCA (indirect immunofluorescence assay)	1 : 20	<1 : 20
PR3	26.2 kU/L	
MPO	1.4 kU/L	
Anti-GBM Ab	0.9 U/mL	

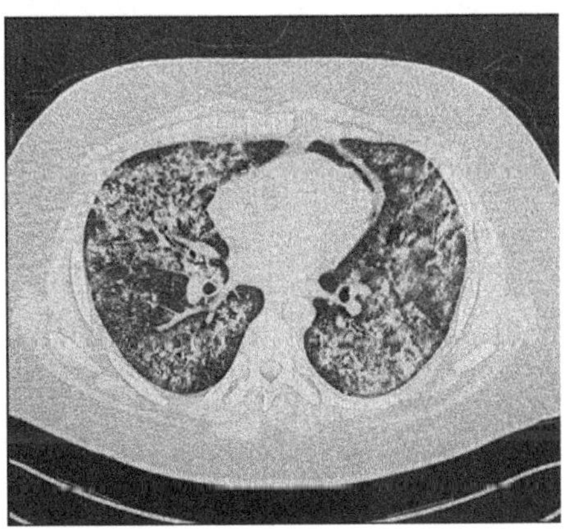

FIGURE 4: Pretreatment high resolution computed tomography.

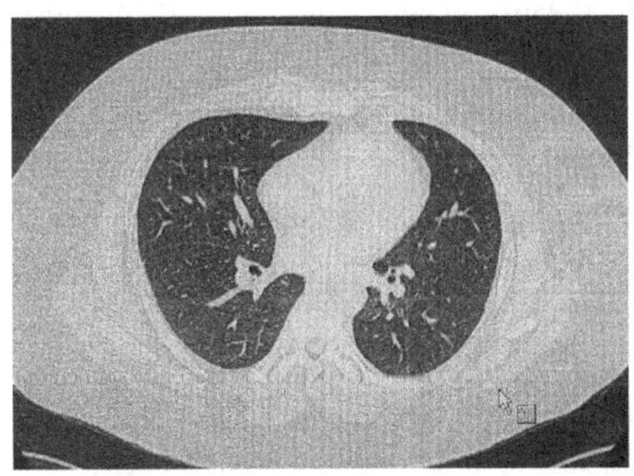

FIGURE 5: Posttreatment high resolution computed tomography.

pattern of GPA lung involvement is the article by Cordier et al. [4]. The authors had characterized the patterns and frequencies of pulmonary findings in 77 patients with biopsy proven GPA. Of this population of patients, 53 "69%" had presented with nodular manifestations, while the occurrence of infiltrates was found in 41 patients "53%." The incidence of pleural effusions was established in 9 patients "12%," and only 3 patients "4%" had developed atelectasis. Furthermore, alveolar hemorrhage as a presenting symptom was only reported in 6 patients (8%), and in contrast to our case report findings, pneumomediastinum had not developed in any of these cases.

Pneumomediastinum is the presence of air in the mediastinum. This phenomenon may occur either due to an underlying precipitant or even with the lack thereof. Trauma, infections, and procedures are all known culprits [6]. At the time of our patient's presentation, he had none of these well-described secondary causes. Caceres et al. [6] had further described a different set of factors that could predispose to the development of spontaneous pneumomediastinum. These factors include smoking, inhaled drugs, and airway lung disease such as asthma and chronic obstructive pulmonary disease, as well as idiopathic pulmonary fibrosis. Although smoking was present in our case and might have been a contributing factor to the patient's development of pneumomediastinum, a direct causality relationship cannot be substantiated as the patient had also presented with an active vasculitic lung pathology.

Associations between pneumomediastinum and autoimmune diseases have been scarcely mentioned in the literature. These associations were mainly seen in conditions with a predilection for the development of interstitial lung disease. There have been a few case reports linking pneumomediastinum with systemic sclerosis, systemic lupus erythematosus, and rheumatoid arthritis [9–11]. Pneumomediastinum was also found to be predictive of poor prognosis in patients with dermatomyositis [12]. However, regarding associations with ANCA vasculitis, the only report found was in a patient with a preexisting interstitial pneumonia who developed microscopic polyangitis [8].

Histopathological features of vasculitic pulmonary affection had been delineated by Homma et al. [13] who had studied 31 patients with myeloperoxidase ANCA-associated vasculitis and pulmonary fibrosis. Findings included vasculitic changes in pulmonary arteries and arterioles in three cases each and in capillaries presenting with alveolar hemorrhages in two cases. The characteristic histological features of vasculitis found in pulmonary arterioles were leukocytoclastic angiitis, intimal elastofibrosis with destroyed elastic fibers, and granulomatous angiitis, each in one of the three cases mentioned. Proposed underlying mechanisms for pneumomediastinum on the other hand may include mucosal necrosis in the airways as a result of vasculitic processes at the level of bronchial arterioles, a process that may also manifest with cutaneous vasculopathy, suggest Kono et al. who had studied patients with dermatomyositis and pneumomediastinum [14]. Based on previously laid data, we can extrapolate the pathological pathway of our case, which may have started with mucosal necrosis secondary to GPA vasculitis and subsequent rupture of vulnerable alveolar connective tissue leading to the development of pneumomediastinum.

We hope to further enrich the medical literature with our addition of the first documented association of GPA and pneumomediastinum and to pave the way for more research in this field.

References

[1] D. A. Bloch, B. A. Michel, G. G. Hunder et al., "The American college of rheumatology 1990 criteria for the classification of vasculitis: patients and methods," *Arthritis & Rheumatism*, vol. 33, pp. 1068–1073, 1990.

[2] J. C. Jennette, R. J. Falk, P. A. Bacon et al., "2012 revised international Chapel Hill Consensus conference nomenclature of vasculitides," *Arthritis & Rheumatism*, vol. 65, no. 1, pp. 1-11, 2013.

[3] R. J. Falk, W. L. Gross, L. Guillevin et al., "Granulomatosis with polyangiitis (Wegener's): an alternative name for Wegener's granulomatosis," *Arthritis & Rheumatism*, vol. 63, no. 4, pp. 863-864, 2011, þ.

[4] J.-F. Cordier, D. Valeyre, L. Guillevin, R. Loire, and J.-M. Brechot, "Pulmonary Wegener's granulomatosis," *Chest*, vol. 97, no. 4, pp. 906–912, 1990.

[5] M. Yates, R. A. Watts, I. M. Bajema et al., "EULAR/ERA-EDTA recommendations for the management of ANCA-associated vasculitis," *Annals of the Rheumatic Diseases*, vol. 75, no. 9, pp. 1583–1594, 2016.

[6] M. Caceres, S. Z. Ali, R. Braud, D. Weiman, and H. E. Garrett, "Spontaneous pneumomediastinum: a comparative study and review of the literature," *The Annals of Thoracic Surgery*, vol. 86, no. 3, pp. 962–966, 2008.

[7] E. J. Dein, K. Lee, H. Timlin, and L. Hummers, "Spontaneous pneumomediastinum in limited cutaneous systemic sclerosis and myositis overlap," *BMJ Case Reports*, vol. 2018, pp. bcr-2018, 2018.

[8] K. Isoda, T. Takeuchi, T. Ishida, S. Makino, and T. Hanafusa, "Pneumomediastinum in a patient with microscopic polyangiitis preceded by interstitial pneumonia," *Internal Medicine*, vol. 53, no. 8, pp. 891–893, 2014.

[9] M. Haroon, P. McLaughlin, M. Henry, and S. Harney, "Spontaneous pneumomediastinum in a patient with anti-centromere antibody-positive limited scleroderma," *Journal of Clinical Rheumatology*, vol. 17, no. 1, pp. 42-43, 2011.

[10] S. O. Paria and S. Roverano, "Bilateral pneumothorax and mediastinal emphysema in systemic lupus erythematosus," *Clinical Rheumatology*, vol. 11, no. 4, pp. 571–573, 1992.

[11] A. Patel, B. Kesler, and R. A. Wise, "Persistent pneumomediastinum in interstitial fibrosis associated with rheumatoid arthritis," *Chest*, vol. 117, no. 6, pp. 1809–1813, 2000.

[12] B. Le Goff, P. Chérin, A. Cantagrel et al., "Pneumomediastinum in interstitial lung disease associated with dermatomyositis and polymyositis," *Arthritis Care & Research*, vol. 61, no. 1, pp. 108–118, 2008.

[13] S. Homma, H. Matsushita, and K. Nakata, "Pulmonary fibrosis in myeloperoxidase antineutrophil cytoplasmic antibody-associated vasculitides," *Respirology*, vol. 9, no. 2, pp. 190–196, 2004.

[14] H. Kono, S. Inokuma, H. Nakayama, and M. Suzuki, "Pneumomediastinum in dermatomyositis: association with cutaneous vasculopathy," *Annals of the Rheumatic Diseases*, vol. 59, no. 5, pp. 372–376, 2000.

27

A Case Report of Statin-Induced Immune-Mediated Necrotizing Myopathy Treatment Challenges

Anwar I. Joudeh[1] **Mhd Kutaiba Albuni,**[2] **Sara Seife Hassen,**[2] **Phool Iqbal,**[2,3] **Elsaid Mohamed Aziz Bedair,**[4] **and Salah Mahdi**[1]

[1]*Department of Internal Medicine, Al-Khor Hospital, Hamad Medical Corporation, Doha, Postcode 3050, Qatar*
[2]*Department of Internal Medicine, Hamad General Hospital, Hamad Medical Corporation, Doha, Postcode 3050, Qatar*
[3]*Department of Critical Care, Hamad General Hospital, Hamad Medical Corporation, Doha, Postcode 3050, Qatar*
[4]*Department of Radiology, Al-Khor Hospital, Hamad Medical Corporation, Doha, Postcode 3050, Qatar*

Correspondence should be addressed to Anwar I. Joudeh; anwarjoudeh@gmail.com

Academic Editor: Mario Salazar-Paramo

Statin-induced necrotizing autoimmune myopathy is an immune-mediated necrotizing myopathy related to the use of statins. It is a very rare disease, which usually presents with proximal muscle weakness and frank elevation in creatine kinase levels. Stopping statin and the use of immunosuppressive therapy are considered the mainstay therapy. Use of steroids in patients with inflammatory myopathy can be complicated by steroid-induced myopathy. Herein, we present a case of a 55-year-old patient with statin-induced necrotizing autoimmune myopathy based on the presence of proximal muscle weakness, magnetic resonance findings, suggestive muscle biopsy features, and positive anti-HMGCR autoantibodies. The patient was treated with triple immunosuppressive therapy with a particularly good response to intravenous immunoglobulin. This report highlights the importance of timely diagnosis and early use of combined immunosuppressive therapy to improve patients' outcome affected by this rare disease.

1. Introduction

Statins are among the most commonly prescribed medications for primary and secondary prevention of cardiovascular disease in eligible patients. Statin-associated muscle symptoms represent a wide spectrum of clinical manifestations ranging from nonspecific muscle aches to severe necrotizing myositis [1]. Statin-induced immune-mediated necrotizing myopathy (IMNM) is a distinctive disease that persists and sometimes progresses after withdrawal of the statin [2]. The exact pathophysiological mechanism of this condition is not fully understood, but it is postulated that development of anti-3-hydroxy-3-methylglutaryl-coenzyme A reductase (anti-HMGCR) autoantibodies is linked to statin exposure in genetically susceptible patients particularly those with class II major histocompatibility complex (MHC) allele DRB1*11:01 [3]. In vivo studies also supported the pathogenic effect of anti-HMGCR antibodies on myofiber injury through a complement-mediated mechanism which makes complement-targeting therapies and plasma exchange plausible treatment options [4]. Herein, we describe treatment challenges of a 55-year-old man who developed statin-induced IMNM 30 months after starting atorvastatin.

2. Case Presentation

A 55-year-old male patient with a history of type 2 diabetes mellitus, hypertension, and dyslipidemia presented to the family clinic for a periodic review. He was noticed to have high liver enzymes; therefore, the general practitioner stopped atorvastatin 20 mg which was originally prescribed two and a half year ago. Upon further questioning, he reported a history of fatigability with a 7-kilogram weight loss over the past 1 year. Ultrasound abdomen done at that time was only remarkable for mild fatty infiltration of the liver, and his hepatitis profile was negative. Five months later, the patient presented to the emergency department complaining of progressive muscle weakness with pain and a difficulty in standing up from the sitting position and holding his arms above the head. He had no anorexia, difficulty of swallowing, diplopia, numbness, or lower limb claudication. He had no skin rash, joint pain, or morning stiffness, and there was no family history of malignancy, autoimmune diseases, or neuromuscular disorders. His current medications included only metformin and lisinopril.

On initial assessment, his vital signs were within the normal range. Musculoskeletal examination revealed proximal muscle weakness that is greater in the lower extremities (upper limb power 4/5 proximally and 5/5 distally, lower limb power 2/5 proximally and 4/5 distally). He had normal muscle tone, reflexes, and sensory examination. The rest of systemic examination was also noncontributory. Laboratory investigations revealed a significant rise in creatinine kinase (CK) 11029 IU, aspartate aminotransferase (AST) 275 U/L, alanine aminotransferase (ALT) 365 U/L, lactic dehydrogenase (LDH) 799 U/L, and myoglobin 1822 ng/ml. However, gamma-glutamyltransferase (GGT), alkaline phosphatase (ALP), thyroid-stimulating hormone, renal functions, serum electrolytes, haemoglobin A1C, full blood count, and vitamin D and B12 levels were all within the normal range.

Computed tomography of the chest, abdomen, and pelvis was performed to rule out any associated occult malignancy, and it was unremarkable. Magnetic resonance imaging of both thighs showed diffuse signal changes exhibiting hyperintense signal on T2 and STIR sequences involving bilateral adductor groups and posterior compartment muscles of the thighs giving the picture of myositis (Figure 1).

Electromyography (EMG) study reported irritable myopathy with severe involvement of the proximal muscles suggestive of immune-mediated necrotizing myopathy. Subsequently, a muscle biopsy was performed which showed rare necrotic fibers without regenerating fibers or inflammatory changes. We checked anti-HMGCR antibodies' level which came back positive with a value of 208.1 CU (normal: less than 20). The rest of autoimmune workup for myositis was negative including anti-SSA 52KD antibody, ANA, anti-Jo-1, anti-La, anti-Scl70, anti-U1 RNP, anti-U2 RNP, anti-U3 RNP, anti-PL-12, anti-PL-7, anti-OJ, anti-EJ, anti-SRP, anti-Ku, anti-PM/SCL100, anti-Mi-2, anti-TIF-1, anti-MDA5, and anti-NXP-2 antibodies.

Based on the above discussion, the patient was diagnosed to have statin-induced IMNM and was started on pulse steroid therapy with intravenous methylprednisolone at 1000 mg daily for 3 days followed by prednisolone 60 mg daily together with intravenous immunoglobulin (IVIG) at 0.4 gm/kg daily for 5 days. He showed significant improvement of muscle strength, and CK dropped from 14866 U/L on the day of starting immunosuppressive therapy to 4800 U/L five days later. With the help of intensive physiotherapy, he was able to ambulate without assistance and was discharged home on oral prednisolone 40 mg daily in a tapering dose.

Despite the initial improvement in this patient clinical status, he presented 3 weeks after discharge from hospital with worsening muscle weakness without increase in muscle enzymes (CK = 2350 U/L). Upon further inquiry, the patient stated that he used a double dose of oral steroids without tapering by mistake. In the assumption of possible steroid-induced myopathy, he was admitted again for gradual tapering of steroids and introduction of methotrexate as a steroid-sparing agent. His blood glucose readings remained within the acceptable range during his readmission, and he was commenced on another cycle of IVIG for 5 days together with intensive physiotherapy. Thereafter, the patient was transferred to a long-term rehabilitation facility for around four weeks and was maintained on prednisolone 10 mg daily, methotrexate 20 mg weekly, folic acid 5 mg once weekly, and monthly IVIG at 1 gm/kg.

During the subsequent six months, the patient had recurrent relapses of muscle weakness alongside increase in muscle enzymes each time prednisolone dose was tapered to less than 10 mg daily despite keeping him on monthly IVIG and a weekly dose of methotrexate at 20 mg orally. Therefore, 1 gm of intravenous rituximab infusion was given after counseling the patient about its associated pros and cons, and a repeated dose was given two weeks later. Nevertheless, the patient was still requiring monthly infusion of IVIG for relapsing muscle weakness on the subsequent six months of rituximab use.

3. Discussion

Statin-induced IMNM is a rare side effect of statin intake that complicates their use in two to three patients for every 100,000 individuals exposed to statin [5]. It is considered as a pure autoimmune myopathy that does not improve after withdrawal of the medication and responds to immunosuppressive therapy [6]. Patients with statin-induced IMNM usually have progressive proximal muscle weakness, high serum muscle enzyme levels (CK levels ranging between 2,000 and 20,000 IU/L), myopathic features on electromyography, and muscle fiber necrosis and regeneration with scarce inflammation [7].

Unlike self-limited forms of statin myotoxicity, the pharmacological properties of statins (being hydrophilic or lipophilic, dose of statin used) do not seem to be associated with the development of statin-induced IMNM. However, atorvastatin, simvastatin, and pravastatin were linked to confirmed cases of statin-induced IMNM although this association could be linked to prescribing practice and do not necessarily indicate a causal relationship [8–10]. In a case series by Grable-Esposito et al. on twenty-five patients with statin-induced IMNM, the average duration of treatment with statin prior to onset of symptoms was three years with a range of two months to ten years [9]. The patient in our case was diagnosed with this condition 30 months after using atorvastatin although he started to develop symptoms around one year prior to diagnosis.

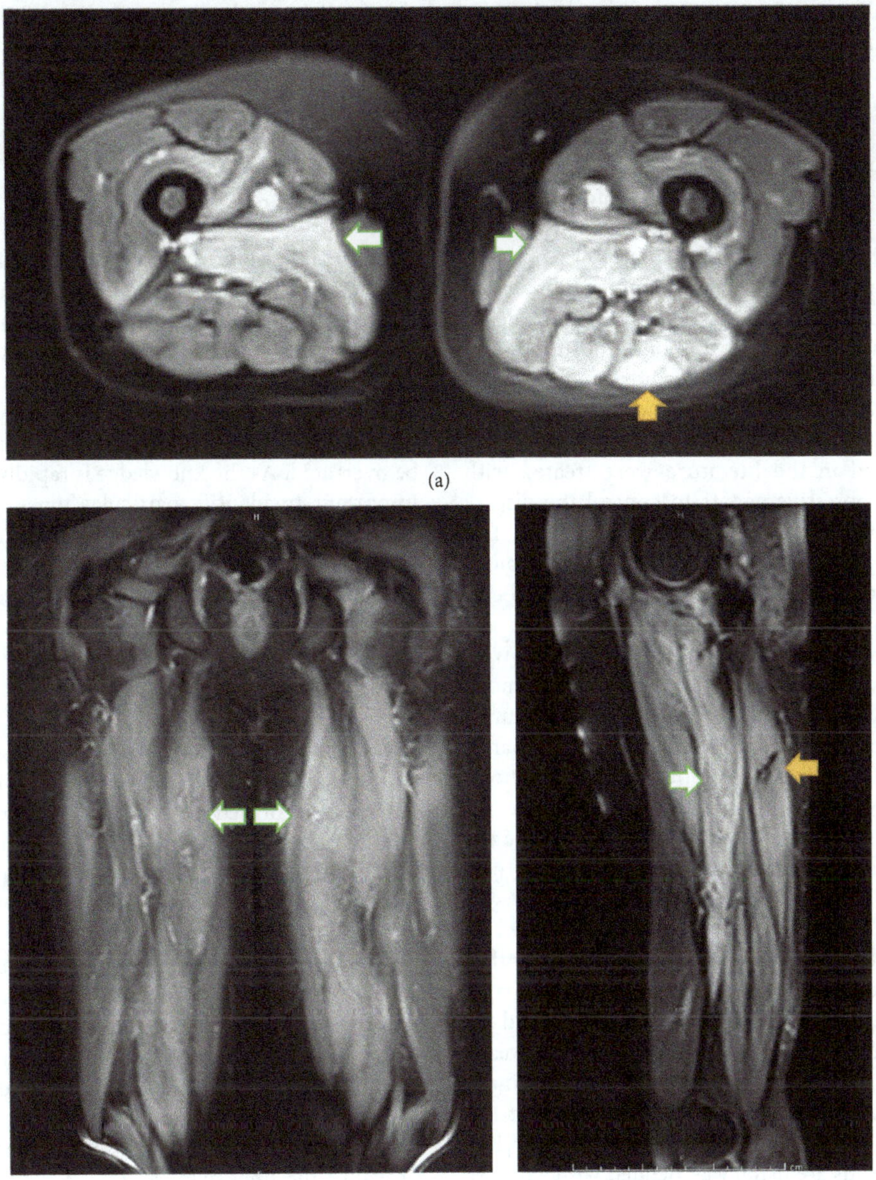

(a)

(b) (c)

FIGURE 1: MRI of both thighs ((a) T2 tse fat sat axial, (b) T2-tirm-fs coronal, and (c) T2 tse-fs sagittal left thigh) showing a considerable degree of slightly heterogenous relative hyperintensity of the adductor muscles of both thighs (white arrows) as well as the hamstring muscles of the left thigh (yellow arrows) with no gross increased volume of the muscles appearance. These findings raise the possibility of partial atrophy and intrasubstance edema possibly due to the effects of chronic myositis/myopathy with secondary early muscle atrophic changes.

Identification of anti-HMGCR antibodies supports the diagnosis of statin-induced IMNM in the appropriate clinical settings with a high sensitivity and specificity (94.4% and 99.3%, respectively) [6, 11]. Nevertheless, not all patients with positive anti-HMGCR antibodies were exposed to statins [12]. According to Mammen et al., around one-third of patients with anti-HMGCR-positive IMNM were not exposed to statin before and those patients were characteristically younger with higher levels of inflammation [12]. In fact, IMNM is considered a heterogenous disease. In 2016, the European Neuromuscular Center categorized IMNM into three subtypes: anti-signal recognition particle (anti-SRP) myopathy, anti-HMGCR myopathy (statin-exposed and nonstatin exposed), and antibody-negative IMNM. Although these subtypes share many common clinicopathological features, they are distinct categories with variable degrees of muscle involvement severity, extramuscular involvement, and response to individual therapies [13].

Werner et al. studied the association of anti-HMGCR antibodies with disease activity and serum muscle enzyme level in 55 patients with anti-HMGCR-positive IMNM (including 40 patients exposed to statin). The authors found that the initial levels of anti-HMGCR antibodies correlated with serum muscle enzyme levels and muscle weakness in all patients, and they found declining antibody titers and improved muscle strength with immunosuppressive therapy.

However, statistically significant improvement was only noticed in statin-induced anti-HMGCR-positive IMNM suggesting a phenotypically different disease between statin-induced and statin-unexposed anti-HMGCR-positive patients [14].

Till date, there are no clinical trials to guide management of statin-induced IMNM. Most treatment recommendations were mainly based on observational evidence, case series, and previous experience of other inflammatory myopathies [7, 15]. However, early identification, stopping statin, and a combination of immunosuppressive therapy are considered the mainstay of treatment [16]. Several immunosuppressive agents were used including corticosteroids, methotrexate, azathioprine, calcineurin antagonists and mycophenolate mofetil, intravenous immunoglobulin, and rituximab [13]. Most cases described in the literature were treated with multiple immunosuppressive agents to control the disease activity including two oral agents plus IVIG [13, 14, 17]. Expert opinions suggested that intravenous immunoglobulin could be particularly useful in patients with diabetes mellitus [5, 18]. However, glucocorticoids alone are not usually adequate and should be used in combination with another immunomodulatory agent. Similarly, IVIG monotherapy is not always effective, and additional immunosuppressive agents are frequently required for maintenance therapy [13, 14, 17]. In this case report, the patient was improving clinically and biochemically each time he received a dose of IVIG but he frequently relapsed despite the use of rituximab, methotrexate, and a low dose of oral steroids.

Management of this patient was further complicated by steroid-induced myopathy which is a clinical diagnosis that requires a high index of suspicion. Steroid-induced myopathy in patients with inflammatory myopathy should be suspected when patients develop worsening muscle weakness accompanied by declining or static creatine kinase levels. Clinical improvement three to four weeks after the discontinuation of steroids can also be supportive [19]. Higher doses of steroids are usually associated with a higher risk of developing myopathy which could present in an acute or a chronic form [19]. In our case, the patient took a double dose of oral steroid (40–80 mg), and his laboratory investigations showed downtrending CK levels with normal inflammatory markers and serum electrolyte levels. This highlights the importance of comprehensive clinical assessment in evaluating patients with complex medical conditions as in this case.

3.1. Patient Perspective. The patient has kindly shared his insights and thoughts on the management and impact of this disease on his life. He believes that maintaining effective and regular patient-physician communication was the main factor that helped him to get through this disease process. He thinks that it was extremely difficult for him to become dependent on his family who took good care of him, but that deeply affected his morals and he developed clinical depression for more than one year. Regarding statin use, patients stated that he did not receive enough education on this medicine at the time of starting this treatment nor at the subsequent follow-up visits in primary care clinics. He believes that family medicine physicians should be more vigilant in providing education to patients and in recognizing statin-associated muscle symptoms.

4. Conclusion

In summary, we presented a case of statin-induced IMNM diagnosis and treatment challenges. Although this disease is a rare side effect of statin use, physicians should maintain high index of suspicion for this rare entity in patients with statin-associated muscle symptoms who do not improve after stopping the medication. Prompt diagnosis and early use of combination of immunosuppressive therapy cannot be overrated. As the knowledge is rapidly accumulating, it is important to identify particular types of statin associated with this potentially serious side effect and build prediction tools to avoid their use in high-risk patients. Finally, patient education is the cornerstone of successful management in patients with chronic diseases.

Authors' Contributions

SM was responsible for case selection, case identification and conceptualization, literature review, manuscript writing, obtaining informed written consent, prescribing medicine, and clinical follow-up. AJ involved in manuscript writing and editing, literature review, and approval of the final manuscript. MA took part in manuscript writing, literature review, and approval of the final manuscript. SH performed history and physical observations, manuscript writing and editing, case identification and conceptualization, literature review, and approval of the final manuscript. PI carried out history and physical observations, manuscript writing, case identification and conceptualization, literature review, and approval of the final manuscript. EB contributed to literature review, manuscript writing, MRI report writing, and approval of the final manuscript.

Acknowledgments

Open Access funding was provided by Qatar National Library. The authors appreciate the support of Dr. Dhabia Al Mohannadi, Internal Medicine Residency Program Director.

References

[1] R. S. Rosenson, S. K. Baker, T. A. Jacobson, S. L. Kopecky, and B. A. Parker, "An assessment by the statin muscle safety task force: 2014 update," *Journal of Clinical Lipidology*, vol. 8, no. 3, pp. S58–S71, 2014.

[2] M. Needham, V. Fabian, W. Knezevic, P. Panegyres, P. Zilko, and F. L. Mastaglia, "Progressive myopathy with up-regulation of MHC-I associated with statin therapy," *Neuromuscular Disorders*, vol. 17, no. 2, pp. 194–200, 2007.

[3] I. Pinal-Fernandez, M. Casal-Dominguez, and A. L. Mammen, "Immune-mediated necrotizing myopathy," *Current Rheumatology Reports*, vol. 20, no. 4, pp. 1–0, 2018.

[4] C. Bergua, H. Chiavelli, Y. Allenbach et al., "In vivo pathogenicity of IgG from patients with anti-SRP or anti-HMGCR autoantibodies in immune-mediated necrotising myopathy," *Annals of the Rheumatic Diseases*, vol. 78, no. 1, pp. 131–139, 2019.

[5] A. L. Mammen, "Statin-associated autoimmune myopathy," *New England Journal of Medicine*, vol. 374, no. 7, pp. 664–669, 2016.

[6] P. D. H. Hamann, R. G. Cooper, N. J. McHugh, and H. Chinoy, "Statin-induced necrotizing myositis - A discrete autoimmune entity within the "statin-induced myopathy spectrum"," *Autoimmunity Reviews*, vol. 12, no. 12, pp. 1177–1181, 2013.

[7] A. Selva-O'Callaghan, M. Alvarado-Cardenas, I. Pinal-Fernández et al., "Statin-induced myalgia and myositis an update on pathogenesis and clinical recommendations," *Expert Review of Clinical Immunology*, vol. 14, no. 3, pp. 215–224, 2018.

[8] M. Molokhia, P. McKeigue, V. Curcin, and A. Majeed, "Statin Induced Myopathy and Myalgia Time Trend Analysis and Comparison of Risk Associated with Statin Class from 1991-2006," *PLoS One*, vol. 3, no. 6, Article ID e2522, 2008.

[9] P. Grable-Esposito, H. D. Katzberg, S. A. Greenberg, J. Srinivasan, J. Katz, and A. A. Amato, "Immune-mediated necrotizing myopathy associated with statins," *Muscle & Nerve Official Journal of the American Association of Electrodiagnostic Medicine*, vol. 41, no. 2, pp. 185–190, 2010.

[10] L. Nichols, K. Pfeifer, A. L. Mammen, N. Shahnoor, and C. G. Konersman, "An unusual case of statin-induced myopathy: anti-HMGCoA necrotizing autoimmune myopathy," *Journal of General Internal Medicine*, vol. 30, no. 12, pp. 1879 1883, 2015.

[11] A. L. Mammen, K. Pak, E. K. Williams et al., "Rarity of anti-3-hydroxy-3-methylglutaryl-coenzyme A reductase antibodies in statin users, including those with self-limited musculoskeletal side effects," *Arthritis Care & Research*, vol. 64, no. 2, pp. 269–272, 2012.

[12] A. L. Mammen, T. Chung, L. Christopher-Stine et al., "Autoantibodies against 3-hydroxy-3-methylglutaryl-coenzyme A reductase in patients with statin-associated autoimmune myopathy," *Arthritis & Rheumatism*, vol. 63, no. 3, pp. 713–721, 2011.

[13] Y. Allenbach, A. L. Mammen, O. Benveniste et al., "224th ENMC International Workshop," *Neuromuscular Disorders*, vol. 28, no. 1, pp. 87–99, 2018.

[14] J. L. Werner, L. Christopher-Stine, S. R. Ghazarian et al., "Antibody levels correlate with creatine kinase levels and strength in anti-3-hydroxy-3-methylglutaryl-coenzyme A reductase-associated autoimmune myopathy," *Arthritis & Rheumatism*, vol. 64, no. 12, pp. 4087–4093, 2012.

[15] JA Day and V. Limaye, "Immune-mediated necrotising myopathy: a critical review of current concepts," *Seminars in Arthritis and Rheumatism*, vol. 49, no. 3, pp. 420–429, 2019.

[16] S. Babu and Y. Li, "Statin induced necrotizing autoimmune myopathy," *Journal of the Neurological Sciences*, vol. 351, no. 1-2, pp. 13–17, 2015.

[17] I. Pinal-Fernandez and A. L. Mammen, "Spectrum of immune-mediated necrotizing myopathies and their treatments," *Current Opinion in Rheumatology*, vol. 28, no. 6, pp. 619–624, 2016.

[18] A. L. Mammen and E. Tiniakou, "Intravenous immune globulin for statin-triggered autoimmune myopathy," *New England Journal of Medicine*, vol. 373, no. 17, pp. 1680–1682, 2015.

[19] R. M. R. Pereira and J. Freire de Carvalho, "Glucocorticoid-induced myopathy," *Joint Bone Spine*, vol. 78, no. 1, pp. 41–44, 2011.

Transient Pneumonitis as a Possible Adverse Reaction to the BNT162b2 COVID-19 mRNA Vaccine in a Patient with Rheumatoid Arthritis: A Case Report and Review of the Literature

Yusuke Ohkubo, Shin-ichiro Ohmura, Ryuhei Ishihara, and Toshiaki Miyamoto

Department of Rheumatology, Seirei Hamamatsu General Hospital, Hamamatsu, Shizuoka, Japan

Correspondence should be addressed to Shin-ichiro Ohmura; s-omura0018@sis.seirei.or.jp

Academic Editor: Mario Salazar-Paramo

The coronavirus disease (COVID-19) pandemic caused by severe acute respiratory syndrome coronavirus 2 has led to rapid progress in vaccine development to prevent the spread of the disease. Although COVID-19 vaccines have excellent effectiveness in reducing morbidity and disease severity with minor adverse reactions, some patients develop late hypersensitivity events as autoimmune reactions such as rheumatoid arthritis, lupus nephritis, and vasculitis following COVID-19 vaccination. Herein, we describe a case of pneumonitis following COVID-19 mRNA vaccination in a patient with rheumatoid arthritis, which resolved spontaneously.

1. Introduction

The development of coronavirus disease (COVID-19) vaccines has progressed rapidly. Several vaccines have been reported to be effective in reducing morbidity and disease severity [1, 2]. In Japan, the mRNA vaccines BNT162b2 (Pfizer-BioNTech) and mRNA-1273 (Moderna) have been approved. Although minor adverse reactions are common, few serious adverse reactions have been reported [1, 2]. In addition, there have been late hypersensitivity events as autoimmune reactions such as rheumatoid arthritis (RA), lupus nephritis, and vasculitis following COVID-19 vaccination [3–6]. Herein, we describe a case of pneumonitis following COVID-19 mRNA vaccine, thought to be due to an autoimmune reaction, in a patient with RA, which resolved spontaneously.

2. Case Presentation

A 76-year-old woman with stable RA developed malaise and a high-grade fever (>39.0°C) 5 days after receiving a second dose of BNT162b2 mRNA vaccine. Ten days after vaccination, she developed a persistent cough and dyspnea. Seventeen days after vaccination, she was admitted to another hospital because of persistent fever. Blood tests showed a white blood cell (WBC) count of 4990/μL and lactate dehydrogenase (LDH) and C-reactive protein (CRP) levels of 477 U/L and 6.4 mg/dL, respectively. Although the antigen test for SARS, serum B-D glucan, and blood culture was negative, tests for *Mycoplasma*, *Chlamydia*, and sputum culture were not examined. Chest computed tomography (CT) showed infiltration and ground glass opacites (GGOs) in all lung fields (Figure 1(a)). The patient was provisionally diagnosed with interstitial lung disease (ILD) and was transferred to our hospital 21 days after vaccination.

Prior to the onset of her symptoms, the patient's RA had been stable on methotrexate treatment (12 mg/week), which she had taken for 15 years.

On admission, her body temperature, blood pressure, pulse, respiratory rate, and SpO_2 were 36.5°C, 110/60 mmHg, 65 beats/min, 18 breaths/min, and 98% (in room air), respectively. Her arthritis was stable and showed no changes of note since a previous check-up one month earlier. The results of blood tests were as follows: WBC, 5420/μL; red

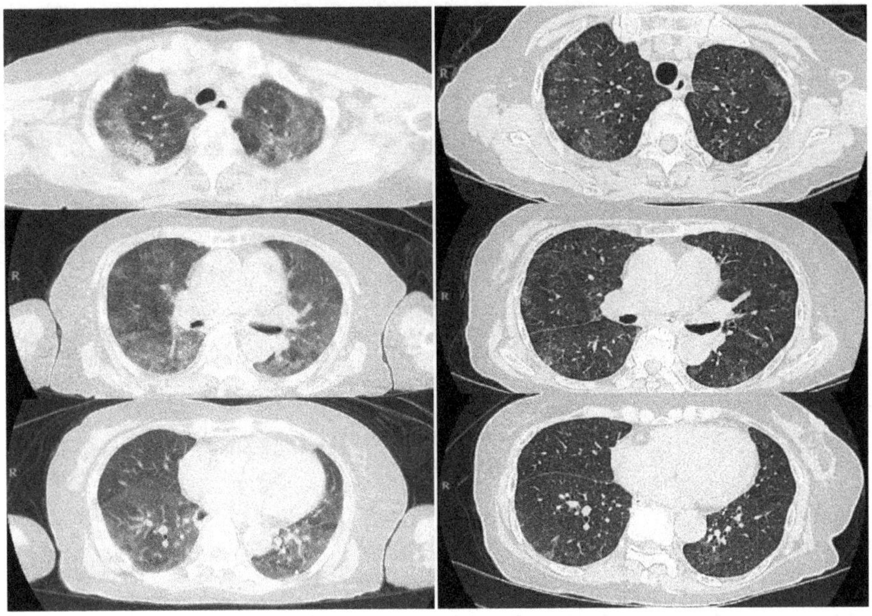

Days after vaccination day17 day21

(a) (b)

FIGURE 1: Chest computed tomography scans showing changes in the lung lesions. (a) CT scan performed on Day 17. (b) CT scan performed on Day 21. The second CT scan shows a clear improvement compared to the CT scan performed 4 days earlier. CT: computed tomography.

blood cells (RBC), $377 \times 10^4/\mu L$; hemoglobin (Hb), 11.2 g/dL; hematocrit, 35.5%; platelets, $40.4 \times 10^4/\mu L$; CRP 1.47 mg/dL; LDH, 311 U/L; Krebs von den Lungen-6 (KL-6), 452.4 U/mL; and surfactant protein D (SP-D), 226 ng/mL. Her rheumatoid factor, anti-cyclic citrullinated peptide antibody, and antinuclear antibody were negative.

Tests for *Mycoplasma*, *Chlamydia*, and *tuberculosis* (T-Spot), and antigen tests for *Cryptococcus*, *Candida*, *Aspergillus*, cytomegalovirus antigen, and SARS-CoV-2 antigen were negative. Serum β-D glucan, blood culture, and polymerase chain reaction testing of respiratory samples for *Pneumocystis jirovecii* DNA were also negative. Chest CT showed a significant improvement compared to the chest CT performed 4 days earlier (Figure 1(b)). The patient was treated conservatively and did not receive antibiotics or immunosuppressive drugs during hospitalization. Her cough, dyspnea, and fever resolved spontaneously, and she was discharged from hospital after 7 days. Her final diagnosis was transient pneumonitis induced by a COVID-19 mRNA vaccine. At the 3-month follow-up, she had not experienced a relapse of pneumonitis and her blood test results had improved: CRP, 0.06 mg/dL (from 1.47 mg/dL); LDH, 189 U/L (from 311 U/L); KL-6, 165.1 U/mL (from 452.4 U/mL); and SP-D, 102 ng/mL (from 226 ng/mL).

3. Discussion

To the best of our knowledge, this is the first report of transient pneumonitis following COVID-19 mRNA vaccination in a patient with RA. The patient's CT scan showed bilateral GGOs, which was consistent with ILD. The diagnosis of ILD in patients with RA is challenging because ILD has several causes, including bacterial pneumonia, viral pneumonia, *Pneumocystis* pneumonia, RA, and certain drugs. Drug-induced ILD is particularly difficult to diagnose because the clinical, radiological, and histological findings are non-specific and other causes of ILD must be excluded [11]. Bronchoscopy is required to diagnose drug-induced ILD. However, the Japan Society for Respiratory Endoscopy recommends that unnecessary bronchoscopy should be avoided during the COVID-19 pandemic [7]. In our patient, we did not perform bronchoscopy based on the Japan Society for Respiratory Endoscopy recommendation because blood tests did not show any sign of infection, including *Mycoplasma*, *Chlamydia*, or *Pneumocystis* infection, and her blood culture was negative. The patient had been taking the same drugs for 15 years, and the only new medication that she had received was the COVID-19 mRNA vaccine. Furthermore, her symptoms developed 5 days after the vaccination and the pneumonitis improved spontaneously with decreasing serum KL-6 and SP-D, without any relapse. These findings suggest that the COVID-19 mRNA vaccine induced transient pneumonitis. However, several investigators reported that the serum KL-6 and SP-D is associated with pulmonary diseases with alveolar inflammation, not only in ILD but also in respiratory infections, such as *Pneumocystis* pneumonia, COVID-19, and viral bronchitis [8–10, 12]. We could not exclude all respiratory diseases including infectious pneumonia because of the lack of bronchoscopic confirmation and tests for all respiratory infections with increasing KL-6 and SP-D.

The BNT162b2 mRNA vaccine contains RNA, lipids including polyethylene glycol (PEG), and a buffer, but unlike

Table 1: Characteristics of patients with ILD after COVID-19 vaccination.

	Case 1	Case 2	Case 3	Case 4	Case 5
Age (years)	86	65	60	66	76
Sex	M	M	M	M	F
Comorbidities	HT, DM, CKD	OMI, HL, HT	ACO, HT	None	RA, HT, myoma
Smoking	Never	Ex-smoker	Ex-smoker	NS	Never
Allergy history	NS	None	None	NS	Hay fever
Vaccine type	Pfizer-BioNTech	Pfizer-BioNTech	Pfizer-BioNTech	Pfizer-BioNTech	Pfizer-BioNTech
Dose	First	First	Second	Second	Second
Time from vaccination to symptom onset (days)	1	5	4	2	5
Symptoms	Fever, cough, dyspnea	Fever, dyspnea	Dyspnea	Fever, cough, dyspnea	Fever, cough
CRP (mg/dL)	11.4	5.5	10.9	8.7	6.4
Bilateral GGO on chest CT	Yes	Yes	Yes	Yes	Yes
Immunosuppressive therapy	Yes	Yes	Yes	Yes	No
Outcome	Survived	Survived	Survived	Survived	Survived
Reference	[7]	[8]	[9]	[10]	Current case

Note. ACO: asthma and chronic obstructive pulmonary disease overlap; CKD: chronic kidney disease; CRP: C-reactive protein; CT: computed tomography; DM: diabetes mellitus; F: female; GGO: grand glass opacity; HL: hyperlipidemia; HT: hypertension; ILD: interstitial lung disease; M: male; NS: not specified; OMI: old myocardial infarction; RA: rheumatoid arthritis.

other vaccines, it contains no adjuvants or preservatives. Compared to conventional vaccines, mRNA vaccines have several advantages: they are non-infectious, do not contain cellular components, induce cellular immunity, do not require adjuvants, are simple to produce, and are inexpensive [2, 13]. The spike protein of the virus adsorbs to cell membranes covered with lipid bilayers and receptor-binding proteins on the body's immune cells, which react with these proteins to produce neutralising antibodies. PEG, one of the components of the vaccine, can cause anaphylactic reactions [14]. The overall risk of anaphylaxis following vaccination with COVID-19 mRNA vaccines is low, and almost all adverse reactions are minor [15]. However, severe adverse reactions, including ILD, have been reported following vaccination [16, 17].

We conducted a literature search for studies published up to October 2021 to determine the characteristics of patients who developed pneumonitis after the COVID-19 mRNA vaccination and found four case reports (Table 1) [16–19]. All patients had received the BNT162b2 vaccine. Of the five patients (the four previously reported cases and our patient), pneumonitis developed in two patients after the first dose and in three patients after the second dose. All patients developed the symptoms within five days after vaccination. The median age was 66 years (range, 60–86 years), and four of the five patients were male. Chest CT showed bilateral GGOs in all patients. Four patients received immunosuppressive therapy, and all patients survived. Our patient developed symptoms five days after vaccination with the BNT162b2 vaccine, which is consistent with the other cases. Notably, unlike the other cases, our patient's pneumonitis resolved spontaneously without the use of immunosuppressive therapy.

The mechanism of pneumonitis development following COVID-19 vaccination is unclear. In contrast, in patients with pneumonitis after influenza vaccination, two major mechanisms are involved: cytotoxicity of the vaccine itself and an autoimmune response to the vaccine [20]. As with patients who develop pneumonitis following COVID-19 vaccination, almost all patients with pneumonitis after influenza vaccination develop bilateral GGOs on chest CT within 10 days and recover after immunosuppressive therapy [16, 21]. The risk factors for developing pneumonitis after vaccination are unknown. According to the World Health Organization, there is no association between vaccination and the development of autoimmune diseases in patients with no underlying disease [22]. Several investigators have reported that systemic rheumatic diseases (SRD) did not worsen after influenza, pneumococcal, or human papillomavirus vaccination [23–25]. According to the 2019 European League against Rheumatic Diseases (EULAR) recommendations for vaccination in adult patients with autoimmune inflammatory rheumatic diseases, influenza vaccination is recommended for patients with RA [26]. In addition, the American College of Rheumatology and EULAR recommend COVID-19 vaccination for patients with SRD.

It is difficult to predict severe adverse reactions to COVID-19 mRNA vaccines because they are the first mRNA vaccines to be developed. Although serious adverse reactions, such as thrombosis with thrombocytopenia, myocarditis, and Guillain–Barré syndrome, have been reported after COVID-19 vaccination [27–29], risk factors for these adverse reactions have not been identified. Further prospective studies are warranted to investigate severe adverse reactions following COVID-19 vaccination, including pneumonitis.

In conclusion, COVID-19 mRNA vaccines may induce autoimmune diseases, including pneumonitis, and clinicians should be aware of the possibility of these diseases following COVID-19 vaccination.

Authors' Contributions

All authors approved the final version of this article. YO had full access to all of the data. SO was responsible for the organization and coordination of the case.

References

[1] F. P. Polack, S. J. Thomas, N. Kitchin et al., "Safety and Efficacy of the BNT162b2 mRNA Covid-19 vaccine," *New England Journal of Medicine*, vol. 383, pp. 2603–2615, 2020.

[2] L. R. Baden, H. M. El Sahly, B. Essink et al., "Efficacy and safety of the mRNA-1273 SARS-CoV-2 vaccine," *New England Journal of Medicine*, vol. 384, no. 5, pp. 403–416, 2021.

[3] C. Baimukhamedov, S. Makhmudov, and A. Botabekova, "Seropositive rheumatoid arthritis after vaccination against SARS-CoV-2 infection," *International Journal of Rheumatics Diseases*, vol. 24, no. 11, pp. 1440-1441, 2021.

[4] M. F. Zavala-Miranda, S. G. González-Ibarra, A. A. Pérez-Arias, N. O. Uribe-Uribe, and J. M. Mejia-Vilet, "New-onset systemic lupus erythematosus beginning as class V lupus nephritis after COVID-19 vaccination," *Kidney International*, vol. 100, no. 6, pp. 1340-1341, 2021.

[5] A. Prabhahar, G. S. R. S. N. K. Naidu, P. Chauhan et al., "ANCA-associated vasculitis following ChAdOx1 nCoV19 vaccination: case-based review," *Rheumatology International*, vol. 42, no. 4, pp. 749–758, 2022.

[6] M. E. Grossman, G. Appel, A. J. Little, and C. J. Ko, "Post-COVID-19 vaccination IgA vasculitis in an adult," *Journal of Cutaneous Pathology*, vol. 49, no. 4, pp. 385–387, 2022.

[7] The Japan Society for Respiratory Endoscopy, "Urgent Recommendations on Corona Virus Disease on 2019 (COVID-19)," 2019, http://www.jsre.org/info/200217_corona_teigen.pdf.

[8] D. T. Arnold, C. Donald, M. Lyon et al., "Krebs von den Lungen 6 (KL-6) as a marker for disease severity and persistent radiological abnormalities following COVID-19 infection at 12 weeks," *PLoS One*, vol. 16, no. 4, Article ID e0249607, 2021.

[9] N. Nathani, G. D. Perkins, W. Tunnicliffe, N. Murphy, M. Manji, and D. R. Thickett, "Kerbs von Lungren 6 antigen is a marker of alveolar inflammation but not of infection In patients with acute respiratory distress syndrome," *Critical Care*, vol. 12, no. 1, 2008.

[10] H. Nakamura, M. Tateyama, D. Tasato et al., "Clinical utility of serum beta-D-glucan and KL-6 levels in Pneumocystis jirovecii pneumonia," *Internal Medicine*, vol. 48, no. 4, pp. 195–202, 2009.

[11] M. Schwaiblmair, W. Behr, T. Haeckel, B. Märkl, W. Foerg, and T. Berghaus, "Drug induced interstitial lung disease," *The Open Respiratory Medicine Journal*, vol. 6, pp. 63–74, 2012.

[12] Y. Kawasaki, Y. Aoyagi, Y. Abe et al., "Serum KL-6 levels as a biomarker of lung injury in respiratory syncytial virus bronchiolitis," *Journal of Medical Virology*, vol. 81, no. 12, pp. 2104–2108, 2009.

[13] A. Wadhwa, A. Aljabbari, A. Lokras, C. Foged, and A. Thakur, "Opportunities and challenges in the delivery of mRNA-based vaccines," *Pharmaceutics*, vol. 12, no. 2, p. E102, 2020.

[14] K. G. Blumenthal, L. B. Robinson, C. A. Camargo et al., "Acute allergic reactions to mRNA COVID-19 vaccines," *JAMA*, vol. 325, no. 15, pp. 1562–1565, 2021.

[15] M. H. Kim, S. Y. Lee, S. E. Lee et al., "Anaphylaxis to iodinated contrast media: clinical characteristics related with development of anaphylactic shock," *PLoS One*, vol. 9, no. 6, Article ID e100154, 2014.

[16] J. Y. Park, J. H. Kim, I. J. Lee et al., "COVID-19 vaccine-related interstitial lung disease: a case study," *Thorax*, vol. 77, no. 1, pp. 102–104, 2022.

[17] S. Matsuzaki, H. Kamiya, I. Inoshima, Y. Hirasawa, O. Tago, and M. Arai, "COVID-19 mRNA vaccine-induced pneumonitis," *Internal Medicine*, vol. 61, no. 1, pp. 8310–8316, 2022.

[18] A. Yoshifuji, K. Ishioka, Y. Masuzawa et al., "COVID-19 vaccine induced interstitial lung disease," *Journal of Infection and Chemotherapy*, vol. 28, no. 1, pp. 95–98, 2022.

[19] A. Kono, R. Yoshioka, P. Hawk et al., "A case of severe interstitial lung disease after COVID-19 vaccination," *QJM: International Journal of Medicine*, vol. 114, no. 11, pp. 805-806, 2022.

[20] O. Matsuno, "Drug-induced interstitial lung disease: mechanisms and best diagnostic approaches," *Respiratory Research*, vol. 13, 2012.

[21] T. Okusaki and K. Fukuhara, "Exacerbation of connective tissue disease-associated interstitial lung disease due to influenza vaccination," *Respiratory Medicine Case Reports*, vol. 33, Article ID 101463, 2021.

[22] L. Conklin, A. Hviid, W. A. Orenstein, A. J. Pollard, M. Wharton, and P. Zuber, "Vaccine safety issues at the turn of the 21st century," *BMJ Glob Health*, vol. 6, no. Suppl 2, Article ID e004898, 2021.

[23] A. Chalmers, D. Scheifele, C. Patterson et al., "Immunization of patients with rheumatoid arthritis against influenza: a study of vaccine safety and immunogenicity," *Journal of Rheumatology*, vol. 21, no. 7, pp. 1203–1206, 1994.

[24] F. Del Porto, B. Laganà, R. Biselli et al., "Influenza vaccine administration in patients with systemic lupus erythematosus and rheumatoid arthritis. Safety and immunogenicity," *Vaccine*, vol. 24, no. 16, pp. 3217–3223, 2006.

[25] O. Elkayam, D. Paran, D. Caspi et al., "Immunogenicity and safety of pneumococcal vaccination in patients with rheumatoid arthritis or systemic lupus erythematosus," *Clinical Infectious Diseases*, vol. 34, no. 2, pp. 147–153, 2002.

[26] V. Furer, C. Rondaan, M. W. Heijstek et al., "2019 update of EULAR recommendations for vaccination in adult patients with autoimmune inflammatory rheumatic diseases," *Annals of the Rheumatic Diseases*, vol. 79, no. 1, pp. 39–52, 2020.

[27] H. Akiyama, S. Kakiuchi, J. Rikitake et al., "Immune thrombocytopenia associated with Pfizer-BioNTech's BNT162b2 mRNA COVID-19 vaccine," *IDCases*, vol. 25, Article ID e01245, 2021.

[28] B. Singh, P. Kaur, L. Cedeno et al., "COVID-19 mRNA vaccine and myocarditis," *European Journal of Case Report International Medicine*, vol. 8, no. 7, Article ID 002681, 2022.

[29] M. García-Grimshaw, A. Michel-Chávez, J. M. Vera-Zertuche et al., "Guillain–Barré syndrome is infrequent among recipients of the BNT162b2 mRNA COVID-19 vaccine," *Clinical Immunology*, vol. 230, Article ID 108818, 2021.

29

Doxycycline-Induced Antinuclear Antibody and Antineutrophil Cytoplasmic Antibody Associated Vasculitis: A Case Report and Literature Review

Davisson J. Wriston,[1] **Evan R. Norfolk**,[2] **Lindsay M. Smith**,[2] **Guoli Chen**,[3] **and David H. Bulbin**[4]

[1]*Department of Internal Medicine, Geisinger Medical Center, Danville, Pennsylvania, USA*
[2]*Department of Nephrology, Geisinger Medical Center, Danville, Pennsylvania, USA*
[3]*Department of Pathology, Geisinger Medical Center, Danville, Pennsylvania, USA*
[4]*Department of Rheumatology, Geisinger Medical Center, Danville, Pennsylvania, USA*

Correspondence should be addressed to Davisson J. Wriston; dwriston1@geisinger.edu

Academic Editor: Franco Schiavon

Drug-induced antineutrophil cytoplasmic antibody (ANCA)-associated vasculitis (AAV) has been increasingly recognized in the literature with numerous medications listed as causative agents in disease pathology. Doxycycline is a commonly prescribed medication within the United States which is a synthetic, broad-spectrum antibiotic with antimicrobial properties and at low doses exhibits anti-inflammatory effects. In this report, we describe a case of doxycycline-induced ANCA-associated vasculitis with laboratory and biopsy findings supporting the diagnosis, which to the best of our knowledge is the first described case of doxycycline-induced AAV in the literature. The patient was started on doxycycline for treatment of potential Lyme disease. She began to develop progressively worsening myasthenia, erythematous macular rash, anorexia, anemia, and fatigue for several weeks following the course of doxycycline with initial concern of a paraneoplastic process. Ultimately, the patient was discovered to be positive for antinuclear antibody (ANA), perinuclear antineutrophil cytoplasmic antibody (pANCA), and myeloperoxidase (MPO) antibody for which she was treated with a course of prednisone leading to complete remission of disease. A brief review of the pathogenesis of ANCA vasculitides will also be discussed within this article.

1. Introduction

Drug-induced antineutrophil cytoplasmic antibody (ANCA)-associated vasculitis is a unique subset of the ANCA-associated vasculitides which are classified as small vessel vasculitides. Small vessel vasculitis was divided into ANCA-associated vasculitis (AAV) and immune complex vasculitis in the 2012 revised Chapel Hill Consensus Conference. The division was made due to a higher level of confidence that ANCAs are directly involved in the pathogenesis of AAV which has been confirmed in follow-up literature [1, 2]. ANCA-associated vasculitis is a disease entity comprising microscopic polyangiitis (MPA), granulomatosis with polyangiitis (GPA), and eosinophilic granulomatous with polyangiitis (EGPA) that are all ANCA positive. There are several antigens to ANCA that have been discovered; however, there are two in particular that are part of diagnostic criteria for MPA, GPA, and EGPA. These antigens are proteinase 3 (PR3) and myeloperoxidase (MPO) which are almost exclusively found in neutrophils and monocytes [3]. ANCA indirect immunofluorescence against PR3 results in a diffuse cytoplasmic (cANCA) staining pattern, whereas indirect immunofluorescence staining against MPO results in a perinuclear pattern (pANCA). A perinuclear ANCA pattern can be seen with several other proteins such as elastase, cathepsin, β-glucuronidase, or lactoferrin [4]. A cytoplasmic ANCA pattern is almost exclusively caused by PR3.

AAV pathogenesis is multifactorial, comprising genetic factors, epigenetic factors, and environmental factors [5]. Environmental factors specifically include drugs or infections. Drug-induced AAV pathogenesis can be based on the medication's direct effects such as sulfasalazine causing necroptosis or the metabolites of the drugs that accumulate within the neutrophil binding to specific proteins, thereby making the proteins immunogenic [6]. Pathogenic ANCAs cause excessive neutrophil activation which leads to the persistent formation of neutrophil extracellular traps (NETs). NETs are used to trap and kill bacteria. NETs likely occur at a stable rate of production and degradation under homeostatic conditions [7]. However, persistent formation of NETs ultimately leads to damage of small vessels. ANCA production is also caused by NETs which leads to an unrelenting vicious cycle of ongoing inflammation [5]. There is still significant information to learn in regard to the exact pathogenesis of drug-induced AAV as some medications including minocycline, which is a tetracycline in the same class as doxycycline, do not appear to directly induce NET formation or inhibit NET degradation raising the question if another mechanism is at work for causing the drug-induced AAV [8].

Drug-induced ANCA-associated vasculitis presents similarly to primary AAV with clinical and serological profiles [9]. However, there are certain characteristics that drug-induced AAV alone seems to display. Most data on the subject are from retrospective studies with antithyroid drug-induced AAV compared to primary AAV. These data appear to be consistent with case reports consisting of other medications causing AAV. Specifically, patients with antithyroid drug-induced AAV, when compared to primary AAV, more often have skin damage, positive ANA, and good prognosis with high likelihood of disease remission [9, 10]. Kidney involvement is less common in antithyroid drug-induced AAV compared to primary AAV [11].

Doxycycline is a synthetic, broad-spectrum antibiotic with antimicrobial properties and at low doses exhibits anti-inflammatory effects [12]. Doxycycline and minocycline are part of the class of antibiotics called tetracyclines. There have been several case reports of minocycline-induced systemic erythematous lupus (SLE) and minocycline-induced AAV over the last 20 years. A single case report of doxycycline-induced subacute cutaneous lupus erythematous was reported in 2011 found on a Medline literature search [13]. However, there have been no previous cases reports of doxycycline-induced AAV.

2. Case Presentation

A 56-year-old woman with medical history notable only for lower extremity deep vein thrombosis in her 20s while being on oral contraceptive pills, 35 pack-year former smoker initially presented to her general practitioner for evaluation of jaw trismus which occurred a couple of days after she found a tick on her body. It was the first week of May and the patient resided an area with a high incidence of Lyme disease; therefore, her general practitioner prescribed a 3-week prescription doxycycline for treatment of potential Lyme disease. Soon after beginning the doxycycline, she began to experience worsening conjunctivitis, myalgias, generalized muscle weakness, erythematous rash, fatigue, weight loss, and anorexia. Doxycycline was continued by her general practitioner until day 18. Ultimately, the patient's Lyme titers were negative. The patient continued to experience worsening symptoms of muscle weakness, anorexia associated with weight loss, and fatigue with spontaneous resolution of conjunctivitis. She was seen in the emergency department for evaluation of symptoms at which time laboratory investigations revealed anemia with a hemoglobin of 10.4 g/dL. A repeat Lyme test was performed that also resulted as negative.

The patient was discharged home from the emergency department; however, one week later she was admitted in mid-June with nausea in addition to the aforementioned symptoms. Workup revealed microcytic anemia, ferritin of 478 ng/mL, erythrocyte sedimentation rate (ESR) > 120mm/hr, and rheumatoid factor of 52 IU/mL. The patient had further decline in hemoglobin with a negative fecal occult blood test. Hemolytic investigations were unrevealing. Anti-mitochondrial antibody and anti-smooth muscle antibody were both negative. ANA titer, anti-CCP IgG antibody, and anti-cardiolipin antibodies were pending at the time of discharge. The patient was informed to follow-up with her general practitioner for concern of underlying autoimmune disease.

The patient was seen at the rheumatology clinic two weeks following hospital discharge which was five weeks since stopping her doxycycline. She had worsening arthralgia, rash, 12 kilograms of unintentional weight loss, proximal weakness limiting her ability to ambulate with bloodwork from previous hospitalization revealing positive ANA 1 : 40 titer, anti-cyclic citrullinated antibody negative, and positive anti-phospholipid antibodies. The patient was hospitalized directly from the clinic as there was concern for an underlying paraneoplastic process, but other differentials included systemic lupus erythematosus and dermatomyositis. The patient underwent gastroscopy and colonoscopy to investigate for possible gastrointestinal malignancy which was unremarkable. She also had an echocardiogram to explore for possible myxoma which was also unremarkable. Admission laboratory work was notable for ESR > 120 mm/hr, CRP 237 mg/L, ANA titer of 1: 2,560, pANCA positive with confirmatory MPO resulting as 69.3 Units, creatinine of 1.0, and urinalysis (UA) reporting moderate blood with 5–9 white blood cells (WBCs) and 30–49 red blood cells (RBCs). Nephrology was consulted about obtaining a kidney biopsy given kidney involvement would mean exposing her to significant immunosuppressive agents. Repeat serial UAs consistently resulted in 5–9 RBCs without dysmorphic RBCs. Kidney biopsy was deferred given low suspicion of glomerulonephritis. The patient was started on IV methylprednisolone 500 mg daily for 3 days and transitioned to oral prednisone 60 mg daily with significant improvement in symptoms. The working diagnosis at the time of discharge was microscopic polyangiitis. She was discharged on prednisone 60 mg daily with a slow taper, azathioprine 100 mg daily,

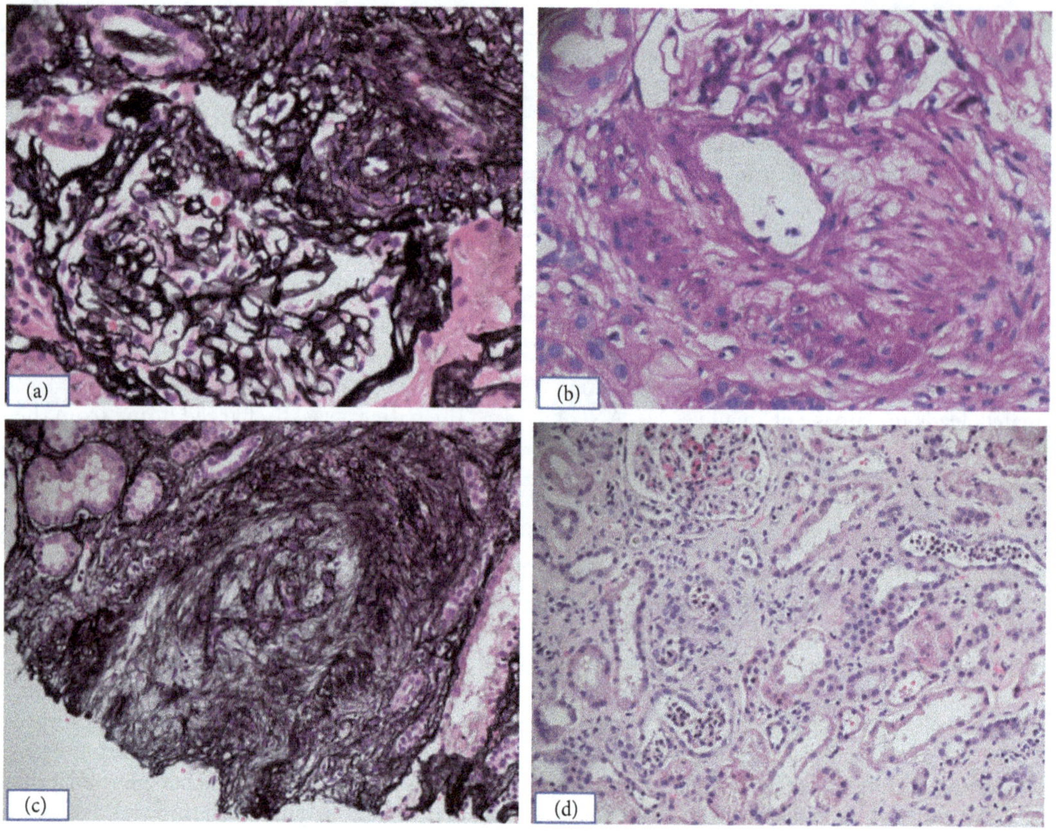

FIGURE 1: Representative images of histological/pathological findings in a renal biopsy specimen from the patient. (a) Jones silver stain shows a glomerulus in a relatively normal morphology, with no crescents or necrosis noted; adjacent is an arterial with medial hypertrophy. (b) An arterial and PAS stain shows marked intimal thickening/fibrosis. (c) Jones silver stain demonstrates an artery with fibrous obliteration/complete luminal occlusion. (d) H&E stain shows focal intraluminal neutrophilic casts/debris in the tubules, which can be seen in infections or other types of tubular interstitial nephritis. No immune complexes were present in the glomeruli.

and omeprazole as well as follow-up appointments with nephrology and rheumatology.

At her follow-up rheumatology visit one month after hospital discharge, she was noted to have new mildly pruritic, erythematous papular rash on her upper and lower extremities; however, her previous systemic symptoms of fatigue, anorexia, and myasthenia were resolving. The new rash was concerning for drug eruption from azathioprine versus leukocytoclastic vasculitis from MPA. She was able to be sent directly to the dermatology clinic for skin biopsy. The patient was continued on azathioprine and prednisone until biopsy results showed the rash to be consistent with drug eruption without any evidence of vasculitis. Azathioprine was discontinued, and the rash resolved without further intervention.

The patient had follow-up with nephrology given concern about her abnormal UAs in the setting of suspected MPA. Her creatinine remained slightly elevated at 1.1 with mildly elevated protein/creatinine ratio ranging from 0.17 to 0.90 (normal limit <0.14). Ultimately, the patient underwent a kidney biopsy in mid-August without complications. Biopsy did not show active signs of vasculitis but did have signs that may be representative of previous sequelae of vasculitis. Urine cultures obtained during this time period were all negative. Biopsy results are shown in Figure 1.

She had complete resolution of symptoms noted at follow-up rheumatology visits after the kidney biopsy. The prednisone taper ended the first week of October without any relapse of symptoms. She had serial blood work that demonstrated disease resolution, listed in Table 1, confirming the diagnosis of doxycycline-induced AAV. The patient continues to be seen annually and is doing well. Spring 2020 marked 5 years since her episode of doxycycline-induced AAV.

The following laboratory results are included for reference but will not be discussed in further detail as they did not directly affect the patient's clinical course. Complement levels were normal in July with a mildly decreased complement C4 of 81 noted on mid-August at the time of kidney biopsy. Anti-beta 2 glycoprotein IgA and anti-beta 2 glycoprotein IgM were 103.4 and >150, respectively, at the time of the first admission. Anti-double stranded DNA, ribonucleoprotein antibody, anti-Ro antibody, and anti-La antibody were all negative.

3. Discussion

Tetracycline-induced vasculitis is a rare entity that should be explored in a patient presenting with symptoms concerning for the underlying autoimmune process and reporting a

TABLE 1: Antinuclear antibodies (ANA), perinuclear-antineutrophil cytoplasmic antibodies (pANCA), and anti-myeloperoxidase antibody (anti-MPO AB).

	Reference range	6/18/15	7/1/15	11/23/15	12/26/15
ANA dilution	Normal < 40 titer	40	2,560	1,280	640
pANCA	Normal titer negative		pANCA positive	pANCA positive	Negative
Anti-MPO AB	Normal < 20.1 units		69.3 units	5.4 units	
CRP	Normal 0–5 mg/L		235 mg/L	10 mg/L	

recent medication change. Previously, studies have investigated if duration and dosage of the offending drug play an increased role in drug-induced lupus. It was shown that long-term minocycline users had increased risk of drug-induced lupus [14]. It seems likely that drug-induced AAV would follow a similar pattern.

Our patient had an 18-day exposure to doxycycline with systemic symptoms that continued to worsen for several weeks upon discontinuation of the medication. It is not possible to say if her vasculitis would have resolved without treatment of immunosuppressants had the doxycycline been discontinued immediately upon her development of symptoms. She may have had spontaneous resolution of AAV if doxycycline was discontinued at her first sign of symptoms. Fortunately, she had a great response to prednisone with resolution of disease.

A kidney biopsy was not pursued in conjunction with symptoms. Additionally, she had been on oral prednisone 60 mg daily for over 40 days before kidney biopsy was obtained. This is likely why the biopsy did not show evidence of active vasculitis but had findings that were consistent with sequelae of vasculitis. Her UAs never showed dysmorphic RBCs which are specific for glomerulonephritis but not sensitive [15]. Urinalysis resulted in RBCs (highest value 30–49 per high power field) during the period of time when she had symptoms, significantly elevated ANA titer, and MPO antibodies with resolution of RBCs in follow-up UAs when her symptoms were resolved.

An investigation in 2019 by Dam et al. studied neutrophil stimulation from SLE patient's serum and AAV patient's serum, specifically examining the mechanisms of NET formation and composition. The kinetics, induction pathways, and composition of the NETs were distinct in SLE compared to AAV [16]. This study potentially raises the question of whether the particular characteristics of drug-induced AAV and primary AAV may be in part due to intrinsically different NET formation.

This is the first case to be described in literature of doxycycline-induced AAV. It is reported that approximately 5 million prescriptions of doxycycline are made annually, thereby making doxycycline a top 150 most commonly prescribed medication within the United States [17]. We postulate that the rarity of doxycycline-induced autoimmune pathology is due to it having no significant metabolism and no known metabolites found in humans [18, 19]. This is in stark contrast to minocycline which has up to six metabolites reported with numerous confirmed cases of drug-induced lupus and drug-induced AAV [18, 20, 21].

4. Conclusion

Tetracycline-induced vasculitis is rare but should be recognized by providers as a potential cause of autoimmune disease symptomatology. The pathogenesis of AAV is still not fully understood, but there is a foundation of knowledge that is continuing to be built upon. Drug-induced AAV patients typically respond well with discontinuation of offending medication; however, they may also need steroids for immunosuppression. Doxycycline is not typically associated with autoimmune pathology likely because it has no known metabolites. Per our literature search, this is the first reported case of doxycycline-induced antineutrophil cytoplasmic antibody vasculitis with the patient having complete remission of disease following a tapered course of prednisone.

References

[1] J. C. Jennette, R. J. Falk, P. A. Bacon et al., "2012 revised international chapel hill consensus conference nomenclature of vasculitides," *Arthritis & Rheumatism*, vol. 65, no. 1, pp. 1–11, 2013.

[2] J. C. Jennette, R. J. Falk, P. Hu, and H. Xiao, "Pathogenesis of antineutrophil cytoplasmic autoantibody-associated small-vessel vasculitis," *Annual Review of Pathology: Mechanisms of Disease*, vol. 8, no. 1, pp. 139–160, 2013.

[3] L. A. Charles, R. J. Falk, and J. C. Jennette, "Reactivity of antineutrophil cytoplasmic autoantibodies with mononuclear phagocytes," *Journal of Leukocyte Biology*, vol. 51, no. 1, pp. 65–68, 1992.

[4] A. Radice and R. A. Sinico, "Antineutrophil cytoplasmic antibodies (ANCA)," *Autoimmunity*, vol. 38, no. 1, pp. 93–103, 2005.

[5] D. Nakazawa, S. Masuda, U. Tomaru, and A. Ishizu, "Pathogenesis and therapeutic interventions for ANCA-associated vasculitis," *Nature Reviews Rheumatology*, vol. 15, no. 2, pp. 91–101, 2019.

[6] X. Jiang, G. Khursigara, and R. Rubin, "Transformation of lupus-inducing drugs to cytotoxic products by activated neutrophils," *Science*, vol. 266, no. 5186, pp. 810–813, 1994.

[7] D. Soderberg and M. Segelmark, "Neutrophil extracellular traps in ANCA-associated vasculitis," *Frontiers in Immunology*, vol. 7, pp. 1–9, 2016.

[8] J. A. Irizarry-Caro, C. Carmona-Rivera, D. M. Schwartz, S. S. Khaznadar, M. J. Kaplan, and P. C. Grayson, "Brief report: drugs implicated in systemic autoimmunity modulate neutrophil extracellular trap formation," *Arthritis & Rheumatology*, vol. 70, no. 3, pp. 468–474, 2018.

[9] B. Bonaci-Nikolic, M. M. Nikolic, S. Andrejevic, S. Zoric, and

M. Bukilica, "Antineutrophil cytoplasmic antibody (ANCA)-associated autoimmune diseases induced by antithyroid drugs: comparison with idiopathic ANCA vasculitides," *Arthritis Research & Therapy*, vol. 7, no. 5, pp. R1072–R1081, 2005.

[10] A. Wiik, "Clinical and laboratory characteristics of drug-induced vasculitic syndromes," *Arthritis Research & Therapy*, vol. 7, no. 5, pp. 191-192, 2005.

[11] Y.-X. Chen, W. Zhang, X.-N. Chen et al., "Propylthiouracil-induced antineutrophil cytoplasmic antibody (ANCA)-associated renal vasculitis versus primary ANCA-associated renal vasculitis: a comparative study," *The Journal of Rheumatology*, vol. 39, no. 3, pp. 558–563, 2012.

[12] B. Sloan and N. Scheinfeld, "The use and safety of doxycycline hyclate and other second-generation tetracyclines," *Expert Opinion on Drug Safety*, vol. 7, no. 5, pp. 571–577, 2008.

[13] K. K. Miller, J. Chu, R. Patel, and H. Kamino, "Drug-induced subacute cutaneous lupus erythematosus related to doxycycline," *Dermatology Online Journal*, vol. 17, no. 10, p. 3, 2011.

[14] M. C. J. M. Sturkenboom, C. R. Meier, H. Jick, and B. H. C. Stricker, "Minocycline and lupuslike syndrome in acne patients," *Archives of Internal Medicine*, vol. 159, no. 5, pp. 493–497, 1999.

[15] A. M. Hamadah, K. Gharaibeh, K. C. Mara et al., "Urinalysis for the diagnosis of glomerulonephritis: role of dysmorphic red blood cells," *Nephrology Dialysis Transplantation*, vol. 33, no. 8, pp. 1397–1403, 2018.

[16] L. S. Dam, T. Kraaij, S. W. A. Kamerling et al., "Intrinsically distinct role of neutrophil extracellular trap formation in antineutrophil cytoplasmic antibody-associated vasculitis compared to systemic lupus erythematosus," *Arthritis & Rheumatology*, vol. 71, no. 12, pp. 2047–2058, 2019.

[17] Agency for Healthcare Research and Quality, "Doxycycline drug dosage statistics, United States," Medical Expenditure Panel Survey (MEPS) 2007–2017, Agency for Healthcare Research and Quality, Rockville, MA, USA, https://clincalc.com/DrugStats/Drugs/Doxycycline.

[18] K. N. Agwuh and A. MacGowan, "Pharmacokinetics and pharmacodynamics of the tetracyclines including glycylcyclines," *Journal of Antimicrobial Chemotherapy*, vol. 58, no. 2, pp. 256–265, 2006.

[19] S. Saivin and G. Houin, "Clinical pharmacokinetics of doxycycline and minocycline," *Clinical Pharmacokinetics*, vol. 15, no. 6, pp. 355–366, 1988.

[20] O. Elkayam, D. Levartovsky, C. Brautbar et al., "Clinical and immunological study of 7 patients with minocycline-induced autoimmune phenomena," *The American Journal of Medicine*, vol. 105, no. 6, pp. 484–487, 1998.

[21] A. Gough, S. Chapman, K. Wagstaff, P. Emery, and E. Elias, "Minocycline induced autoimmune hepatitis and systemic lupus erythematosus-like syndrome," *BMJ*, vol. 312, no. 7024, pp. 169–172, 1996.

30

PL-7 Antisynthetase Syndrome in Association with Sjögren's, Systemic Lupus Erythematosus and Rheumatoid Arthritis

Mehrin Jawaid, Yael Ross, and Mohammad Kamran

WellStar Kennestone Regional Medical Center, Marietta, GA 30060, USA

Correspondence should be addressed to Mehrin Jawaid; mehrin.jawaid@wellstar.org

Academic Editor: George S. Habib

We present a rare case of PL-7 antisynthetase syndrome (ASS) in association with Sjögren's, systemic lupus erythematosus (SLE), and seropositive rheumatoid arthritis (RA). Initially, the patient was diagnosed with Sjögren's followed by Sjögren's/SLE overlap and then Sjögren's/SLE/RA overlap. She was eventually diagnosed with Sjögren's/SLE/RA overlap with PL-7 ASS with interstitial lung disease (ILD). ILD was discovered after complaints of pleuritic chest pain with subsequent workup with coronary computed tomography (CT) revealing pulmonary fibrosis. This case demonstrates the ambiguity with which symptoms of ASS can present; given the high respiratory morbidity and mortality of ASS especially in non-Jo-1 patients, those who present with Raynaud's, myositis, or joint pain, whether together or in isolation, should be assessed for presence of additional features of ASS and potentially undergo testing for ASS antibodies if appropriate.

1. Introduction

Antisynthetase syndrome (ASS) is a subgroup of idiopathic inflammatory myopathies (IIM) characterized by the presence of antisynthetase antibodies and at least one of the following: myositis, ILD, and inflammatory arthritis. Raynaud's, mechanic's hands, and fevers may be present as well. Given the lack of specific classification criteria, often ASS can be confused with arthritis or other connective tissue diseases. Various antisynthetase antibodies include anti-Jo-1, anti-PL-12, anti-PL-7, anti-OJ, anti-EJ, anti-KS, anti-Zo, and anti-YRS [1]. Prevalence of ASS remains unknown; however, IIM, which includes the ASS subset, has a prevalence of 10 per 100, 000 individuals [2]. Anti-Jo-1 is the most common ASS antibody with prevalence of 20–25% in IIM, and the remaining are very rare with prevalence between <1% and 5% [3].

2. Case Presentation

A 41-year-old African American female presented with complaints of fatigue, xerostomia, xerophthalmia, and mild polyarthralgias with less than ten minutes of morning stiffness. The patient denied fevers, unintentional weight loss, photosensitivity, alopecia, oral ulcers, serositis, blood clots, or unusual headaches. She had never been pregnant, was a life time nonsmoker, worked in an office setting, and did not take any medications. Family history was significant for rheumatoid arthritis in her father.

On physical exam, she exhibited dry oral mucosa. She did not exhibit any rashes, synovitis, or joint tenderness. Examination of all other organ systems was unremarkable. An antinuclear antibody by immunofluorescence was positive (1 : 160) with nucleolar pattern (ref >1 : 80 elevated). Double-stranded DNA (DsDNA), Smith, and ribonucleoprotein antibodies were negative. C3 was 89 mg/dL (ref 90–180). C4 was 10 mg/dL (ref 16–47). Sjögren's antibody (SSA) was 6.7 (ref <1), serum protein electrophoresis was normal, and rheumatoid factor negative. She was diagnosed with Sjögren's syndrome based on the symptoms of xerostomia and xerophthalmia, positive SSA antibody, and fatigue. Xerophthalmia was confirmed by her ophthalmologist via positive Schirmer test.

Approximately 18 months after her initial diagnosis, the patient developed photosensitivity with rash, headaches, increased hair loss, alopecia, and increased fatigue. She continued to experience xerostomia, xerophthalmia, and Raynaud's. Repeat serologies showed DsDNA antibodies were now positive at a titer of 1 : 10, (ref <1 : 10). Complements were low with C3 84 mg/dL and C4 8 mg/dL. Smith and ribonucleoprotein antibodies, complete blood count, complete metabolic panel, urinalysis, and antiphospholipid antibodies were normal. At that time, a diagnosis of Sjögren's/SLE overlap was made. She was started on hydroxychloroquine 200 mg twice daily.

She remained stable on hydroxychloroquine for over a year. On a follow-up visit, she complained of increased joint pain and swelling in her hands and knees associated with morning stiffness for more than two hours over the previous two months. On physical exam, she exhibited tenderness and synovitis of bilateral wrists, bilateral metacarpophalangeal, and bilateral proximal interphalangeal joints. Repeat serologies revealed rheumatoid factor (RF) of 167 IU/mL (ref < 14) and anticyclic citrullinated peptide antibody (CCP) > 250 (ref > 59 strong positive). Hand X-rays showed no erosions. The patient met the 2010 American College of Rheumatology criteria for the diagnosis of RA in addition to already diagnosed overlap of Sjögren's/SLE. Recommendation was made to start methotrexate, but she declined due to concern over side effect profile. She was unable to tolerate sulfasalazine and leflunomide due to symptoms of lightheadedness and hair loss, respectively, and was reluctant to initiate biologic agents due to concern over side effect profile. She managed her symptoms on hydroxychloroquine 200 mg twice daily and ibuprofen 200–400 mg three times daily as needed for pain. The patient did take a prednisone taper initially for 3 weeks and stopped thereafter.

Due to complaints of pleuritic chest pain, the patient underwent workup which included a coronary CT scan, which revealed lung fibrosis. Follow-up high-resolution CT (HRCT) revealed multiple, noncalcified pulmonary nodules, the largest measuring 7 mm and mild honeycombing in the peripheries in a usual interstitial pneumonia (UIP) pattern (Figures 1–3). Given the findings on her CT scan, an ILD/myositis panel was ordered. Anti-PL-7 antibody was positive, 79 (ref < 11). An echocardiogram showed mild tricuspid regurgitation; pulmonary artery pressure was 26. Pulmonary function testing (PFT) was normal. A diagnosis of PL-7-positive antisynthetase syndrome with Sjögren's/SLE/RA overlap was made. Rituximab or mycophenolate was recommended; however, patient declined due to concern over side effect profile. On follow-up five months later, PFTs revealed moderately reduced diffusion lung capacity for carbon monoxide. She was evaluated at an ILD clinic at a university hospital where the diagnosis and treatment plan were agreed upon. After initial hesitation about starting medications, the patient agreed to start mycophenolate.

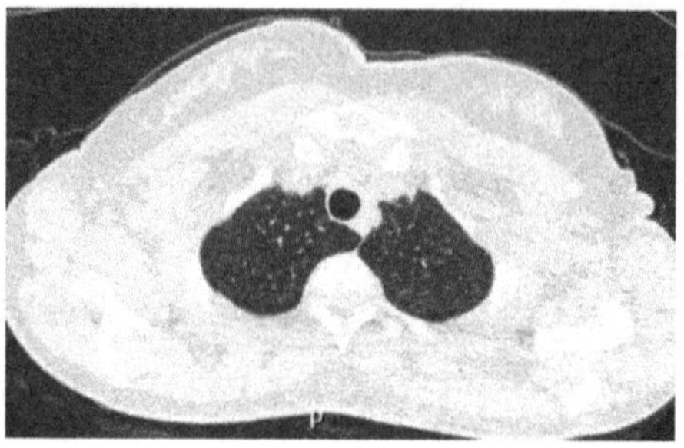

Figure 1: HRCT chest, prone image, and apical view.

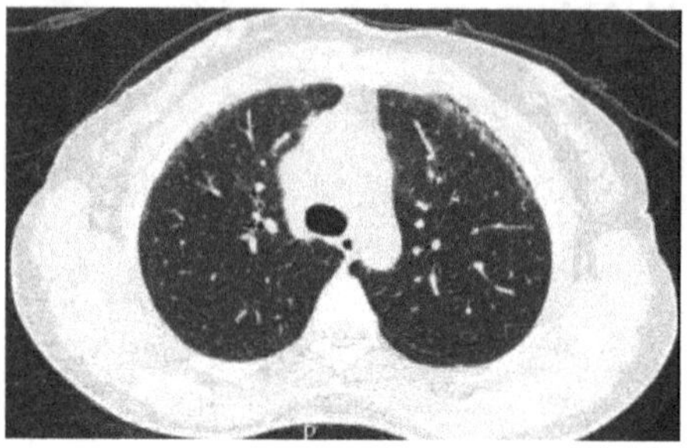

Figure 2: HRCT chest, prone image, and honeycombing in the anterior upper lobes.

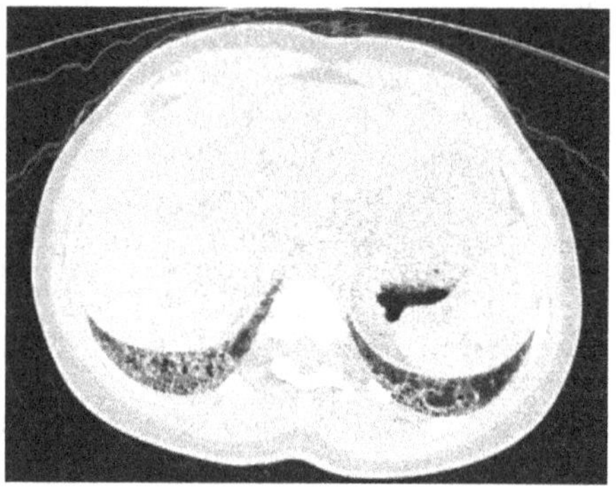

Figure 3: HRCT chest, prone image, honeycombing, and reticulation peripheral lung bases.

3. Discussion

This is an interesting rare case of overlap syndrome with PL-7 ASS, Sjögren's, systemic lupus erythematosus, and rheumatoid arthritis with evolving symptoms over time. ASS has often been reported in overlap with polymyositis, dermatomyositis, systemic sclerosis, Sjögren's, and RA [4–7].

Clinical heterogeneity is a feature of ASS with variable symptoms among different ASS antibody subgroups. Muscle involvement has been shown to be milder in patients with PL-7 antibodies compared to those with Jo-1 antibodies, including in those patients who have ASS in overlap with polymyositis/dermatomyositis [4, 5, 8]. There have also been reports of lower prevalence of mechanics hands and joint symptoms in PL-7 patients compared to Jo-1 patients [8, 9]. Pulmonary involvement can present as a spectrum from asymptomatic to progressive or acute lung disease. Pericardial disease, intestinal peudo-obstruction, and malignancy have been reported in ASS as well [9].

Interstitial lung disease is the largest contributor toward morbidity and mortality in ASS, especially in non-Jo-1 patients. It has been demonstrated that survival from time of diagnosis is significantly poorer in non-Jo-1 patients, and these patients also have increased pulmonary morbidity and mortality compared to Jo-1 positive patients [8]. In Marie et al.'s cohort of 15 anti-PL-7 patients, none of the patients had resolution of ILD. 35.7% of patients experienced deterioration of ILD with worsened functional status, and 7.1% died from lung complications [9]. Besides the presence of the non-Jo-1 antibody, concurrent presence of the Ro52 antibody, older age, and elevated serum ferritin have been associated with more rapidly progressive interstitial lung disease (RPILD) [10]. Those with the UIP pattern by HRCT have also demonstrated decreased steroid responsiveness and RPILD [9].

Nonspecific interstitial pneumonia (NSIP) and organizing pneumonia are the predominant HRCT patterns that have been reported in ASS [11, 12]; however, cases of ASS with UIP pattern have also been reported as with Marie et al.'s cohort of 15 patients of which 42.9% demonstrated UIP, 42.9% NSIP, and 14.2% with organizing pneumonia [9]. Yousem et al. also highlight the presence of the UIP pattern in biopsies of PL-7 patients [13].

Furthermore, the onset of ILD and initial presenting symptoms can vary in ASS. It has been shown in PL-7 patients that ILD could present either before, simultaneously, or after myositis presentation [9, 14]. Overall, in comparison to Jo-1 positive patients, non-Jo-1 patients tend to present with nonspecific connective tissue disease symptoms. There have also been cases where PL-7 patients have presented in overlap with various other diagnoses and as in our case, in overlap with Sjögren's, SLE, and RA. Thus, PL-7 ASS or other non-Jo-1 antibody syndromes could present at least initially, as idiopathic ILD, undifferentiated connective tissue disease, and/or evolve into or present as an overlap syndrome.

Our case demonstrates the ambiguity of initial presenting symptoms of non-Jo-1 patients, which is in line with the literature for presentation of most non-Jo-1 patients. Our patient initially presented with Raynaud's during her teenage years; then, in her 40s, she developed Sjögren's followed by Sjögren's/SLE overlap and then Sjögren's/SLE/RA overlap. She was eventually diagnosed with Sjögren's/SLE/RA in overlap with PL-7 ASS after complaints of pleuritic chest pain and CT revealing ILD with a positive ASS panel. The ambiguity of presenting symptoms is thought to contribute to delayed diagnosis and treatment of ASS which increases pulmonary morbidity and mortality, especially in non-Jo-1 patients, and contributes to poor survival [8]. When evaluating patients with connective tissue disease, careful attention should be paid to identifying features of ASS and potentially testing appropriate patients with ASS antibodies even in patients with rheumatoid arthritis with positive RF, CCP antibodies, and erosive changes on X-ray [15, 16].

Immunosuppressive agents treat manifestations of antisynthetase syndrome. Frequently used agents include azathioprine, mycophenolate mofetil, tacrolimus, rituximab, and cyclophosphamide, though there is little consensus on a single preferred age. The use of these agents to treat antisynthetase syndrome-related ILD is off-label [17]. In a recent 2018 retrospective review of 25 ASS patients treated with rituximab, in most patients, improvement or stability was demonstrated on chest CT and PFTs. Glucocorticoid requirements decreased, and the medication was well tolerated in most patients [18]. Rituximab was also found to be beneficial in ASS and seropositive RA overlap syndrome with joint efficacy and extra-articular improvement and or stability. On the contrary, in few patients, TNF alpha inhibitors resulted in exacerbation of myositis and respiratory status [7].

4. Learning Points

(i) ASS especially non-Jo-1 cases can present ambiguously as idiopathic ILD, undifferentiated connective tissue disease, and/or evolve into or present as an overlap syndrome; we present a unique case of PL-7 ASS in overlap with Sjögren's, RA, and SLE.

(ii) Given the high respiratory morbidity and mortality of ASS patients, when evaluating patients with ILD, arthralgias, Raynaud's, or myositis, careful attention should be paid to identifying features of ASS, and the appropriate patients should be screened for ASS antibodies.

References

[1] M. Cojocaru, I. M. Cojocaru, and B. Chicos, "New insights into antisynthetase syndrome," *Maedica*, vol. 11, no. 2, pp. 130–135, 2016.

[2] I. E. Lundberg, F. W. Miller, A. Tjärnlund, and M. Bottai, "Diagnosis and classification of idiopathic inflammatory myopathies," *Journal of Internal Medicine*, vol. 280, no. 1, pp. 39–51, 2016.

[3] B. Hervier and O. Benveniste, "Clinical heterogeneity and outcomes of antisynthetase syndrome," *Current Rheumatology Reports*, vol. 15, pp. 2–12, 2013.

[4] Y. Yamasaki, H. Yamada, T. Nozaki et al., "Unusually high frequency of autoantibodies to PL-7 associated with milder muscle disease in Japanese patients with polymyositis/dermatomyositis," *Arthritis & Rheumatism*, vol. 54, no. 6, pp. 2004–2009, 2006.

[5] B. Hervier, Y. Uzunhan, E. Hachulla et al., "Antisynthetase syndrome positive for anti-threonyl-tRNA synthetase (anti-PL7) antibodies," *European Respiratory Journal*, vol. 37, no. 3, pp. 714–717, 2011.

[6] S. Sato, M. Hirakata, M. Kuwana et al., "Clinical characteristics of Japanese patients with anti-PL-7 (anti-threonyl-tRNA synthetase) autoantibodies," *Clinical and Experimental Rheumatology*, vol. 23, pp. 609–615, 2005.

[7] A. Meyer, G. Lefevre, G. Bierry et al., "In antisynthetase syndrome, ACPA are associated with severe and erosive arthritis," *Medicine*, vol. 94, no. 20, p. e523, 2015.

[8] R. Aggarwal, E. Cassidy, N. Fertig et al., "Patients with non-Jo-1 anti-tRNA-synthetase autoantibodies have worse survival than Jo-1 positive patients," *Annals of the Rheumatic Diseases*, vol. 73, no. 1, pp. 227–232, 2014.

[9] I. Marie, S. Josse, O. Decaux et al., "Clinical manifestations and outcome of anti-PL7 positive patients with antisynthetase syndrome," *European Journal of Internal Medicine*, vol. 24, no. 5, pp. 474–479, 2013.

[10] J. Shi, S. Li, H. Yang et al., "Clinical profiles and prognosis of patients with distinct antisynthetase autoantibodies," *The Journal of Rheumatology*, vol. 44, no. 7, pp. 1051–1057, 2017.

[11] M. Tomonaga, N. Sakamoto, Y. Ishimatsu et al., "Comparison of pulmonary involvement between patients expressing anti-PL-7 and anti-Jo-1 antibodies," *Lung*, vol. 193, no. 1, pp. 79–83, 2015.

[12] M.-P. Debray, R. Borie, M.-P. Revel et al., "Interstitial lung disease in anti-synthetase syndrome: initial and follow-up CT findings," *European Journal of Radiology*, vol. 84, no. 3, pp. 516–523, 2015.

[13] S. A. Yousem, F. Schneider, D. Bi, C. V. Oddis, K. Gibson, and R. Aggarwal, "The pulmonary histopathologic manifestations of the anti-PL7/antithreonyl transfer RNA synthetase syndrome," *Human Pathology*, vol. 45, no. 6, pp. 1199–1204, 2014.

[14] A. Labirua-Iturburu, A. Selva-O'Callaghan, M. Vincze et al., "Anti-PL-7 (anti-threonyl-tRNA synthetase) antisynthetase syndrome," *Medicine*, vol. 91, no. 4, pp. 206–211, 2012.

[15] M. González-Gay, C. Montecucco, A. Selva-O'Callaghan et al., "Timing of onset affects arthritis presentation in anti-synthetase syndrome," *Clinical and Experimental Rheumatology*, vol. 36, pp. 44–49, 2018.

[16] L. Cavagna, L. Nuño, C. A. Scirè et al., "Serum Jo-1 autoantibody and isolated arthritis in the antisynthetase syndrome: review of the literature and report of the experience of AENEAS collaborative group," *Clinical Reviews in Allergy & Immunology*, vol. 52, no. 1, pp. 71–80, 2017.

[17] L. J. Witt, J. J. Curran, and M. E. Strek, "The diagnosis and treatment of antisynthetase syndrome," *Clinical Pulmonary Medicine*, vol. 23, no. 5, pp. 218–226, 2016.

[18] T. J. Doyle, N. Dhillon, R. Madan et al., "Rituximab in the treatment of interstitial lung disease associated with anti-synthetase syndrome: a multicenter retrospective case review," *The Journal of Rheumatology*, vol. 45, no. 6, pp. 841–850, 2018.

31

Abatacept in the Treatment of Juvenile Dermatomyositis-Associated Calcifications in a 16-Year-Old Girl

Sukesh Sukumaran[1] **and Vini Vijayan**[2]

[1]*Division of Rheumatology, Department of Pediatrics, Valley Children's Hospital, Madera, CA, USA*
[2]*Division of Infectious Diseases, Department of Pediatrics, Valley Children's Hospital, Madera, CA, USA*

Correspondence should be addressed to Sukesh Sukumaran; ssukumaran@valleychildrens.org

Academic Editor: Syuichi Koarada

Calcinosis is a feared complication of JDM that may be seen in up to 40% of children with JDM. It is associated with negative impact on the patients' quality of life due to weakness, functional disability, joint contractures, muscle atrophy, skin ulcers, and secondary infections. Calcinosis can present as superficial nodules or plaques, larger nodular deposits extending into deeper tissue layers, accumulation of calcifications along the fascial planes of muscles or tendons, or an exoskeleton of calcium leading to limitations in mobility and joint contractures. Currently, there are no known effective treatments for calcinosis and current therapy is based on anecdotal retrospective studies and cases series. We report the case of a child with JDM-associated calcinosis with extensive intramuscular calcifications who failed conventional therapies but demonstrated improvement as evident by decrease in calcinosis and improved physical function with use of abatacept. We found that use of abatacept was associated with improvement in functional outcome and recurrence did not occur. This case suggests use of abatacept as a safe and effective treatment option for calcinosis due to JDM. Furthermore, large-scale clinical studies are needed to validate our findings and to evaluate the long-term outcomes.

1. Introduction

Juvenile dermatomyositis (JDM) is the most common inflammatory myopathy of childhood, with an estimated incidence of 3.2 children per million per year [1]. The disease is characterized by proximal muscle weakness and characteristic rashes. Multiple organ systems including the gastrointestinal, cardiac, and pulmonary systems can be involved and contribute to the morbidity and mortality associated with JDM. Previously, the prognosis of JDM was poor with a reported mortality of 30% [1, 2]. However, with the advent of new treatments for JDM, survival and functional outcomes have improved considerably and the reported mortality has declined and is currently estimated to be 2% [3, 4]. Despite the many progresses in the treatment of JDM, calcinosis continues to be a feared complication of the disease [5, 6].

In this report, we describe the case of a 16-year-old girl with refractory JDM and skin ulcerations as well as extensive intramuscular calcifications that were poorly responsive to conventional therapy but were subsequently successfully treated with abatacept. The purpose of this report is to share our experience to rheumatologists regarding the use of abatacept as a potential treatment option for refractory calcinosis due to JDM.

2. Case

A 16-year-old Caucasian female was diagnosed with juvenile dermatomyositis (JDM) at the age of 7 when she presented with moderate weakness of the proximal muscles, heliotrope rash, Gottron's papules overlying the elbows, knees, and extensor aspect of the fingers, and periungual telangiectasia. She had an elevated aldolase of 15 U/L (normal 3.4–8.6 U/L) and elevated lactate dehydrogenase (LDH) of 1100 (normal 470–750 U/L), and her creatinine kinase was 506 U/L (normal 22–198 U/L). Her aspartate aminotransferase (AST) and alanine transaminase (ALT) were 115 U/L and 110 U/L, respectively. Antinuclear antibodies, human leukocyte antigen B-27, angiotensin converting enzyme, and anti-neutrophil cytoplasmic antibodies were negative. Magnetic resonance imaging (MRI) demonstrated diffuse muscle edema and myositis. Child was started on pulse methylprednisolone (30 mg/kg/day) for three doses followed by tapering doses of oral steroids 2 mg/kg/day and methotrexate subcutaneously weekly (15 mg/m^2). She also received monthly intravenous immunoglobulin (IVIG). She showed gradual improvement in her muscle weakness then resolution of her rash. Her disease remained relatively quiescent on hydroxychloroquine and mycophenolate mofetil.

At 9 years into her disease course, she presented with a 3-month history of hard masses over the buttocks and lower extremities and multiple painful, ulcerative lesions with foul smelling drainage. She denied fever, cough, difficulty swallowing, or abdominal pain but reported generalized fatigue and muscle weakness. She admitted being poorly compliant with her medications. On examination, bony hard masses ranging between 2.5 cm and 3.5 cm in diameter were palpable on her lower extremities and extended along the length of thigh to the ankle. She also had multiple ulcerative lesions over her buttocks and the posterior aspect of her thighs. Musculoskeletal examination showed symmetrical proximal muscle weakness of her pelvic and pectoral muscles, and limited range of motion of the bilateral hip, knee, and ankles. She also had lipodystrophy and muscle atrophy of her lower extremities. Laboratory investigations revealed AST 65 U/L, aldolase 12 U/L, LDH 470, and creatinine kinase 29 U/L. The rest of the physical examination were unremarkable. Her initial Childhood Myositis Assessment Scale (CMAS) score was 28 out of 52, and Childhood Health Assessment Questionnaire (CHAQ) score was 0.75. MRI of the pelvis and thighs showed extensive calcifications in her skin, in the facial planes, and muscle edema around her thighs and buttocks bilaterally. She also had muscle edema (Figure1).

Child was started on cyclophosphamide 750 mg/m^2 in addition to high dose steroids and methotrexate. Due to the continued extension of the calcifications despite 6 months of this regimen, colchicine and probenecid were attempted with no improvement in ulcerations, calcinosis, or muscle strength. Child underwent surgical excision of the calcium deposits but continued to develop new areas of calcification and skin ulcers, and hence cyclophosphamide was discontinued. High-dose corticosteroids and IVIG were continued and, in addition, she was started on abatacept intravenously (IV) at 10 mg/kg/dose at 0, 2, and 4 weeks and then every 4 weeks. Three months after initiation of abatacept, child's cutaneous ulcerations completely healed. Her calcifications became softer and she demonstrated increased range of motion in her hip and knee joints. Her CMAS score improved to 45 out of 52, and the CHAQ score improved to 0.5 at 6 months of therapy. Her oral steroid dose was decreased by 50% at her 6-month follow-up. Nine months after starting abatacept, she was weaned off steroids completely. Plain X-rays and MRI of her lower extremities confirmed lack of progression of calcinosis, and no new lesions were detected after 1 year of treatment. She did not develop any adverse effects from abatacept.

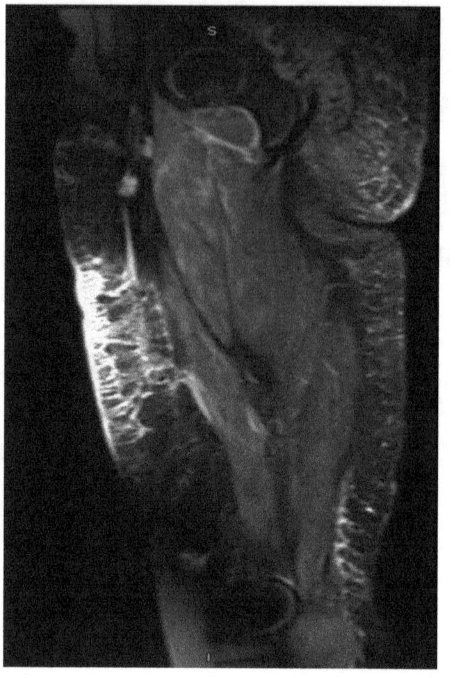

FIGURE 1: MRI imaging of thigh. Sagittal fat suppressed T2-weighted images revealing muscle edema and calcifications in the fascial planes.

3. Discussion

Calcinosis is a known contributor to the morbidity associated with JDM and can have a negative impact on the patients' quality of life, causing weakness, functional disability, joint contractures, muscle atrophy, skin ulcers, and secondary infections. Calcinosis may be seen in up to 40% of children with JDM, but the prevalence ranges anywhere from 10 to 70%. Calcinosis usually appears 1–3 years after onset of JDM but has reported to occur at onset of the disease to as long as 20 years after disease onset [6–8]. Risk factors for the development of calcinosis include a delay in the diagnosis, delay in initiating treatment or inadequate treatment, tumor necrosis factor (TNF) alpha-308A genotype, presence of autoantibodies against nuclear matrix protein 2 (NXP2), and younger age at disease onset [9, 10].

The phenotypical presentations of calcinosis are diverse. It can present as superficial nodules or plaques, larger nodular deposits extending into deeper tissue layers, accumulation of calcifications along the fascial planes of muscles or tendons, or an exoskeleton of calcium leading to limitations in mobility and joint contractures. Although calcinosis is often painless, these lesions can ulcerate and become infected. The most commonly affected sites are the buttocks, trunk, hands, feet, elbows, and knees, but lesions can develop at any site. The presentation of calcinosis differs from adults wherein calcinosis occurs in only 20% of patients and the lesions occur primarily on the extremities [6–10].

The pathogenesis of calcinosis in JDM is unknown but calcinosis also appears to occur more frequently in patients with ongoing inflammation. This finding is supported by reports indicating the presence of cells and proinflammatory cytokines such as IL-1 and TNF-alpha and a variety of proteins related to mineralization at the calcinosis site. Cytokines such as IL-6, IL-1β, TNF-α, IL-1β, and IL-6 were also detected in serum, suggesting the role of activated macrophages in JDM-associated calcinosis. It has also been associated with the presence of antibodies against the 140 kDa protein and with TNF-alpha-308A polymorphism [10–12].

There are no standardized recommendations for the treatment of calcinosis due to JDM, but the overarching goal of treatment is to minimize symptoms and alleviate functional limitations. Although calcium channel blockers, probenicid, and intralesional corticosteroids have been used, none of these agents have demonstrated a consistently reliable response. Many studies have reported both treatment success and failure of colchicine for calcinosis cutis. Surgical intervention can be considered in areas of noninflammatory calcinosis for treatment of pain, functional impairment, and/or skin ulceration due to calcinosis, although some reports have suggested the possibility for recurrence when underlying JDM disease activity is not well controlled [12]. Considering the high levels of TNF-alpha in patients with calcinosis, anti-TNF therapy may play a role in treating calcinosis. In 2008, Riley et al. reported a case series of five patients successfully treated with the TNF-alpha inhibitor, infliximab, for calcinosis and JDM refractory to standard therapy [13]. Given the increasing information regarding the importance of novel autoantibodies in the pathogenesis of JDM, B-cell depletion with agents such as rituximab may also prove to be effective. However, reports have suggested the possibility for recurrence when underlying JDM disease activity is not well controlled and hence control of the underlying disease process is of utmost importance.

Abatacept is a fully human soluble fusion of cytotoxic T lymphocyte antigen-4 and the Fc portion of immunoglobulin. Cytotoxic T lymphocyte antigen-4 inhibits costimulation of T-cell activation by blocking the binding of CD28 on T cells with CD80/86 on antigen-presenting cells, thereby exerting an antiinflammatory effect. Abatacept is used in the treatment of adult rheumatoid arthritis and juvenile idiopathic arthritis, but there are very limited data regarding its use for calcinosis due to juvenile dermatomyositis [14]. The mechanism of action of abatacept in JDM-associated calcinosis may be due to the inhibition of macrophages and consequent decrease in proinflammatory cytokines [14]. Arabshahi et al. reported the successful use of abatacept and sodium thiosulfate in a patient with severe recalcitrant juvenile dermatomyositis complicated by ulcerative skin disease and progressive calcinosis. This combination therapy resulted in significant reductions in muscle and skin inflammation, decreased corticosteroid dependence, and halted the progression of calcinosis. In their study, topical sodium thiosulfate was used based on its property to dissolve calcium deposits. It was not possible to determine if their patient improved due to the combination of abatacept and sodium thiosulfate or due to the sodium thiosulfate alone [15]. Our case differs in that we did not use sodium thiosulfate and hence provides further evidence for the efficacy of abatacept in calcinosis with objective radiological improvement.

In conclusion, we describe a case of refractory JDM with skin ulcerations and extensive intramuscular calcifications that were poorly responsive to conventional therapy but were subsequently successfully treated with abatacept. Our patient initially underwent surgical excision and increase in immunomodulation, but her calcinosis continued to progress which prompted use of abatacept. We found that use of abatacept was associated with improvement in her functional outcome and recurrence did not occur. As treatment late in the course of JDM has been associated with a greater amount of dystrophic calcium salt deposition, rheumatologists should explore use of abatacept early on in disease course. Further studies are needed to validate the use of abatacept for treatment of calcinosis in children with JDM and to evaluate the long-term outcomes.

Disclosure

This case was presented as a poster at the 21st Asia Pacific League of Associations for Rheumatology Congress in Brisbane, Australia, April 8–11, 2019.

References

[1] E. P. Mendez, R. Lipton, R. Ramsey-Goldman et al., "US incidence of juvenile dermatomyositis, 1995–1998: results from the national institute of arthritis and musculoskeletal and skin diseases registry," *Arthritis & Rheumatism*, vol. 49, no. 3, pp. 300–305, 2003.

[2] A. Bohan and J. B. Peter, "Polymyosistis and dermatomyositis," *The New England Journal of Medicine*, vol. 292, pp. 344–403, 1975.

[3] A. M. Huber, B. Lang, C. M. A. LeBlanc et al., "Medium- and long-term functional outcomes in a multicenter cohort of children with juvenile dermatomyositis," *Arthritis & Rheumatism*, vol. 43, no. 3, pp. 541–549, 2000.

[4] N. Martin, C. K. Li, and L. R. Wedderburn, "Juvenile dermatomyositis: new insights and new treatment strategies," *Therapeutic Advances in Musculoskeletal Disease*, vol. 4, no. 1, pp. 41–50, 2012.

[5] A. V. Ramanan and B. M. Feldman, "Clinical outcomes in juvenile dermatomyositis," *Current Opinion in Rheumatology*, vol. 14, no. 6, pp. 658–662, 2002.

[6] M. F. Hoeltzel, E. J. Oberle, A. B. Robinson, A. Agarwal, and L. G. Rider, "The presentation, assessment, pathogenesis, and treatment of calcinosis in juvenile dermatomyositis," *Current Rheumatology Reports*, vol. 16, no. 12, 2014.

[7] C. E. Blance, S. J. White, E. M. Braunstein et al., "Patterns of calcification in childhood dermatomyositis," *American Journal of Roentgenology*, vol. 142, pp. 397–400, 1984.

[8] L. G. Rider, "Calcinosis in juvenile dermatomyositis: pathogenesis and current therapies," *Pediatric Rheumatology*, vol. 1, p. 2, 2003.

[9] S. L. Bowyer, C. E. Blane, D. B. Sullivan, and J. T. Cassidy, "Childhood dermatomyositis: factors predicting functional outcome and development of dystrophic calcification," *The Journal of Pediatrics*, vol. 103, no. 6, pp. 882–888, 1983.

[10] L. M. Pachman, M. R. Liotta-Davis, D. K. Hong et al., "TNFα-308A allele in juvenile dermatomyositis: association with increased production of tumor necrosis factor α, disease duration, and pathologic calcifications," *Arthritis & Rheumatism*, vol. 43, no. 10, pp. 2368–2377, 2000.
[11] M. Mukamel, G. Horev, and M. Mimouni, "New insight into calcinosis of juvenile dermatomyositis: a study of composition and treatment," *The Journal of Pediatrics*, vol. 138, no. 5, pp. 763–766, 2001.
[12] L. M. Pachman, A. Veis, S. Stock et al., "Composition of calcifications in children with juvenile dermatomyositis: association with chronic cutaneous inflammation," *Arthritis & Rheumatism*, vol. 54, no. 10, pp. 3345–3350, 2006.
[13] P. Riley, L. J. Mccann, S. M. Maillard, P. Woo, K. J. Murray, and C. A. Pilkington, "Effectiveness of infliximab in the treatment of refractory juvenile dermatomyositis with calcinosis," *Rheumatology*, vol. 47, no. 6, pp. 877–880, 2008.
[14] U. Fiocco, P. Sfriso, F. Oliviero et al., "Co-stimulatory modulation in rheumatoid arthritis: the role of (CTLA4-Ig) abatacept," *Autoimmunity Reviews*, vol. 8, no. 1, pp. 76–82, 2008.
[15] B. Arabshahi, R. A. Silverman, O. Y. Jones, and L. G. Rider, "Abatacept and sodium thiosulfate for treatment of recalcitrant juvenile dermatomyositis complicated by ulceration and calcinosis," *The Journal of Pediatrics*, vol. 160, no. 3, pp. 520–522, 2012.

32

Treatment of Down Syndrome-Associated Arthritis with JAK Inhibition

Jordan T. Jones[1,2,3]

[1]*Department of Pediatrics, Children's Mercy Kansas City, Kansas, MO, USA*
[2]*University of Missouri-Kansas City School of Medicine, Kansas, MO, USA*
[3]*University of Kansas School of Medicine, Kansas, KS, USA*

Correspondence should be addressed to Jordan T. Jones; jtjones@cmh.edu

Academic Editor: Syuichi Koarada

Down syndrome (DS) results from a trisomy of chromosome 21, which causes immune dysregulation that leads to hyperactivation of interferon and Janus kinase (JAK) signaling. This results in complex medical abnormalities in the immune system and an increase in autoimmune and autoinflammatory conditions such as down syndrome-associated arthritis (DA). DA is an aggressive, destructive, inflammatory arthritis that is easily misdiagnosed and difficult to treat. Treatment commonly includes immunosuppressive therapy, but these are often associated with adverse effects and ineffectiveness. This case report outlines a 6-year-old male with DA that was successfully treated with the JAK inhibitor tofacitinib. Due to the aggressive nature of DA and poor response to many immunosuppressive therapies, this case report was created to increase awareness of JAK inhibition as an effective, well-tolerated treatment for DA.

1. Introduction

Down syndrome (DS) is one of the most common birth defects in the United States [1] and the most common genomic disorder that results from a trisomy of human chromosome 21 [2]. The trisomy 21 results in an increased prevalence of hypothyroidism, congenital heart disease, hematologic disorders, and autoimmune disease such as celiac disease, diabetes mellitus, and down syndrome-associated arthritis (DA) [3]. It has been established that there is immune dysregulation in those with DS that contributes to elevated levels of the tumor necrosis factor (TNF) and interferon (IFN) [4] as the trisomy 21 causes hyperactivation of IFN and Janus kinase (JAK) signaling [5, 6] and may be responsible for the cause of DA. Most children with DA present with polyarticular (five or more joints with arthritis at presentation), rheumatoid factor (RF), and antinuclear antibody (ANA) negative disease that is aggressive with bone and joint damage at presentation. There is also a long delay in diagnosis due to lack of screening guidance and misdiagnosis due to common mechanical issues seen in those with DS such as pes planus, hypermobility, and hypotonia [3]. Once diagnosed, and despite aggressive immunosuppressive therapy, the disease burden remains high, and therapeutic challenges are common due to an increase in adverse effects and ineffectiveness of therapy [7]. Synthetic and biologic disease modifying antirheumatic drugs (DMARDs) have not been as successful as a therapeutic option for DA compared to other forms of arthritis due to poor disease control and adverse effects [3]. With the hyperactivation of IFN and JAK signaling seen in DS, JAK inhibition is an appealing option for disease control. This report describes the first reported case of a pediatric patient with DA who was successfully treated to clinically inactive disease with the JAK inhibitor tofacitinib.

2. Case Presentation

A 6-year-old male with trisomy 21 (meiotic nondisjunction), hypothyroidism (with negative thyroid peroxidase and thyroid globulin antibodies), and a history of frequent bacterial, viral, and topical fungal infections with hypogammaglobulinemia requiring IVIg was seen in the rheumatology clinic in July of 2017 for a 12-month history of bilateral foot and ankle pain. There was right ankle swelling and limitation that had been present for the previous three months, which was thought to be correlated to an increase in activity over that time frame with starting school and a new dance class. The right ankle swelling fluctuated in severity but never completely resolved, and there were 20 minutes of morning stiffness daily. The swelling and limitation did improve with ibuprofen (10 mg/kg every 6 hours as needed) but never resolved. On physical exam, the patient was noted to have swelling and limitation of bilateral ankles with antalgic gait along with generalized joint hypermobility (Beighton score of 8/9) and bilateral pes planus. His initial laboratory evaluation revealed a normal C-reactive protein (CRP; <0.5 mg/dL), erythrocyte sedimentation rate (ESR; 8 mm/h), complete blood count (without any cytosis or cytopenia), negative ANA, RF, and human leukocyte antigen B-27. He had low immunoglobulin G (602 mg/dL), immunoglobulin M (44 mg/dL), and normal immunoglobulin A (81 mg/dL). An ultrasound of bilateral ankles and feet showed the fluid surrounding the bilateral extensor digitorum longus, left peroneal brevis and longus tendons, and left extensor hallucis longus tendon consistent with tenosynovitis. He was started on naproxen (10 mg/kg twice daily), and after eight weeks, he showed minimal improvement in pain, swelling, and limitation. The family was hesitant to start immunosuppressive therapy due to his history of recurrent infections with hypogammaglobulinemia, and so he was switched to meloxicam (0.25 mg/kg daily). After an eight-week course, there was no improvement in ankle and foot pain and swelling, and he continued to have antalgic gait. His morning stiffness persisted and increased to 30 minutes daily. He also developed swelling and discomfort in his bilateral second and third metacarpophalangeal joints. His family remained hesitant about immunosuppression but was interested in additional therapy, and hydroxychloroquine (3.5 mg/kg daily) was added. The combination of meloxicam and hydroxychloroquine did result in mild improvement in ankle, foot, and hand swelling and limitation over the next five months; however, none of the symptoms resolved. There were plans to start IV abatacept for continued evidence of active arthritis; however, the patient developed seizures and regression with oral intake, eating, toileting, and weight loss, and the family wanted to prioritize evaluation and treatment of neurodevelopmental and behavioral issues, so the patient was continued on the combination of meloxicam and hydroxychloroquine. The medications were inconsistently used due to the other health issues related to DS until April 2020 when he developed an upper respiratory infection with fever and had worsened joint pain, limitation, and swelling in bilateral ankles, feet, and metacarpophalangeal joints. In addition, he developed swelling and limitation in the bilateral knees. After resolution of the febrile illness he continued with pain, swelling, limitation, and antalgic gait. He did not want to engage in activities he usually enjoyed and would avoid physical activities as well. After his febrile illness resolved, laboratory tests showed normal platelets (429×10^3/mcL) and hemoglobin (13.3 gm/dL) with low white blood cells (4.1×10^3/mcL), elevated ESR (18 mm/h), and normal CRP (<0.5 mg/dL). With the increase in inflammatory arthritis symptoms and impact on quality of life, the family decided they were ready to escalate to immunosuppressive therapy. A discussion of risks and benefits was undertaken to outline additional therapy options. We decided to avoid corticosteroids due to the common adverse effects such as weight gain that is commonly experienced in children with DS [8]. We also avoided synthetic DMARDs such as methotrexate due to the increased intolerance and adverse effects experienced in children with DS [9]. In addition, evidence shows that many patients with DA have poor response to biologic DMARDs such as anti-TNF inhibitors [7], so we looked for another option for treatment. Since trisomy 21 causes elevated levels of IFN through JAK signaling, a JAK inhibitor such as tofacitinib was determined to be an appealing possible therapeutic option. In addition, the family was worried about administration of injectable synthetic and biologic DMARDs, which can be challenging in the pediatric population. Furthermore, the patient was under investigation for autism due to behavioral changes and regression, and the family felt an injectable therapy would be difficult to administer regularly. At the time (April 2020), no JAK inhibitor was approved by the United States Food and Drug Administration (FDA) for arthritis in children, but it was under investigation in clinical trials and was approved for use in adults with inflammatory arthritis. JAK inhibition was determined to have good potential for disease control, and so tofacitinib was initiated at 2.5 mg orally, twice daily. There was a rapid improvement in joint swelling, limitation, and stiffness. There was no more morning stiffness or antalgic gait. The patient was noted to be more active with improved mood, and there was complete resolution of arthritis two months after initiation of tofacitinib. The laboratory tests (CRP and ESR) continued to be normal, and there were no adverse effects or serious infections reported since initiation approximately 28 months ago.

3. Discussion

Down syndrome-associated arthritis (DA) is an aggressive, destructive, inflammatory arthritis that has long delay in time from symptom onset to diagnosis that can be up to three years due to being underrecognized [9]. In addition, those with DS commonly have hypotonia, hypermobility, pes planus, and autism, which may mislead providers and further delay diagnosis. Patients with DA commonly present with bone and joint damage at presentation; however, the patient reported here was diagnosed earlier than usual as the down syndrome clinic at our institution has a brief musculoskeletal screen given to all patients seen in the DS clinic, which includes focused questions about musculoskeletal pain and limitation with positive screens that trigger additional evaluation and referral as appropriate [10]. This does provide support for regular musculoskeletal screening for patients with DS as DA has a prevalence of 10 per 1000 patients [3]; however, the optimal timing and interval of screening is unclear.

Once diagnosed, the therapeutic approach to DA has been similar to juvenile idiopathic arthritis (JIA) [11], which is the most common rheumatic disease in childhood. JIA is an autoimmune disease that results in arthritis in children, and studies have shown differences in clinical presentation and pathogenesis between DA and JIA. A study that evaluated the adaptive immune system of individuals with DA and JIA found that those with DA had expansion of IgM-only memory B cells and decreased number of transitional B cells. It was also noted that those with DA have increased proinflammatory cytokines TNF and INF compared to those with JIA. It is thought that the proinflammatory cytokine response is associated with increased T cell plasticity in those with DA [12]. There have also been findings to suggest that the synovial tissue inflammation is different between those with DA and JIA with increased infiltration of T and B cells in the inflamed synovium in DA [12]. The immune dysregulation in DA is likely in part caused by the four IFN receptors encoded on chromosome 21, which leads to hypersensitivity of IFN ligands, increased JAK signaling, and increase in proinflammatory autoimmune and autoinflammatory disease [5, 6, 13]. Evidence continues to build that shows a connection among increased IFN, JAK signaling, and inflammatory disease in those with DS. In September 2020, the JAK inhibitor tofacitinib was approved by the FDA for treatment of polyarticular JIA in children of 2 years of age and older. This approval may make it easier for those with DA to obtain this medication now, as some view DA and JIA as the same disease [11], despite growing evidence to suggest otherwise [3]. In addition, JAK inhibition has also been used to successfully treat psoriatic arthritis in an adult with DS [14] with rapid improvement in skin and joint disease and no adverse effects. This further supports JAK inhibition for inflammatory conditions seen in DS.

DA is an aggressive, destructive, inflammatory joint disease in those with DS that is poorly understood; however, as awareness of DA improves and as more individuals with DS are diagnosed, we will need better therapies and therapeutic approaches that are tailored to those with DA. The current therapeutic options for DA, which have been borrowed from JIA, come with more adverse effects and less effectiveness; however, JAK inhibition may become a preferred option for those with DA as it is oral medication, has proven effective for arthritis treatment, and targets the immune dysregulation seen in those with DS.

Authors' Contributions

JJ developed conception, drafting, and final version of the whole manuscript. All authors read and approved the final manuscript.

References

[1] G. de Graaf, F. Buckley, and B. G. Skotko, "Estimates of the live births, natural losses, and elective terminations with Down syndrome in the United States," *American Journal of Medical Genetics, Part A*, vol. 167, no. 4, pp. 756–767, Apr 2015.

[2] S. E. Antonarakis, B. G. Skotko, M. S. Rafii et al., "Down syndrome," *Nature Reviews Disease Primers*, vol. 6, no. 1, p. 9, 2020, https://pubmed.ncbi.nlm.nih.gov/32029743/.

[3] J. T. Jones, J. Kitchen, and N. Talib, "Down syndrome-associated arthritis (DA): diagnostic and management challenges," *Pediatric Health, Medicine and Therapeutics*, vol. 13, pp. 53–62, 2022.

[4] M. N. Rostami, M. Douraghi, A. M. Mohammadi, and B. Nikmanesh, "Altered serum pro-inflammatory cytokines in children with Down's syndrome," *European Cytokine Network*, vol. 23, no. 2, pp. 64–67, 2012.

[5] K. D. Sullivan, H. C. Lewis, A. A. Hill et al., "Trisomy 21 consistently activates the interferon response," *Elife*, vol. 5, Article ID e16220, 2016.

[6] K. A. Waugh, P. Araya, A. Pandey et al., "Mass cytometry reveals global immune remodeling with multi-lineage hypersensitivity to type I interferon in Down syndrome," *Cell Reports*, vol. 29, no. 7, pp. 1893–1908, 2019.

[7] J. T. Jones, C. Smith, M. L. Becker, D. Lovell, and C. R. Investigators, "The Down syndrome-associated arthritis cohort in the new childhood arthritis and rheumatology research alliance (CARRA) registry: clinical characteristics, treatment and outcomes," *Arthritis Care & Research*, vol. 73, 2020.

[8] J. T. Jones, C. Smith, and N. Talib, "Assessment of Down syndrome-associated arthritis: a survey of Down syndrome clinic providers," *Global Pediatric Health*, vol. 8, 2021.

[9] J. T. Jones, N. Talib, D. Lovell, and M. L. Becker, "Clinical features and treatment of Down syndrome arthropathy: experience from two US tertiary hospitals," *Pediatric Drugs*, vol. 21, no. 1, pp. 33–39, 2019.

[10] J. T. Jones, C. Smith, and N. Talib, "Brief musculoskeletal screen and patient education for Down syndrome-associated arthritis," *Global Pediatric Health*, vol. 8, 2021.

[11] A. Nicek, N. Talib, D. Lovell, C. Smith, M. L. Becker, and J. T. Jones, "Assessment and treatment of Down syndrome-associated arthritis: a survey of pediatric rheumatologists," *Pediatric Rheumatology*, vol. 18, no. 1, p. 57, 2020.

[12] C. Foley, A. Floudas, M. Canavan, M. Biniecka et al., Increased T cell plasticity with dysregulation of follicular helper T, peripheral helper T, and treg cell responses in children with juvenile idiopathic arthritis and Down syndrome-associated arthritis," *Arthritis & Rheumatology*, vol. 72, no. 4, pp. 677–686, 2019.

[13] R. K. Powers, R. Culp-Hill, M. P. Ludwig et al., "Trisomy 21 activates the kynurenine pathway via increased dosage of interferon receptors," *Nature Communications*, vol. 10, no. 1, 2019.

[14] A. T. Pham, A. L. Rachubinski, B. Enriquez-Estrada, K. Worek, M. Griffith, and J. M. Espinosa, "JAK inhibition for treatment of psoriatic arthritis in Down syndrome," *Rheumatology*, vol. 60, no. 9, pp. e309–e311, 1 2021.

A Case of Granulomatosis with Polyangiitis with Various Breast Lesions as the Initial Symptoms: A Case-Based Review

Masatoshi Kawataka,[1] Toshiki Kido,[1] Reina Tsuda,[1] Takafumi Onose,[1] Ryoko Asano,[1] Miho Yamazaki,[1] Naonori Sugishita,[1] Hiroyuki Hounoki,[1] Toshiko Kakiuchi,[2] Koichiro Shinoda,[1] and Kazuyuki Tobe[1]

[1]*First Department of Internal Medicine, University of Toyama, Toyama, Japan*
[2]*Department of Diagnostic Pathology, University of Toyama, Toyama, Japan*

Correspondence should be addressed to Koichiro Shinoda; koichiro@med.u-toyama.ac.jp

Academic Editor: Gregory J. Tsay

A 44-year-old woman presenting with pus-like discharge from the nipples visited our hospital for scleritis. Subcutaneous induration and ulceration were found on her breast. She was diagnosed with granulomatosis with polyangiitis (GPA) considering scleritis, sinusitis, cutaneous granuloma formation, and antiproteinase 3-antineutrophil cytoplasmic antibodies and was successfully treated with glucocorticoids. Fifteen months later, she developed pulmonary consolidation and a right breast nodule. Biopsies of the breast nodule showed granulomatous vasculitis, and she was treated with rituximab. While breast involvement in GPA is rare, unilateral breast mass is a typical clinical feature; thus, GPA should be considered in such cases.

1. Introduction

Granulomatosis with polyangiitis (GPA) is a systemic necrotizing vasculitis associated with the presence of antiproteinase 3-antineutrophil cytoplasmic antibodies (PR3-ANCA). The most common sites of organ involvement are the upper and lower respiratory tracts and kidneys, and clinical manifestations are granulomatous and necrotizing inflammatory lesions and rapidly progressive pauci-immune glomerulonephritis [1]. By contrast, breast involvement in GPA is rare [2–4]; as far as we could find in the English literature, only one case has been reported in Japan [5]. A unilateral breast tumor-like lesion is a typical clinical and imaging feature and is sometimes misdiagnosed as breast cancer. We, herein, report the case of a patient with GPA who presented with bilateral breast lesions as initial symptoms.

2. Case Presentation

A 44-year-old woman visited the department of ophthalmology in our hospital because of hyperemia in both eyes, which had rapidly worsened two months prior. She was diagnosed with bilateral necrotizing scleritis (Figure 1(a)) and was referred to our department to assess the involvement of an autoimmune disease. Her medical history revealed that she had been experiencing pus-like discharge from bilateral nipples for the past three months and had thus visited a dermatologist; she was treated with antibiotics, but there was no improvement. More recently, she had suffered from nasal congestion and discharge. She was afebrile, and auscultation revealed no rales in her lung fields and no abnormal heart sounds. Subcutaneous induration was observed in both breasts, along with discharge from the nipples (Figure 1(b)). Pale erythema and a skin ulcer were found on the right breast (Figure 1(c)). No lymph node enlargement was observed from the neck to the axilla. Laboratory test results showed an elevated white blood cell count (10,730/μL) with high polymorphonuclear neutrophil level (70.1%), normal liver and renal function, C-reactive protein (CRP) in almost normal range (1.2 mg/L), and a slightly elevated erythrocyte sedimentation rate (ESR) (48 mm/h). Immunological tests were negative for rheumatoid factor, antinuclear antibodies, and myeloperoxidase- (MPO-) ANCA; however, PR3-ANCA was slightly elevated (5.9 U/mL;

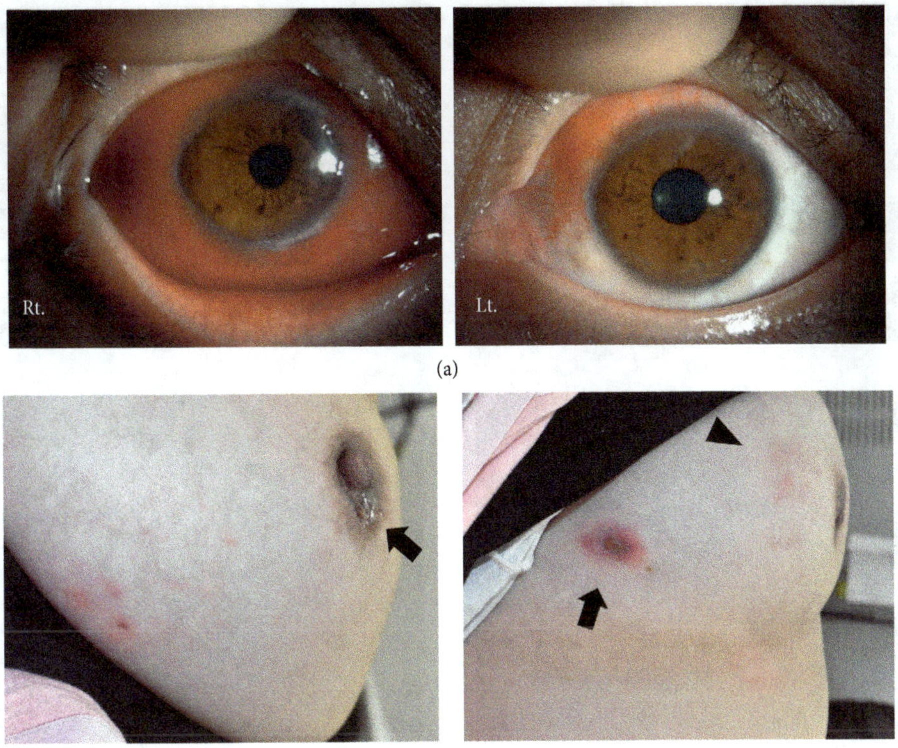

(a) (b) (c)

FIGURE 1: (a) Clinical pictures of the patient's bilateral necrotizing scleritis. (b) Discharge from her nipples (arrow). (c) Pale erythema (arrowhead) and a skin ulcer (arrow) on the right breast.

normal value <2.0 U/mL). The patient tested negative for tuberculosis (TB) in an interferon-γ releasing assay. Urinalysis showed no abnormalities, including hematuria and proteinuria. Computed tomography (CT) of the thorax indicated no abnormalities in the lung fields; however, tumor-like lesions were found in her breasts (Figure 2(a)). CT of the paranasal sinuses showed sinusitis in the right maxillary sinus, and nasopharyngolaryngoscopy demonstrated purulent discharge from the middle meatus. Mammography demonstrated a round, microlobulated, and high-density mass lesion in the right breast, which was classified as category 4, and a 7.5 cm circumscribed, round, and high-density mass lesion in the left breast, which was classified as category 3 (Figure 3). Ultrasonography demonstrated a well-defined, rough-margined, heterogeneous, low-echoic, and unmeasurable giant mass lesion in the left breast and an irregular-shaped, ill-defined, heterogeneous mass lesion in the right breast. Breast cancer, fibroadenoma, sclerosing adenosis, mastitis, and abscess formation were differential diagnoses.

A bacterial culture test and cytological examination of the exudate from the nipples were performed to differentiate between infection and neoplastic lesions. Although a small amount of *Serratia marcescens*, *Corynebacterium* species, *Anaerococcus* species, *Finegoldia magna*, and *Peptoniphilus* species were present in the bacterial culture, infectious mastitis was ruled out considering her clinical course. Cytology revealed infiltration of inflammatory cells, which were mainly lymphocytes and agglomeration of epithelioid cells containing multinucleated giant cells, without malignant cells. Core needle biopsy of her left breast (from the location of the arrow in Figure 2(a)) showed inflammatory cell infiltration consisting of lymphocytes with surrounding fibrotic lesions without vasculitis. A biopsy of a skin ulcer on the right chest wall (from the location of the arrow in Figure 1(c)) showed granuloma formation, including lymphocytes and plasma cells outside the blood vessels without vasculitis. These lesions were suspected as granulomatous mastitis considering breast imaging, nonsignificant bacterial culture, and cytological and pathological examination. Based on the presence of bilateral scleritis, cutaneous granuloma formation, inflammatory breast masses, right maxillary sinusitis, and PR3-ANCA positivity, the patient was diagnosed with a probable case of localized GPA according to the diagnostic criteria of the Ministry of Health, Labor and Welfare of Japan. She was treated with methylprednisolone pulse therapy, followed by a daily dose of 40 mg of prednisolone (PSL) and trimethoprim/sulfamethoxazole. Her symptoms improved, and the titers of CRP, ESR, and PR3-ANCA were normalized. Fifteen months later, when PSL was tapered to 5 mg/day, she complained of cough and nasal discharge. The titer of CRP and ESR had increased to 95.8 mg/L and 80 mm/h. The PR3-ANCA titer had increased to 26.5 U/mL, and whole-body CT revealed pulmonary consolidation in the right lower lobe (Figure 2(b)) and a small nodule in the right breast (Figure 2(c)) as new lesions with recurrence of maxillary sinusitis (Figure 2(d)).

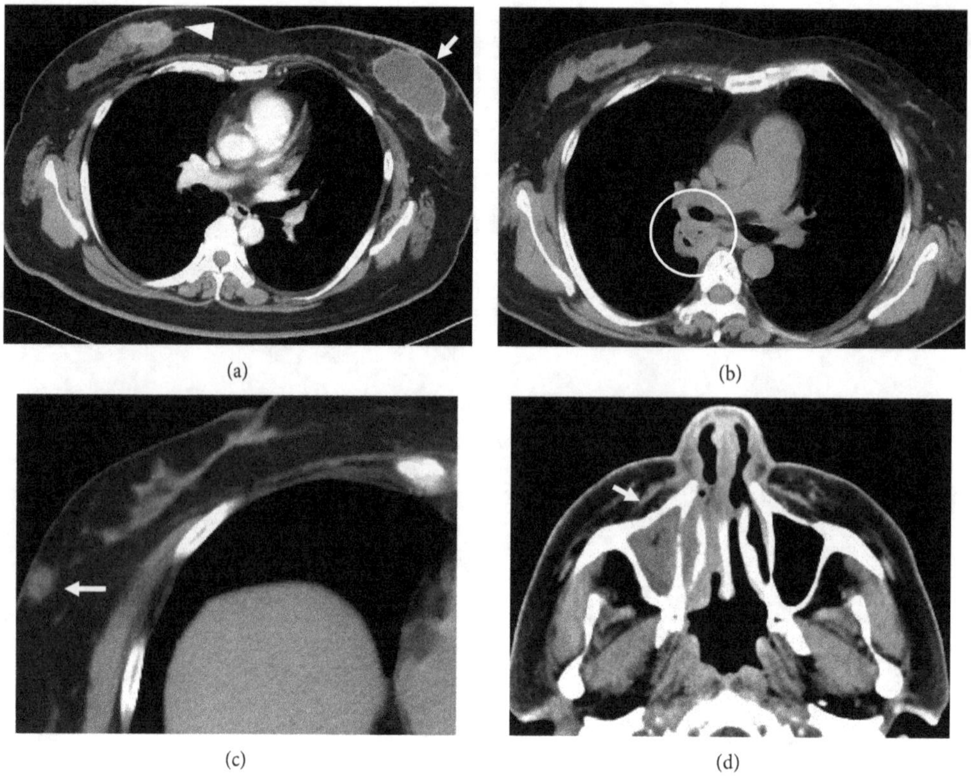

FIGURE 2: (a) Computed tomography showing tumor-like lesions in the patient's breasts (right, arrowhead; left, arrow) on the first admission. (b) Whole-body computed tomography revealing pulmonary consolidation in the right lower lobe (circle). (c) A small nodule in the right breast (arrow), and (d) recurrence of right maxillary sinusitis (arrow) during the second admission.

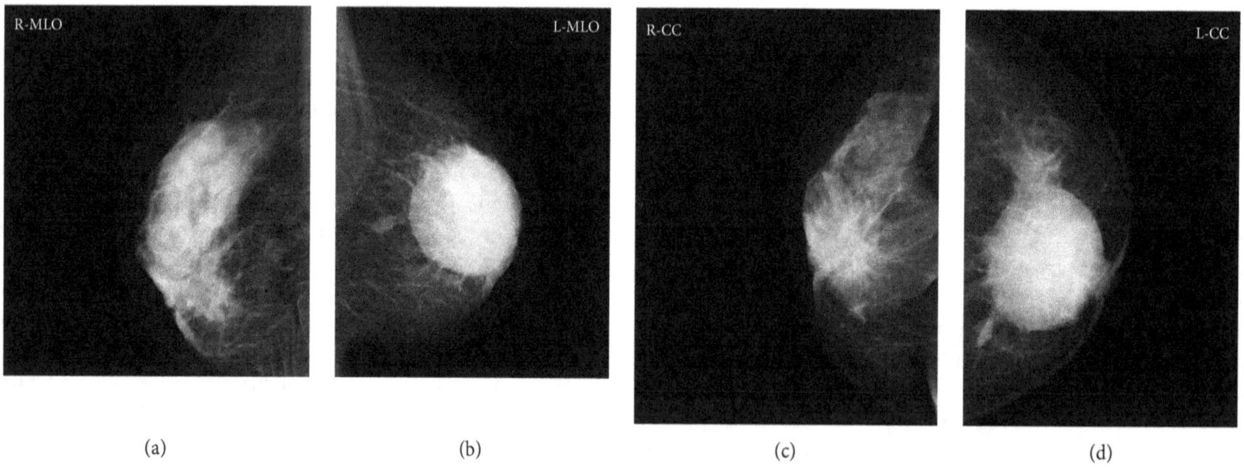

FIGURE 3: Mediolateral oblique (a, b) and craniocaudal (c, d) mammography demonstrates a round, microlobulated, and high-density mass lesion in the right breast (a, c) and circumscribed, round, and high-density mass lesion in the left breast (b, d).

A biopsy of the small nodule in the right breast (from the location of the arrow in Figure 2(c)) showed lymphocyte-dominant inflammatory cell infiltration and granulomas with polynuclear giant cells around the blood vessels in the subcutaneous fat layer, which can be interpreted as necrotizing granulomatous vasculitis (Figures 4(a) and 4(b)). Granulomatous lesions were found in the nasal cavity, and a biopsy of this site showed necrotizing granulomatous inflammation with giant cells. These lesions did not contain caseous necrosis. Thus, the diagnosis was conclusively confirmed as a case of localized GPA; daily PSL was increased to 10 mg, and remission induction therapy for GPA, consisting of four once-weekly doses of 375 mg/m^2 rituximab (RTX), was introduced. After treatment, all symptoms gradually resolved, and the titers of CRP, ESR, and PR3-ANCA normalized.

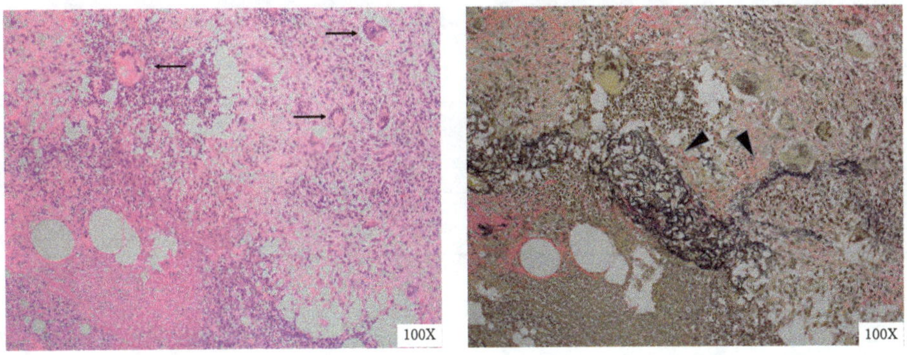

(a) (b)

FIGURE 4: Histopathological findings of the biopsy of the nodule in the right breast. Lymphocyte-dominant inflammatory cell infiltration and granulomas with polynuclear giant cells (arrow) are visible around the blood vessels in the subcutaneous fat layer with hematoxylin and eosin staining (a). Verhoeff's Van Gieson staining shows destruction of the elastic plate (b) (arrowheads).

3. Discussion

Considering the overall clinical course and the positive PR3-ANCA titer, this case was confirmed as a localized form of GPA. However, the initial symptom was pus-like discharge from the nipples that had developed three months prior to hospitalization. Breast lesions in GPA are extremely rare, with 35 cases (clinical and pathological features summarized in Table 1) reported to date since the first report by Elsner in 1969 [4–31]. In brief, the female sex was dominant (33 cases), and only two male patients have been reported with GPA complicated by breast lesions [15]. The age ranged from 28 to 81 years, and the average age was 49 years. Ten cases were either positive for cytoplasmic-ANCA or PR3-ANCA, four cases were negative for ANCA, and no cases were positive for MPO-ANCA. There were 28 cases of unilateral breast lesions, 18 of which were predominant on the right side. Seven cases had bilateral breast lesions, as in our case. Breast lesions were initial symptoms and associated with systemic GPA-related lesions in 19 cases, and in 15 cases, breast lesions developed after GPA diagnosis. Breast lesions were characterized by nodule and mass formation in 31 cases, and only one case had discharge from the nipple [6]; there were also six cases of ulceration. In previous reports, most patients utilized glucocorticoid (28 cases) and/or cyclophosphamide (16 cases) treatment. Four patients reported using RTX, and in all cases, remission was achieved with RTX [26–28, 32]. In our case, sinusitis and pulmonary lesions rapidly improved after RTX administration, and there were no breast lesion recurrences.

Ren et al. reviewed breast lesions in systemic vasculitis and described the characteristics of mammographic and ultrasound findings [2]. Accordingly, mammography revealed increased dense mammary parenchyma, heterogeneous breast tissue, vascular calcification, skin or trabecular thickening, and nodular masses. Meanwhile, breast ultrasonography revealed skin thickening, lesions with or without necrosis or calcifications, hypoechoic mammary parenchyma or infiltration of the breast, and penetration of the blood vessels. However, no radiological and ultrasonographical findings characteristic of vasculitis were described [2]. In our case, although breast cancer, fibroadenoma, sclerosing adenosis, mastitis, and abscess formation were differential diagnoses, a pathological examination was necessary for a definitive diagnosis. In our literature review, of the 34 cases with pathological findings, 25 had necrotizing granulomatous vasculitis that could be definitively diagnosed as GPA, and other pathological findings included inflammatory changes with giant cells, panniculitis, and granulomatous mastitis [4]. According to Allende et al., the pathological diagnosis of breast lesions is challenging because small biopsy materials obtained by core needle biopsy made it difficult to conclusively diagnose vasculitis in breast lesions [4]. Accordingly, the initial core needle biopsy did not reveal vasculitis, but nonspecific inflammatory tissue in our case and cytological examination of the exudate from the nipples revealed an increase in neutrophils, histiocytes, multinucleated giant cells, and epithelial cells, which were evaluated as granulomatous mastitis. In cases where the pathological examination of the breast lesion does not provide a definitive diagnosis, GPA is diagnosed from pathological examination of other tissues (e.g., nasal cavity, kidney, and lung). In the present case, we were able to obtain a definitive pathological diagnosis by excisional biopsy of the subcutaneous nodule in the breast and nasal mucosal biopsy at recurrence. Thus, it is important to biopsy multiple organs during pathological diagnosis of GPA.

Our case was the second reported case of breast involvement with GPA in Japan since Oimomi et al. reported the first case in 1980 [5]. The low number of PR3-ANCA-positive GPA cases in Japan [33, 34] may, therefore, attribute to the subsequent low number of GPA cases associated with breast lesions.

Our case was characterized by various breast lesions: the first was a large bilateral breast mass revealed by mammography, the second was purulent discharges from the bilateral nipples (rarely reported in the literature), the third was a skin ulcer that was not continuous with the breast mass, and the fourth was a necrotizing granulomatous vasculitis appearing as a subcutaneous nodule in the breast at recurrence. Although the mechanism of breast lesion development in GPA is unknown, infection in the mammary

Table 1: Clinical characteristics of 35 cases of breast lesions with GPA.

Mean age ± SD years	49 ± 14 (28–81)
Gender	Male: 2, female: 33
ANCA	PR3(C)-ANCA: 10 Negative: 4 Not described: 21
Location of breast lesion	Bilateral: 7 Unilateral: 28 (right: 18, left: 9, unknown: 1)
Formation of breast lesion	Nodule/tumor: 31 Ulceration: 6 Discharge from nipples: 1
Onset of breast lesion	Initial symptom: 19 Onset after GPA diagnosis: 15
Pathology of breast lesion	Necrotizing granulomatous vasculitis: 25 Granulomatous mastitis: 4 Others (inflammation with giant cells, panniculitis): 5
Treatment	Corticosteroid: 28 Cyclophosphamide: 16 Rituximab: 4

gland, which is connected to the outside through the nipple, may become the trigger of onset, especially because the infection is involved in the development of ANCA-associated vasculitis [35]. Additionally, *Corynebacterium* species, which might be associated with ANCA formation and disease relapse in GPA [36, 37], have been cultured from the nipple discharges in our case. In this case, not only was the mammary gland affected but the skin and subcutaneous fat tissue—which are not continuous with the mammary gland—were also affected. It is unclear why skin lesions are not systemic and, instead, localized on the breast. However, considering that cutaneous vasculitis is more common in the lower extremities, where blood stasis is more likely, and that local pressure is one of the causes of vasculitis, it is possible that the pressure from women's underwear and bras may trigger vasculitis in the skin and subcutaneous areas of the breast in susceptible patients [38].

In conclusion, breast lesions in GPA are extremely rare, and they may present as the first symptom of the disease or of conditions without the clinical symptoms typical of GPA. If unexplained breast masses, ulceration, or other findings such as discharge from the nipples are encountered, GPA should be included in the differential diagnosis.

References

[1] P. Lamprecht, J. Holle, and W. Gross, "Update on clinical, pathophysiological and therapeutic aspects in ANCAAssociated vasculitides," *Current Drug Discovery Technologies*, vol. 6, no. 4, pp. 241-251, 2009.

[2] J. Ren, J. Liu, J. Su, J. Zhang, and J. Zhao, "Systemic vasculitis involving the breast: a case report and literature review," *Rheumatology International*, vol. 39, no. 8, pp. 1447–1455, 2019.

[3] J. T. Lie, "Wegener's granulomatosis: histological documentation of common and uncommon manifestations in 216 patients," *VASA. Zeitschrift fur Gefasskrankheiten*, vol. 26, no. 4, pp. 261–270, 1997.

[4] D. S. Allende and C. N. Booth, "Wegener's granulomatosis of the breast: a rare entity with daily clinical relevance," *Annals of Diagnostic Pathology*, vol. 13, no. 5, pp. 351-357, 2009.

[5] M. Oimomi, I. Suehiro, N. Mizuno et al., "Wegener's granulomatosis with intracerebral granuloma and mammary manifestation," *Archives of Internal Medicine*, vol. 140, no. 6, pp. 853-854, 1980.

[6] B. Elsner and F. B. Harper, "Disseminated Wegener's granulomatosis with breast involvement. Report of a case," *Archives of Pathology*, vol. 87, no. 5, pp. 544–547, 1969.

[7] H. Pambakian and J. R. Tighe, "Breast involvement in Wegener's granulomatosis," *Journal of Clinical Pathology*, vol. 24, no. 4, pp. 343–347, 1971.

[8] H. K. Deininger, "Wegener granulomatosis of the breast," *Radiology*, vol. 154, no. 1, pp. 59-60, 1985.

[9] J. M. Jordan, M. Manning, and N. B. Allen, "Multiple unusual manifestations of Wegener's granulomatosis: breast mass, microangiopathic hemolytic anemia, consumptive coagulopathy, and low erythrocyte sedimentation rate," *Arthritis and Rheumatism*, vol. 29, no. 12, pp. 1527–1531, 1986.

[10] J. M. Jordan, W. T. Rowe, and N. B. Allen, "Wegener's granulomatosis involving the breast," *The American Journal of Medicine*, vol. 83, no. 1, pp. 159–164, 1987.

[11] M. E. Wilson, "Wegener's granulomatosis presenting as breast abscess," *The American Journal of Medicine*, vol. 83, no. 6, p. 1168, 1987.

[12] M. E. Wilson, "Wegener's granulomatosis: another cause of breast masses," *The American Journal of Medicine*, vol. 95, no. 1, pp. 116-117, 1993.

[13] Case Records of the Massachusetts General Hospital, "Case 39-1994. A 69-year-old woman with an orbital mass and an inflammatory mass in the breast," *New England Journal of Medicine*, vol. 331, no. 17, pp. 1143–1149, 1994.

[14] U. Göbel, R. Kettritz, U. Kettritz et al., "Wegener's granulomatosis masquerading as breast cancer," *Archives of Internal Medicine*, vol. 155, no. 2, pp. 205–207, 1995.

[15] R. M. Trüeb, M. Pericin, E. Kohler, J. Barandun, and G. Burg, "Necrotizing granulomatosis of the breast," *British Journal of Dermatology*, vol. 137, no. 5, pp. 799–803, 1997.

[16] I. Stappaerts, C. Colpaert, J. Verbraecken, E. Van Marck, and P. Vermeire, "Granulomatous mastitis as presenting sign of Wegener's granulomatosis," *Acta Clinica Belgica*, vol. 54, no. 4, pp. 207–210, 1999.

[17] M. M. U. Chowdhury and S. Natarajan, "Panniculitis of the breast preceding presentation of Wegener's granulomatosis

by 7 years," *International Journal of Dermatology*, vol. 39, no. 4, pp. 312–320, 2000.
[18] S. M. Naz and K. Fairburn, "Pseudotumor of the breast: an unusual presentation of Wegener's granulomatosis," *Breast Journal*, vol. 11, no. 4, pp. 295-296, 2005.
[19] I. Neralic-Meniga, Z. Ivanovi-Herceg, I. Mazuranic et al., "Wegener's granulomatosis of the breast," *Wien Klin Wochenschr*, vol. 118, no. 3-4, pp. 120–123, 2006.
[20] M. Veerysami, M. Freeth, A. R. Carmichael, and P. Carmichael, "Wegener's granulomatosis of the breast," *Breast Journal*, vol. 12, no. 3, pp. 268–270, 2006.
[21] A. s. G. a.-V. Comas, C. A. Fuster Diana, C. C. Crespo, M. M. Cebollada, M. A. L. LiÃ±Ã¡n, and J. V. Roig Vila, "Wegenerâ s granulomatosis presented as recurrent breast abscess," *Breast Journal*, vol. 16, no. 1, pp. 82–84, 2010.
[22] D. A. Kandiah, "Development of granulomatosis with polyangiitis (wegener)," *Journal of Clinical Rheumatology*, vol. 17, no. 5, pp. 275–277, 2011.
[23] J. Szabo-Moskal, "Wegener's granulomatosis of the breast: a case report," *Polish Journal of Radiology*, vol. 79, pp. 117–119, 2014.
[24] R. Georgescu, M. D. Podeanu, I. Colcer et al., "Wegener's granulomatosis of the breast with peculiar radiological aspect mimicking breast carcinoma," *Breast Journal*, vol. 21, no. 5, pp. 550–552, 2015.
[25] D. Giordano, L. Dardani, and A. Ghidini, "Atypical presentation of granulomatosis with polyangiitis," *Journal of the Belgian Society of Radiology*, vol. 102, no. 1, p. 72, 2018.
[26] Y. Ali, M. Khudadah, M. Alali et al., "Treating granulomatosis with polyangiitis presenting as mastitis with rituximab," *Archives of rheumatology*, vol. 34, no. 2, pp. 241-242, 2019.
[27] P.-A. Jarrot, M.-L. Pelletier, M. Brun et al., "Bilateral breast ulcers: granulomatosis with polyangiitis," *The American Journal of Medicine*, vol. 132, no. 2, pp. 179–181, 2019.
[28] J. Lluch, L. Montserrat Pérez-Tapia, M. d. R. Taco-Sánchez, and J. Narváez, "Breast involvement in granulomatosis with polyangiitis," *Joint Bone Spine*, vol. 86, no. 2, pp. 263-264, 2019.
[29] K. Paley, J. McSorley, F. Azmi et al., "Painful cutaneous ulcer associated with Wegeners granulomatosis," *Dermatology Online Journal*, vol. 13, no. 2, p. 23, 2007.
[30] I. Gallais Sérézal and K. Jennische, "Image Gallery: symmetrical necrosis of the breast as an inaugural manifestation of granulomatosis with polyangiitis (Wegener granulomatosis)," *British Journal of Dermatology*, vol. 175, no. 5, p. e132, 2016.
[31] M. Ryba, A. Konieczny, and Z. Hruby, "Breast involvement in anti-neutrophil cytoplasmic antibodies positive granulomatosis with polyangiitis in a 64-year-old female patient," *Archives of rheumatology*, vol. 32, no. 4, pp. 358–360, 2017.
[32] L. Gadeyne, L. Henckaerts, K. E. Goffin et al., "Granulomatosis with polyangiitis with breast involvement mimicking metastatic cancer: case report and literature review," *European journal of rheumatology*, vol. 7, no. 1, pp. 41–43, 2020.
[33] S. Fujimoto, R. A. Watts, S. Kobayashi et al., "Comparison of the epidemiology of anti-neutrophil cytoplasmic antibody-associated vasculitis between Japan and the UK," *Rheumatology*, vol. 50, no. 10, pp. 1916–1920, 2011.
[34] Y. Tsuchida, M. Shibuya, H. Shoda et al., "Characteristics of granulomatosis with polyangiitis patients in Japan," *Modern Rheumatology*, vol. 25, no. 2, pp. 219–223, 2015.
[35] W. F. Pendergraft 3rd, G. A. Preston, R. R. Shah et al., "Autoimmunity is triggered by cPR-3(105-201), a protein complementary to human autoantigen proteinase-3," *Nature Medicine*, vol. 10, no. 1, pp. 72–79, 2004.
[36] K. N. Konstantinov, C. J. Ulff-Møller, and A. H. Tzamaloukas, "Infections and antineutrophil cytoplasmic antibodies: triggering mechanisms," *Autoimmunity Reviews*, vol. 14, no. 3, pp. 201–203, 2015.
[37] R. L. Rhee, J. Lu, K. Bittinger et al., "Dynamic changes in the nasal microbiome associated with disease activity in patients with granulomatosis with polyangiitis," *Arthritis and Rheumatism*, Article ID 41723, 2021.
[38] J. A. Carlson, L. F. Cavaliere, and J. M. Grant-Kels, "Cutaneous vasculitis: diagnosis and management," *Clinics in Dermatology*, vol. 24, no. 5, pp. 414–429, 2006.

Sensory-Motor Polyneuropathy and Digital Ischemia: A Rare Presentation of Granulomatosis with Polyangiitis

Wasundara Wathurapatha, B. G. A. Rathnamali, and Upul Dissanayake

National Hospital of Sri Lanka, Colombo, Sri Lanka

Correspondence should be addressed to Wasundara Wathurapatha; wsevwandi@hotmail.com

Academic Editor: Gregory J. Tsay

Granulomatosis with polyangiitis (GPA) typically presents with upper or lower respiratory tract symptoms and/or with renal involvement. Although it can affect the peripheral nervous system frequently, with mononeuritis multiplex being the most common pattern, the occurrence of peripheral sensory-motor polyneuropathy as a presenting manifestation is distinctly rare. Prevalence of digital gangrene is also extremely rare in GPA. We describe a 46-year-old woman presenting with severe peripheral sensorimotor polyneuropathy affecting bilateral lower limbs preceded by a purpuric skin rash and multiple painful ulcers confined to the lower limbs. She had evidence of digital ischemia affecting multiple toes and dry gangrene of the left 4th toe. Diagnosis of GPA was made based on skin biopsy, positive ANCA serology, and clinical criteria. She made a good recovery following aggressive immunosuppressive treatment with methylprednisolone and cyclophosphamide and was maintained on prednisolone and azathioprine. This case highlights the importance of suspecting GPA in a patient presenting with sensorimotor polyneuropathy and/or digital ischemia even in the absence of more classic presenting features and underlies the necessity of accurate differential diagnosis in evaluating a case of peripheral neuropathy.

1. Introduction

ANCA-associated vasculitis (AAV) is the commonest primary systemic small-vessel vasculitis (SVV) in adults which consists of granulomatosis with polyangiitis (GPA), eosinophilic granulomatosis with polyangiitis (EGPA), and microscopic polyangiitis (MPA). GPA is characterized by the presence of necrotizing granulomatous inflammation in the absence of asthma and eosinophilia [1]. GPA is a relatively rare disease with a prevalence of 24–152 cases per million [2]. If untreated, the disease usually runs a rapidly fatal course, and 82% of patients die within 1 year [3]. Thus, accurate and prompt diagnosis of GPA is of utmost importance to improve the prognosis.

It mostly affects the upper or lower respiratory tracts and kidneys causing otorhinolaryngological manifestations and crescentic glomerulonephritis [2]. Although significant proportion of patients with GPA develop peripheral nervous system (PNS) involvement during disease course, presentation with peripheral neuropathy is rare, as discussed in the following. Furthermore, according to the published literature, the prevalence of digital ischemia and gangrene in the GPA population is extremely rare as ≤1% [4, 5]. We report a case of GPA presenting with distal sensory-motor polyneuropathy and digital ischemia both of which are atypical and rare presenting features of GPA. The steps in achieving the diagnosis of GPA including the diagnostic criteria are discussed as well as the treatment regimen.

2. Case Report

A 46-year-old woman presented with progressive bilateral lower limb weakness for 2 weeks. This was associated with burning paresthesia and numbness up to the knees. Five days prior to the onset of weakness, she has noticed a skin rash over her soles and multiple painful ulcers over the bilateral lower limb. Concurrently, she has had pain and bluish discoloration of 2nd–5th toes bilaterally which soon evolved

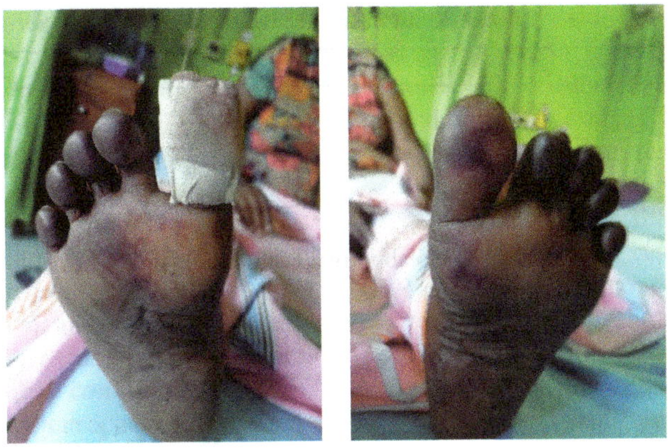

(a) (b)

FIGURE 1: Patient's feet showing retiform purpura and evidence of digital ischemia.

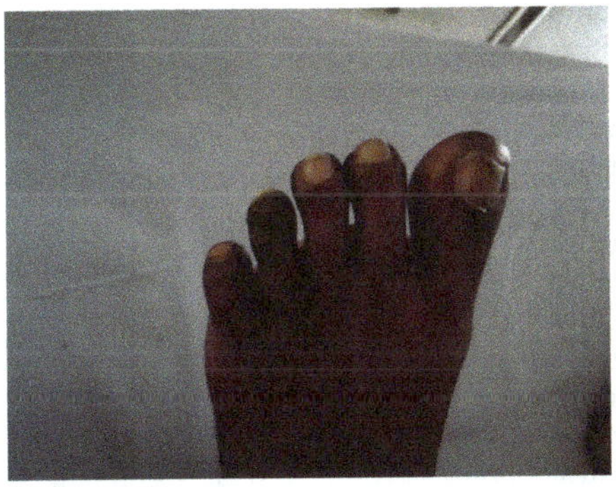

FIGURE 2: Dry gangrene of the left 4th toe.

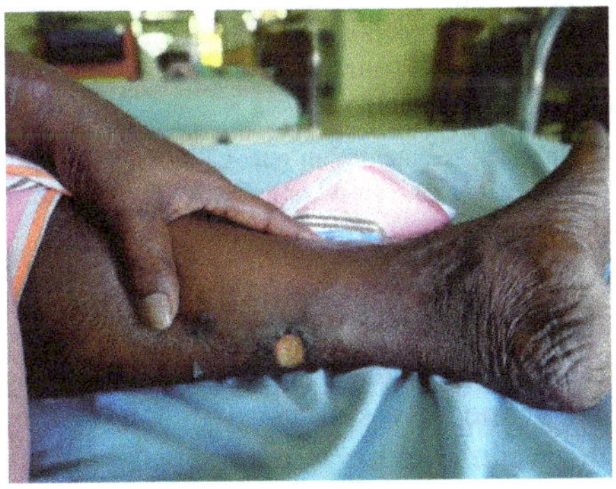

FIGURE 3: Punched out ulcer over the left calf.

into gangrene in the left 4th toe. She had no upper limb, neck, bulbar, or respiratory muscle weakness nor features of dysautonomia. She did not have fever, joint pains, oral ulcers, genital ulcers, or photosensitivity rashes. There was no history of Raynaud phenomenon, hemoptysis, or hematuria. Over the last three years, she has taken medical opinion several times for nasal congestion, symptoms of upper respiratory infections, sinusitis, and one episode of epistaxis. Otherwise, her medical history was insignificant. She was not on any chronic medication. She does not smoke and does not consume alcohol or any illicit substances.

On examination, there were palpable retiform purpuric patches over the plantar surfaces of her feet together with bluish/black discoloration of bilateral 2nd–5th toes (Figure 1) and dry gangrene of the left 4th toe (Figure 2). Few punched out ulcers were present over both legs below the knees (Figure 3). Both posterior tibial and dorsalis pedis pulses were present bilaterally. Skin manifestations were confined to the lower limbs, and there was no involvement of mucosal membranes. She did not have other features suggestive of connective tissue disorders such as malar rash, oral ulcers, photosensitivity, or thickened skin. There was no evidence of active synovitis or deforming arthritis.

Neurological examination revealed bilateral flaccid foot drop, distal motor weakness with grade 2 power, and absent knee and ankle jerks bilaterally. All modalities of sensation were reduced up to the knee in the left leg and up to the midcalf in the right leg. Her upper limbs were neurologically normal, and there was no bladder bowel involvement, postural hypotension, or respiratory compromise. She did not have cerebellar signs, and her higher functions were normal.

Respiratory examination revealed a respiratory rate of 13 breaths per minute, midline trachea, and vesicular breathing with no added sounds. Her heart rate was 80 beats per minute and regular, blood pressure was 140/80 mmHg, and there were no cardiac murmurs. The rest of her examination was unremarkable.

Investigations showed an erythrocyte sedimentation rate (ESR) of 110 mm in the first hour, positive cytoplasmic antineutrophil cytoplasmic antibody (c-ANCA), and associated proteinase 3 ANCA (PR3-ANCA). However, she was negative for perinuclear ANCA (p-ANCA), antinuclear antibody (ANA), rheumatoid factor, and multiple other autoantibodies.

Nerve conduction study (NCS) showed severe sensorimotor axonal polyneuropathy (asymmetrical), and the skin biopsy revealed leukocytoclastic vasculitis with fibrinoid necrosis of vessel walls. There were changes of sinusitis in both maxillary sinuses (Right > left) as shown in her cost, rituximab is restricted for specific circumstances where rituximab is preferred over cyclophosphamide, e.g., for patients who are in their reproductive age. For remission maintenance, low-dose glucocorticoids in combination with either azathioprine, methotrexate, mycophenolate mofetil, or rituximab are recommended with azathioprine being the most preferred. Following induction of remission, maintenance therapy should be continued for at least 24 months [22]. Neuropathies associated with systemic vasculitis should be treated according to the guidelines of the underlying disease [26]. A study involving 40 patients with AAV complicated with VN revealed that all patients who received this aggressive immunosuppressive therapy attained remission of neuropathy within 9 months and 35% of them did not have any long-term sequelae of peripheral neuropathy [11]. As documented in the literature, glucocorticoids and cyclophosphamides are the most commonly used treatment for digital ischemia and gangrene [4]. Our patient was treated with glucocorticoids and cyclophosphamide pulse therapy to achieve remission and subsequently maintained on GC and azathioprine. She made a good recovery with minimal residual disability from peripheral neuropathy, and now, she has remained in remission for more than 1 year.

In conclusion, peripheral sensorimotor polyneuropathy can be a presenting manifestation of systemic SVV. Therefore, patients with peripheral neuropathy of an unclear origin should be investigated thoroughly and closely followed-up to detect a possible underlying GPA. Furthermore, digital ischemia can also be a rare manifestation of GPA despite being a SVV. As both of these conditions warrant aggressive immunosuppressive treatment, early diagnosis is important. Maintaining a high index of suspicion for GPA is important for the physicians to diagnose GPA early, which significantly reduces the morbidity and mortality of this fatal disease.

References

[1] J. C. Jennette and R. J. Falk, "Small-vessel vasculitis," *New England Journal of Medicine*, vol. 337, no. 21, pp. 1512–1523, 1997.

[2] J. Miłkowska-Dymanowska, P. Laskowska, M. Rzuczkowski, A. J. Białas, W. J. Piotrowski, and P. Górski, "Untypical manifestations of granulomatosis with polyangiitis—a review of the literature," *SN Comprehensive Clinical Medicine*, vol. 1, no. 8, pp. 616–626, 2019.

[3] A. Greco, C. Marinelli, M. Fusconi et al., "Clinic manifestations in granulomatosis with polyangiitis," *International Journal of Immunopathology & Pharmacology*, vol. 29, no. 2, pp. 151–159, 2016.

[4] R. A. Lau, R. Bains, D. Suraweera et al., "A rare case of digital ischemia and gangrene in ANCA-associated vasculitis with review of the literature," *Case Reports in Rheumatology*, vol. 2017, Article ID 2421760, 7 pages, 2017.

[5] C. Francès, L. T. H. Du, J.-C. Piette et al., "Wegener's granulomatosis. Dermatological manifestations in 75 cases with clinicopathologic correlation," *Archives of Dermatology*, vol. 130, no. 7, pp. 861–867, 1994.

[6] J. C. Jennette, R. J. Falk, P. Hu, and H. Xiao, "Pathogenesis of antineutrophil cytoplasmic autoantibody-associated small-vessel vasculitis," *Annual Review of Pathology: Mechanisms of Disease*, vol. 8, no. 1, pp. 139–160, 2013.

[7] G. S. Hoffman, G. S. Kerr, R. Y. Leavitt et al., "Wegener granulomatosis: an analysis of 158 patients," *Annals of Internal Medicine*, vol. 116, no. 6, pp. 488–498, 1992.

[8] A. Bischof, V. K. Jaeger, R. D. M. Hadden et al., "Peripheral neuropathy in antineutrophil cytoplasmic antibody-associated vasculitides," *Neurology-Neuroimmunology Neuroinflammation*, vol. 6, no. 6, Article ID e615, 2019.

[9] K. de Groot, D. K. Schmidt, A. C. Arlt, W. L. Gross, and E. Reinhold-Keller, "Standardized neurologic evaluations of 128 patients with wegener granulomatosis," *Archives of Neurology*, vol. 58, no. 8, pp. 1215–1221, 2001.

[10] H. Nishino, F. A. Rubino, R. A. DeRemee, J. W. Swanson, and J. E. Parisi, "Neurological involvement in Wegener's granulomatosis: an analysis of 324 consecutive patients at the Mayo Clinic," *Annals of Neurology*, vol. 33, no. 1, pp. 4–9, 1993.

[11] R. Suppiah, R. D. M. Hadden, R. Batra et al., "Peripheral neuropathy in ANCA-associated vasculitis: outcomes from the European Vasculitis Study Group trials," *Rheumatology*, vol. 50, no. 12, pp. 2214–2222, 2011.

[12] W. Zhang, G. Zhou, Q. Shi, X. Zhang, X. F. Zeng, and F. C. Zhang, "Clinical analysis of nervous system involvement in ANCA-associated systemic vasculitides," *Clinical & Experimental Rheumatology*, vol. 27, no. 1, pp. S65–S69, 2009.

[13] S. Morozumi, H. Koike, M. Tomita et al., "Spatial distribution of nerve fiber pathology and vasculitis in microscopic polyangiitis-associated neuropathy," *Journal of Neuropathology & Experimental Neurology*, vol. 70, no. 5, pp. 340–348, 2011.

[14] M. P. Collins, P. J. B. Dyck, G. S. Gronseth et al., "Peripheral Nerve Society Guideline on the classification, diagnosis, investigation, and immunosuppressive therapy of non-systemic vasculitic neuropathy: executive summary," *Journal of the Peripheral Nervous System*, vol. 15, no. 3, pp. 176–184, 2010.

[15] R. D. M. Hadden, M. P. Collins, S. A. Živković et al., "Vasculitic peripheral neuropathy: case definition and guidelines for collection, analysis, and presentation of immunisation safety data," *Vaccine*, vol. 35, no. 11, pp. 1567–1578, 2017.

[16] M. S. Daoud, L. E. Gibson, R. A. DeRemee, U. Specks, R. A. el-Azhary, and W. P. Daniel Su, "Cutaneous Wegener's granulomatosis: clinical, histopathologic, and immunopathologic features of thirty patients," *Journal of the American Academy of Dermatology*, vol. 31, no. 4, pp. 605–612, 1994.

[17] A. Leung, C. B. Sung, G. Kothari, C. Mack, and C. Fong, "Utilisation of plasma exchange in the treatment of digital infarcts in Wegener's granulomatosis," *International Journal of Rheumatic Diseases*, vol. 13, no. 4, pp. e59–e61, 2010.

[18] R. W. Phillips and M. W. Twiest, "Wegener's granulomatosis and gangrene in the feet," *Annals of Internal Medicine*, vol. 99, no. 4, Article ID 571, 1983.

[19] N. Bessias, K. G. Moulakakis, C. Lioupis et al., "Wegener's granulomatosis presenting during pregnancy with acute limb ischemia," *Journal of Vascular Surgery*, vol. 42, no. 4, pp. 800–804, 2005.

[20] M. Maia, P. Brandão, P. Monteiro et al., "Upper limb ischemia in a patient with Wegener's granulomatosis," *Interactive Cardiovascular and Thoracic Surgery*, vol. 7, no. 6, pp. 1137–1140, 2008.

[21] F. Moosig, P. Lamprecht, and W. L. Gross, "Wegener's granulomatosis: the current view," *Clinical Reviews in Allergy & Immunology*, vol. 35, no. 1-2, pp. 19–21, 2008.

[22] M. Yates, R. A. Watts, I. M. Bajema et al., "EULAR/ERA-EDTA recommendations for the management of ANCA-

associated vasculitis," *Annals of the Rheumatic Diseases*, vol. 75, no. 9, pp. 1583–1594, 2016.

[23] P. Raynaud, R. Garrel, V. Rigau et al., "Comment améliorer la rentabilité diagnostique des biopsies de la sphère oto-rhino-laryngée dans la maladie de Wegener: analyse anatomo-clinique de 49 biopsies chez 21 patients," *Annales de Pathologie*, vol. 25, no. 2, pp. 87–93, 2005.

[24] F. J. van der Woude, N. Rasmussen, S. Lobatto et al., "Autoantibodies against neutrophils and monocytes: tool for diagnosis and marker of disease activity in Wegener's granulomatosis," *The Lancet*, vol. 325, no. 8426, pp. 425–429, 1985.

[25] J. C. Robson, P. C. Grayson, R. Suppiah et al., *American College of Rheumatology and European League against Rheumatism 2017 Provisional Classification Criteria for Granulomatosis with Polyangiitis*, Oxford University Press, Oxford, UK, 2017.

[26] F. Blaes, "Diagnosis and therapeutic options for peripheral vasculitic neuropathy," *Therapeutic Advances in Musculoskeletal Disease*, vol. 7, no. 2, pp. 45–55, 2015.

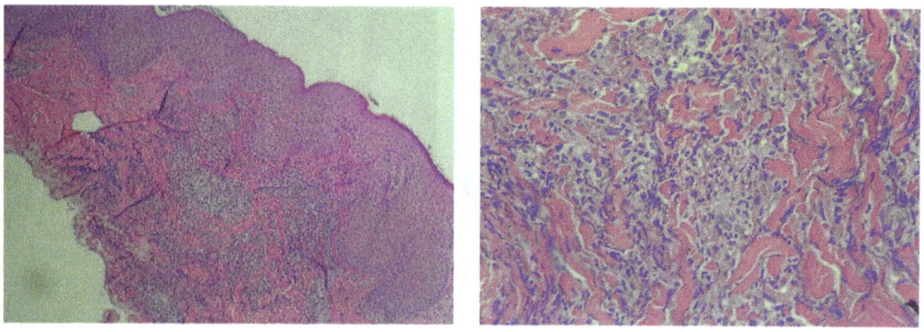

(a) (b)

FIGURE 2: Dermal pathology showing lymphohistiocytic infiltrate and neutrophil granulocytes, consistent with bowel-associated dermatosis-arthritis syndrome (BADAS). Power magnification 40x (a) and 200x (b) of skin slides (hematoxylin-eosin staining).

involved the extremities rather than the trunk, making the diagnosis more challenging. This underscores the importance of considering the diagnosis of BADAS in any patients with inflammatory bowel disease presenting with atypical mucocutaneous presentation and various acute musculoskeletal manifestations.

Currently, little is known about the pathogenesis of BADAS. It has been suggested that intestinal inflammation and bacterial overgrowth may lead to abnormal activation of the immune system, which in turn leads to the deposition of immune complexes on the skin and synovium [3]. The histological appearance of BADAS is not characteristic. Sweet syndrome is histologically identical to BADAS, and the clinical presentation should guide the physician in making the correct diagnosis. Histological biopsy findings of bowel-associated dermato-arthritis syndrome are characterized by predominantly neutrophilic infiltration and lack of fibrinoid necrosis [4]. The bowel-associated dermatosis-arthritis syndrome was reported in both ulcerative colitis and Crohn's diseases in the literature with almost the same extraintestinal presentation. Yet, there was no clear reported predominance of one disease over the other concerning the association with BADAS.

Currently, there is no consensus on the recommended treatment for BADAS. Focusing on treating the underlying disease (i.e., IBD) is essential to control the manifestation of BADAS. In case of bacterial overgrowth or an infectious cause, antibiotics are most frequently used. For patients with an underlying inflammatory bowel disease, controlling disease activity helps to control BADAS. Regaining normal bowel anatomy in bypass surgeries complicated with BADAS has been effective in many cases [5]. The decision to consider the treatment with antibiotics in addition to steroids in this patient was guided by the indeterminate cause of the case since fever and the elevated inflammatory markers can present in inflammation and infectious etiologies. Although BADAS is often overlooked when compiling differential diagnoses for neutrophilic dermatoses, it should be considered in patients with bowel disease or the recent history of bowel surgery. Because this syndrome can recur, early diagnosis can help prevent the recurrence of BADAS [6]. Proper identification and control of BADAS precipitating factors and underlying disease is critical. In our patients, UC disease was not effectively controlled for a long period of time. Recently, successful treatment of BADAS with the interleukin-12 inhibitor ustekinumab has been reported. This underscores the importance of immune complex-mediated pathophysiology as an important role in bowel-associated dermatosis-arthritis syndrome. It suggests that properly controlling the underlying inflammatory bowel disease will play an important role in the management of IBD [7]. The American College of Gastroenterology recommended the surveillance colonoscopies in patient with UC at 1–3-year intervals based on the risk factors to develop a colorectal cancer and the significant findings on the previously done colonoscopy [8]. Arthritis may occur in 25% of patients with UC, and this finding might proceed the diagnosis of the disease [9]. Although the presentation of both conditions can be confusing, extraintestinal manifestations of IBD should be distinguished from BADAS, and the therapeutic strategies will depend entirely on the accurate diagnosis of the patient's condition. Enthesitis is seen in various rheumatic diseases, mainly in spondyloarthropathy, especially with psoriatic arthritis (PsA). Coexistence of PsA and IBD, entities known to share some of the common genetic predisposition, may increase the risk of both disorders (HLA-B27, HLA-DRB1 ∗ 0103, and non-HLA polymorphisms) [10]. The goal of treatment is to achieve low or minimal disease activity in order to control the articular (e.g., enthesitis) and extraarticular manifestations (e.g., IBD).

4. Conclusion

In patients with acute active arthritis, rash, and, as in this case, enthesitis with a history of gastrointestinal disease (e.g., ulcerative colitis and Crohn's disease), it is reasonable to list BADAS as a differential along with extraintestinal manifestations of inflammatory bowel disease. BADAS can recur; therefore, the early recognition of the syndrome and the proper identification and treatment of the underlying cause would result in improvement in the disease burden and the patient's quality of life. Further studies are needed to precisely understand the triggers of the occurrence of BADAS, the best diagnostic tool, as well as the optimal treatment strategy. Preventing the recurrence is crucial for such a rarely occurring disease.

References

[1] J. D. Rosen, O. Stojadinovic, J. D. McBride, R. Rico, J. H. Cho-Vega, and A. J. Nichols, "Bowel-associated dermatosis-arthritis syndrome (BADAS) in a patient with cystic fibrosis," *JAAD Case Reports*, vol. 5, no. 1, pp. 37–39, 2019.

[2] E. M. DeFilippis, C. Magro, and J. L. Jorizzo, "Bowel-associated dermatosis–arthritis syndrome in a patient with ulcerative colitis: an extraintestinal manifestation of inflammatory bowel disease," *Clinical Journal of Gastroenterology*, vol. 7, no. 5, pp. 410–413, 2014.

[3] E. Pereira, P. Estanqueiro, S. Almeida, R. Ferreira, O. Tellechea, and M. Salgado, "Bowel-associated dermatosis-arthritis syndrome in an adolescent with short bowel syndrome," *Journal of Clinical Rheumatology*, vol. 20, no. 6, pp. 322–324, 2014.

[4] C. W. Oldfield, L. A. Heffernan-Stroud, T. S. Buehler-Bota, and J. V. Williams, "Bowel-associated dermatosis-arthritis syndrome (BADAS) in a pediatric patient," *JAAD Case Reports*, vol. 2, no. 3, pp. 272–274, 2016.

[5] N. Hassold, G. Jelin, E. Palazzo et al., "Bowel-associated dermatosis arthritis syndrome: a case report with first positron emission tomography analysis," *JAAD Case Reports*, vol. 5, no. 2, pp. 140–143, 2019.

[6] A. Barland, J. Blackmon, G. Fraga, D. Aires, and R. Chain, "Bowel-Associated Dermatosis-Arthritis syndrome in a patient with Crohn disease," *Cutis*, vol. 97, no. 2, pp. E1–E3, 2016.

[7] M. Heard, M. Zhang, and J. L. Jorizzo, "A case of bowel-associated dermatosis-arthritis syndrome treated with ustekinumab: the importance of targeting underlying gastrointestinal disease," *JAAD Case Reports*, vol. 6, no. 6, pp. 506–508, 2020.

[8] D. T. Rubin, A. N. Ananthakrishnan, C. A. Siegel, B. G. Sauer, and M. D. Long, "ACG clinical guideline: ulcerative colitis in adults," *American Journal of Gastroenterology*, vol. 114, no. 3, pp. 384–413, 2019.

[9] O. Sulima, "Extraintestinal manifestations of ulcerative colitis," *The Opinion of a Rheumatologist and Proctologist*, vol. 11, pp. 159–162, 2020.

[10] A. Y. T. Chia, G. W. X. Ang, A. S. Y. Chan, W. Chan, T. K. Y. Chong, and Y. Y. Leung, "Managing psoriatic arthritis with inflammatory bowel disease and/or uveitis," *Frontiers of Medicine*, vol. 8, 2021.

[11] J. L. Jorizzo, P. Apisarnthanarax, P. Subrt et al., "Bowel-bypass syndrome without bowel bypass: bowel-associated dermatosis-arthritis syndrome," *Archives of Internal Medicine*, vol. 143, no. 3, pp. 457–461, 1983.

Table 1: Comparison of our patient with five published case reports describing RP with concomitant coronary artery disease.

Reference	Age (yrs.)/sex	RP manifestations	Therapy prior to cardiac disease	Cardiac manifestations (duration of RP at the time of onset)	RP disease activity at time of cardiac diagnosis	Therapy	Response to therapy/ clinical outcome
This case report	55/M	Auricular chondritis Nasal deformity Polyarthritis Respiratory chondritis	Adalimumab	Obliterative coronary arteritis	Well-controlled	Methotrexate Etanercept Mycophenolate Mofetil Lefulunomide Minocycline Prednisone Etolac	Sudden cardiac death
Bowness et al. 1991 [8]	33/M	Auricular chondritis Nasal collapse Polyarthritis Respiratory chondritis	Prednisolone (10 mg/day)	Complete heart block (4 wks.) Acute aortic incompetence (8 wks.) Coronary vasculitis detected postmortem	Active: elevated CRP, right auricular chondritis, inflamed vocal cords, hoarseness	Pacemaker AVR Prednisolone (60 mg/day) Cyclophosphamide (oral, 2 mg/kg/day)	Fatal acute heart failure (5 weeks postop.)
Vaidynathan et al. 2006 [12]	26/F	Auricular chondritis Nasal bridge depression	Prednisolone (10 mg/day for 1 year)	Severe aortic regurgitation (2 yrs.) Anterior and lateral wall myocardial infarction with right and left coronary artery ostial stenosis (34 mos.)	Inactive	AVR Prednisolone (20 mg/day)	Fatal cardiac arrest awaiting coronary artery bypass grafting
Stein et al. 2008 [11]	30/M	Auricular chondritis Nasal chondritis Uveitis	Prednisone (30 mg/day for 3 weeks)	Asymmetric proximal aorta and aortic root wall thickening, stenosis of ostium of left and right main coronary arteries, right external iliac artery stenosis (5 yrs.) Positive cardiac stress test (5 yrs.) Critical coronary stenosis (6 yrs.)	Active: auricular chondritis Normal inflammatory markers	AVR CABG Prednisone (1 mg/ kg/day) Cyclophosphamide (oral, 100 mg/ kg/day) Infliximab (5 mg/ kg/dose)	Improvement in symptoms following surgery
McCarthy and Cunnane 2010 [15]	45/M	Auricular deformity Nasal deformity Arthralgia Bilateral sensorineural deafness	Methotrexate Azathioprine Cyclosporine A Infliximab Corticosteroids Rituximab	Severe aortic incompetence, normal aortic root, stenosis of main left and right coronary arteries (16 yrs.)	Active: elevated CRP	AVR CABG Azathioprine	Clinical remission after 18 mos.

Table 1: Continued.

Reference	Age (yrs.)/sex	RP manifestations	Therapy prior to cardiac disease	Cardiac manifestations (duration of RP at the time of onset)	RP disease activity at time of cardiac diagnosis	Therapy	Response to therapy/ clinical outcome
Sugrue et al. 2014 [16]	51/M	Auricular chondritis Arthritis Aortic root dilation	N/A	Aortic root dilation (at time of diagnosis) Femoral bruit (4 mos.) Critical left main stem ostial stenosis (8 mos.) Progression of aortitis (36 mos.)	Active: elevated inflammatory markers that became quiescent with cardiac disease progression	Prednisolone (1 mg/kg) MTX (25 mg/wk) Infliximab (IV 5 mg/kg, 6 weekly initially, increased to 10 mg/kg, 6 weekly)	Normalization of inflammatory markers Asymptomatic after 12 mos.

AVR, aortic valve replacement; CABG, coronary artery bypass grafting; MTX, methotrexate.

described [4, 8]. Such arrhythmias estimated to occur in 4–6% of patients with RP, can be transient or permanent, and may require pacemaker implantation [8, 9]. Treatment of cardiac-related disease in RP can be challenging, as disease may be asymptomatic and progressive despite therapy [3, 10]. Combinations of corticosteroids, methotrexate, azathioprine, infliximab, and cyclophosphamide have been utilized with mixed success, while a recent publication describes successful use of tocilizumab for corticosteroid-resistant RP aortitis [8, 10–13]. When aortic insufficiency and coronary stenosis are severe, surgical treatment with aortic valve repair and coronary artery bypass grafting are indicated, respectively [4].

Coronary artery vasculitis is a rare cause of sudden cardiac death, estimated to account for 12% of non-atherosclerotic-related sudden cardiac death. It is typically associated with an underlying autoimmune or inflammatory condition such as RP, Takayasu arteritis, Kawasaki disease, Behçet's disease, IgG4-related periarteritis, eosinophilic granulomatosis with polyangiitis, granulomatosis with polyangiitis, and polyarteritis nodosa [14]. To date, there are only five case reports describing coronary vasculitis in RP (Table 1) [8, 11, 12, 15, 16]. Notably, cardiac disease was diagnosed during active RP in all four males but only during remission in the female. Furthermore, cardiac disease was diagnosed within 5 years of RP diagnosis in four of the five cases. One patient also experienced progression of cardiac disease despite improvement in symptoms and initiation of methotrexate and infliximab [16]. In contrast, the coronary vasculitis in our male patient was not preceded by any clinical history of great vessel or coronary disease and based on autopsy occurred in the absence of aortic disease. The cardiac event occurred years after diagnosis of RP and during a time of disease remission. Together, these cases underscore the importance for frequent screening for cardiac disease, regardless of symptoms, in patients with RP.

The prominent storiform-type fibrosis in the coronary artery of our patient was reminiscent of IgG4-RD, a chronic inflammatory condition affecting 2.2 per 100,000 individuals and occurring predominantly in middle-aged men. IgG4-RD can affect multiple organs and tissues, with affected tissues characterized by lymphoplasmacytic infiltration, storiform fibrosis, and obliterative phlebitis. IgG4 levels may also be elevated in the serum. Both arterial and venous vasculature can be affected by IgG4-RD, as aortic aneurysms, periaortitis, periarteritis, obliterative arteritis, and obliterative venous phlebitis have all been described [17]. Arteritis, periarteritis, and aneurysmal dilation of the coronary arteries have all been described with relation to IgG4-related cardiac disease. When the coronary arteries are involved, patients may be asymptomatic or minimally symptomatic but remain at risk for myocardial ischemia and sudden cardiac death [18].

Given the rarity of both RP and IgG4-RD, it may seem unlikely for them to coexist; however, three patients have been described: a 67-year-old man with a 20-year history of RP who developed IgG4-RD involving his kidneys and pancreas [19], a 63-year-old man with a 1-year history of RP who developed IgG4-RD of the kidneys and lungs [20], and a 78-year-old man with clinical features of both RP and IgG4-RD [21]. In these cases, the RP predated the onset of IgG4-RD and manifested as auricular chondritis, ocular inflammation, and arthralgia. In addition, we are aware of two other cases suggesting a connection between IgG4 plasma cells and RP, although neither case met the IgG4-RD diagnostic criteria. Within our own institution, a 42-year-old man with psoriatic arthritis recently developed bilateral auricular chondritis and was diagnosed with RP. The auricular cartilage histology showed dense lymphoplasmacytic, cartilaginous, and perichondral inflammation characteristic of RP (Figure 2(a)). Notably, there was a high number of IgG4 plasma cells present albeit below the number required for IgG4-RD diagnosis (Figure 2(b); 216 IgG4 + plasma cells, 601 IgG + plasma cells, IgG4/IgG ratio = 36%). Horai et al. also presented a case of a 79-year-old man with RP with IgG4-expressing plasmacytes present in his left auricular cartilage [22].

These cases of RP and concomitant IgG4-RD suggest that the mechanisms that promote development of IgG4-RD and RP may be shared. A preferential IgG4 subtype of

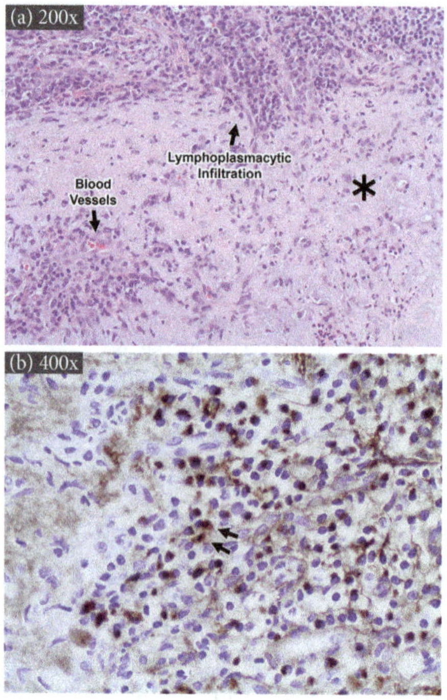

FIGURE 2: Histology of auricular cartilage, and immunohistochemical staining for IgG4 plasma cells from second patient with RP at our institute. (a) High-power magnification of auricular cartilage showing damage to cartilage including cartilage eosinophilia, infiltration by small blood vessels, as well as lymphoplasmacytic infiltration. The asterisk indicates cartilage eosinophilia, and arrows indicate representative small blood vessels and area of lymphoplasmacytic infiltration (H&E, 200x). (b) High-power magnification showing presence of IgG4-positive plasma cells (brown staining) in auricular cartilage, with arrows indicating representative IgG4-positive plasma cells (immunohistochemical staining of IgG4-positive plasma cells, 400x). There were 216 IgG4 + plasma cells and 601 IgG + plasma cells, and the IgG4/IgG ratio was 36%.

immunoglobulin response has been described in other autoimmune diseases such as pemphigus, muscle specific kinase myasthenia gravis, and thrombotic thrombocytopenic purpura [23]. Future studies should assess total and cartilage-specific IgG4 levels in RP. In addition, T-follicular helper cells could also be a driver of IgG4-RD and RP. Importantly, IgG4-RD can mimic some aspects of RP. Both diseases can lead to renal disease, tracheobronchial inflammation, and vasculitis, thus considering the diagnosis of IgG4-RD in some cases thought to be RP is warranted.

4. Conclusion

Cardiac disease and vasculitis in RP pose significant morbidity and mortality to patients. Such disease can be silent and occur even when other disease manifestations, such as chondritis, are inactive. To evaluate for cardiac involvement, patients should routinely be asked about chest pain, dyspnea, palpitations, presyncope, and syncope. Regardless of symptoms, screening for cardiac disease in patients with RP is recommended.

Acknowledgments

This work was supported by the Constance Albrecht Research Fund.

References

[1] C. J. Michet Jr., C. H. McKenna, H. S. Luthra, and W. M. O'Fallon, "Relapsing polychondritis," *Annals of Internal Medicine*, vol. 104, no. 1, pp. 74–78, 1986.

[2] L. P. McAdam, M. A. O'HANLAN, R. Bluestone, and C. M. Pearson, "Relapsing polychondritis," *Medicine*, vol. 55, no. 3, pp. 193–215, 1976.

[3] L. Arnaud, H. Devilliers, S. L. Peng et al., "The relapsing polychondritis disease activity index: development of a disease activity score for relapsing polychondritis," *Autoimmunity Reviews*, vol. 12, no. 2, pp. 204–209, 2012.

[4] A. Mathian, M. Miyara, F. Cohen-Aubart et al., "Relapsing polychondritis: a 2016 update on clinical features, diagnostic tools, treatment and biological drug use," *Best Practice & Research Clinical Rheumatology*, vol. 30, no. 2, pp. 316–333, 2016.

[5] J. H. Buckner, M. Van Landeghen, W. W. Kwok, and L. Tsarknaridis, "Identification of type II collagen peptide 261-273-specific T cell clones in a patient with relapsing polychondritis," *Arthritis & Rheumatism*, vol. 46, no. 1, pp. 238–244, 2002.

[6] J. Dion, N. Costedoat-Chalumeau, D. Sène et al., "Relapsing polychondritis can be characterized by three different clinical phenotypes: analysis of a recent series of 142 patients," *Arthritis & Rheumatology*, vol. 68, no. 12, pp. 2992–3001, 2016.

[7] J. Shimizu, H. Oka, Y. Yamano, K. Yudoh, and N. Suzuki, "Cardiac involvement in relapsing polychondritis in Japan," *Rheumatology (Oxford)*, vol. 55, no. 3, pp. 583-584, 2016.

[8] P. Bowness, I. C. Hawley, T. Morris, A. Dearden, and M. J. Walport, "Complete heart block and severe aortic incompetence in relapsing polychondritis: clinicopathologic findings," *Arthritis & Rheumatism*, vol. 34, no. 1, pp. 97–100, 1991.

[9] B. Hojaili and H. D. Keiser, "Relapsing polychondritis presenting with complete heart block," *JCR: Journal of Clinical Rheumatology*, vol. 14, no. 1, pp. 24–26, 2008.

[10] A.-G. A. Selim, L. G. Fulford, R. H. Mohiaddin, and M. N. Sheppard, "Active aortitis in relapsing polychondritis," *Journal of Clinical Pathology*, vol. 54, no. 11, pp. 890–892, 2001.

[11] J. D. Stein, P. Lee, B. Kuriya et al., "Critical coronary artery stenosis and aortitis in a patient with relapsing polychondritis," *Journal of Rheumatology*, vol. 35, no. 9, pp. 1898–1900, 2008.

[12] R. K. Vaidyanathan, J. R. Byalal, T. Sundaramoorthi et al., "Rapidly progressive coronary ostial stenosis after aortic valve replacement in relapsing polychondritis," *The Journal of Thoracic and Cardiovascular Surgery*, vol. 131, no. 6, pp. 1395-1396, 2006.

[13] G. Elourimi, M. Soussan, U. Warzocha, H. Bugaud, R. Dhôte, and S. Abad, "Efficacy of tocilizumab highlighted by FDG-PET/CT in a patient with relapsing polychondritis-associated aortitis," *Rheumatology International*, vol. 37, no. 11, pp. 1931–1935, 2017.

[14] S. F. Hill and M. N. Sheppard, "Non-atherosclerotic coronary artery disease associated with sudden cardiac death," *Heart*, vol. 96, no. 14, pp. 1119–1125, 2010.

[15] E. M. McCarthy and G. Cunnane, "Treatment of relapsing polychondritis in the era of biological agents," *Rheumatology International*, vol. 30, no. 6, pp. 827-828, 2010.
[16] G. Sugrue, L. Durcan, L. Bell, F. Bolster, S. Donnelly, and E. Kavanagh, "Unsuspected cardiovascular involvement in relapsing polychondritis," *Circulation: Cardiovascular Imaging*, vol. 7, no. 2, pp. 409–411, 2014.
[17] T. Kamisawa, Y. Zen, S. Pillai, and J. H. Stone, "IgG4-related disease," *The Lancet*, vol. 385, no. 9976, pp. 1460–1471, 2015.
[18] N. Oyama-Manabe, S. Yabusaki, O. Manabe, F. Kato, H. Kanno-Okada, and K. Kudo, "IgG4-related cardiovascular disease from the aorta to the coronary arteries: multidetector CT and PET/CT," *Radiographics*, vol. 38, no. 7, pp. 1934–1948, 2018.
[19] Y. Nagayama, M. Takayasu, A. Wakabayashi et al., "New onset of immunoglobulin G4-related disease in a patient with relapsing polychondritis," *Modern Rheumatology*, vol. 27, no. 5, pp. 898–900, 2017.
[20] M. Yamasue, S.-i. Nureki, H. Matsumoto et al., "Corticosteroid therapy for a patient with relapsing polychondritis complicated by IgG4-related disease," *The Tohoku Journal of Experimental Medicine*, vol. 239, no. 3, pp. 223–230, 2016.
[21] A. Le Goueff, F. Vandergheynst, and D. Jayne, "Coincident relapsing polychondritis and IgG4-related disease: a diagnostic challenge," *Polish Archives of Internal Medicine*, vol. 129, no. 7-8, pp. 539–541, 2019.
[22] Y. Horai, T. Miyamura, H. Arase et al., "A case of relapsing polychondritis associated with auricular cartilage infiltration of immunoglobulin G4-positive plasma cells and lung cancer," *Modern Rheumatology*, vol. 21, no. 5, pp. 557–560, 2011.
[23] I. Koneczny, "A new classification system for IgG4 autoantibodies," *Frontiers in Immunology*, vol. 9, p. 97, 2018.

A Patient with Complex Gout with an Autoinflammatory Syndrome and a Sternoclavicular Joint Arthritis as Presenting Symptoms

M. M. Fedeli,[1] **M. Vecchi**,[2] **and P. Rodoni Cassis**[2,3,4]

[1]*Department of Internal Medicine, Ospedale La Carità, Locarno, Switzerland*
[2]*Centro Medico, Chiasso, Switzerland*
[3]*Department of Radiology, Clinica Sant'Anna, Lugano-Sorengo, Switzerland*
[4]*Department of Radiology, Clinica Ars Medica, Gravesano, Switzerland*

Correspondence should be addressed to M. M. Fedeli; marcofedeli89@gmail.com

Academic Editor: James V. Dunne

A 50-year-old man presented to the emergency department with widespread pain, especially at the chest level, fever, and night sweats. Physical examinations revealed a swelling with localized pain in the left sternoclavicular joint. Laboratory tests showed a CPR of 134 mg/l and an ESR of 70 mm/h. The patient's anamnesis is, for a chronic gouty arthritis, poorly controlled type 2 diabetes and a lumbosacral radicular syndrome. Home therapy includes metformin, sitagliptin, gliclazide, naproxen with partial benefit on pain, and febuxostat. Differential diagnoses of sternoclavicular swelling include infection, crystal or psoriatic arthropathy, tumor pathology, SAPHO syndrome, and osteoarthritis. An ultrasound scan performed at the thoracic level showed the presence of effusion in the sternoclavicular joint. A thoracoabdominal CT scan, performed in doubt of neoplasias, shows no masses but osteostructural nonspecific alterations of the sternoclavicular joint. We performed a dual energy CT (DECT) which reports a gouty arthropathy at the sternoclavicular joints (in the literature, only three similar cases are proved). Because of the poor therapeutic effects using febuxostat and systemic corticosteroids, the patient was treated with anakinra, an interleukin 1 receptor antagonist, which led, 6 months after the event, to a total remission.

1. Case Report

R. is a 50-year-old patient who has, since a month, a state of general malaise characterized by widespread pain and intermittent episodes of fever and night sweats. He refers fever with stakes up to 39°C in two days prior to hospitalization at the Department of Rheumatology. The pains are especially at night to the chest level. Despite a home drug therapy with NSAID (nonsteroidal anti-inflammatory drug), symptoms do not regress.

The patient's anamnesis is for a chronic gouty arthritis characterized by the presence of tophi and frequent arthritis; the first gouty attack was in 2011 on the ankles treated with steroids. In 2014, he has undergone surgical operation with the removal of tophaceous masses [1] at the sixth compartment of the right hand because of severe pain and losing range of motion in the affected joint.

He also had high uric acid levels (Figure 1) as he consumed febuxostat (allergic to allopurinol).

He is also known for type 2 diabetes (diagnosis of 2011) in pharmacological treatment with metformin, sitagliptin, and gliclazide poorly controlled because of wrong eating habits without a regular physical activity. In fact, in physiological anamnesis, the patient declares he drinks 2–3 liters of carbonated soft drinks a day.

He has a class 1 obesity (BMI 31.5 Kg/m^2) that is why he underwent gastric banding surgery in 2004 with mediocre success. Another cardiovascular risk factor is a chronic renal failure (Figure 2) G3a (KDIGO, 2012) [2] due to diabetic nephropathy (albuminuria grade A2) [3].

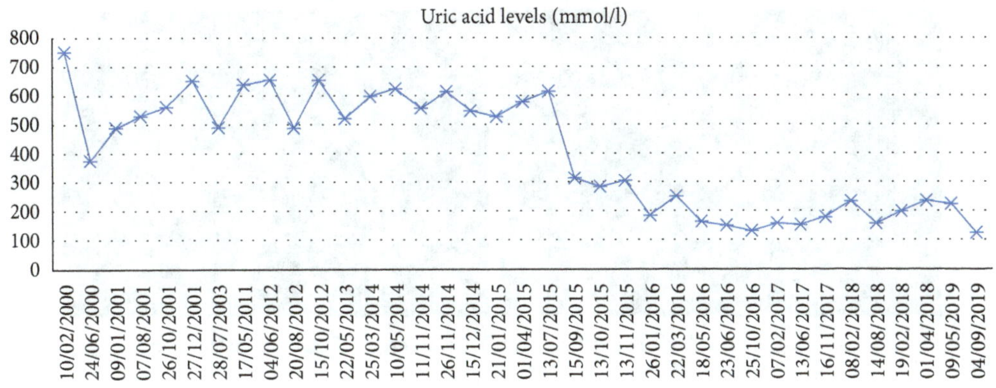

Figure 1: Monitoring uric acid levels over the years.

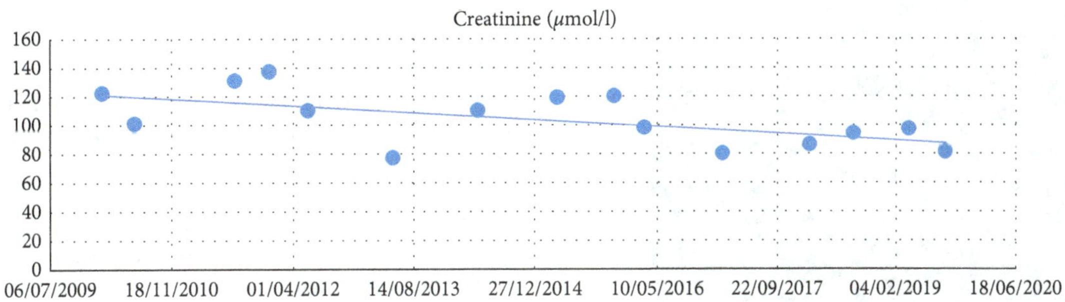

Figure 2: Monitoring renal function levels over the years.

Lastly, he suffered from lumbosacral radicular syndrome, irritative L3 on the left side.

On examination, the patient is in good general condition, 102 kg weight, 180 cm height, with eupnea, normal heart rate, normal heart rhythm, and normal cardiac rhythm. Clinically, there was a florid inflammation at the level of the first metatarsophalangeal joint of the left foot with a swelling of the left ankle without pain on pressure or mobilization. The knees appear bilaterally swollen, warm to thermotouch, aching with the presence of a joint effusion mostly expressed on the left. We deduce inflammation to the metacarpophalangeal joints (II, III, and IV) of the left hand where, in the past, tophi had been removed surgically. The movement in extension of the left elbow is deficient. Lumbar spine mobility is reduced by 1/3 in the lateral-bilateral flexion and in forward flexion with soreness at the lumbosacral level. At chest level, there is a swelling with localized pain in the left sternoclavicular joint. Valid heart sounds, no murmurs were observed. At lung auscultation, there was vesicular murmur spreading ubiquitously. The abdomen is treatable and painless on palpation. No evidence of associated neurological deficits.

The electrocardiogram revealed no significant alterations. Laboratory tests show a CRP of 134 mg/l and an ESR of 70 mm/h. Uric acid is within the normal limit (263 mmol/l).

The differential diagnosis of sternoclavicular swelling:

(i) Infectious arthropathy

(ii) Crystals arthropathy (uric acid or calcium pyrophosphate crystals)

(iii) Tumor pathology

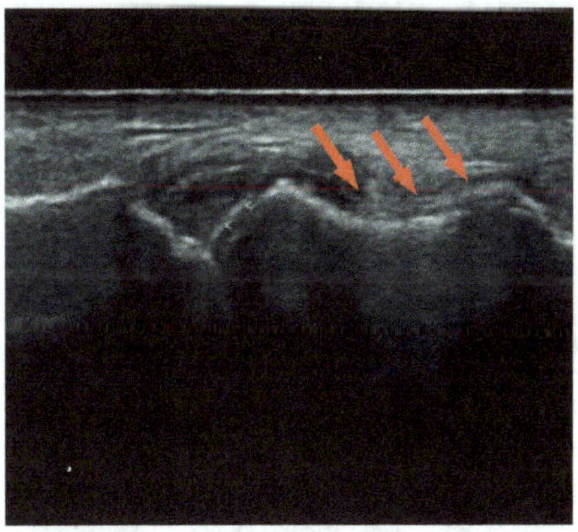

Figure 3: Functional ultrasound scan of the knee.

(iv) Psoriatic arthropathy

(v) SAPHO syndrome (synovitis, acne, pustulosis, hyperostosis, and osteitis)

(vi) Osteoarthritis

Proceeding by elimination, we have eradicated from our list psoriatic arthritis in a patient who showed no skin changes, and with silent family history for this disease. A thoracoabdominal CT scan, performed in doubt of neoplasias, shows no masses but osteostructural nonspecific alterations of the sternoclavicular joint. Procalcitonin is negative reducing the chance of bacterial infection. Trauma was not reported in the recent period. We have also excluded osteoarthritis because of the absence of the classical radiological signs (narrowing of joint space,

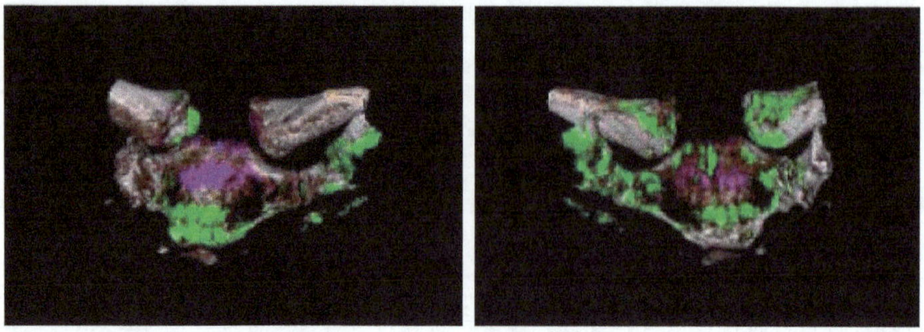

Figure 4: Sternoclavicular details with Dual Energy CT 3D reconstruction.

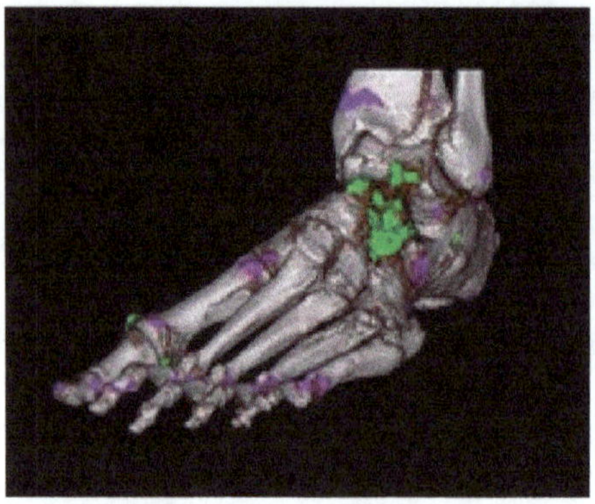

Figure 5: Left foot with Dual energy CT 3D-reconstruction.

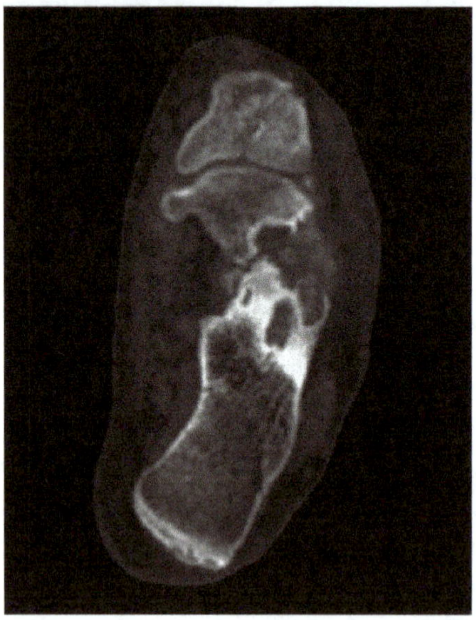

Figure 6: Erosion and intra-articular swelling with tophaceous masses (CT of the left foot).

osteophytes, subchondral bony sclerosis, and subchondral cysts) [4, 5].

Therefore, we continued with a functional ultrasound scan to the knee that showed synovitis with joint effusion and the characteristic double contour that means the presence of deposits of urate at the femoral condyles cartilage level (Figure 3) [1].

The synovial fluid, drawn at the knee level, confirmed this hypothesis given the presence of uric acid crystals.

A chest ultrasound showed the presence of effusion in the sternoclavicular joint and thickening of the synovial capsule.

Because of the lack of joint fluid, we could not carry out arthrocentesis of sternoclavicular joint. We performed a CT with the DUAL ENERGY (DECT) method, which confirmed the suspicion of gout-originated arthropathy at the sternoclavicular joints, explaining the patient's chest symptoms. Specifically, we show the 3D reconstruction of the dual energy CT of the sternoclavicular joints and the foot (Figures 4 and 5) [1]. The uric acid deposits appear in green, while the bone calcium appears in purple.

Our patient has a systemic disease with destructive deforming arthritis. Indeed, it has some tophaceous lesions (Figure 6) [1].

2. Discussion

A gouty arthritis with a sternoclavicular localization is a very rare finding (in the literature, only three similar cases are proved [6]). Classically, imagining a classic case of gout, we thought more frequently to the metatarsophalangeal joint (podagra), to proximal and distal interphalangeal, to elbow and knee [1, 5, 7] Our patient had an intermediate probability of having gout (7.5 points) [8]. In this case, the gold standard for the diagnosis of gout remains arthrocentesis with the detection of uric acid crystals [8]. The diagnostic alternatives include ultrasound, with the classic double contour of the cartilage surface typical of arthropathies with crystal deposits, and the Dual Energy CT [1, 7, 9]. With this method [9], the images are acquired simultaneously, using two different energy levels. Comparing the specific attenuation at 80 and 140 kVp, it is possible to differentiate the chemical composition of tissues subjected to CT. Uric acid crystals are thus differentiated from the bone or from calcium-based dystrophic calcification. Recent studies have shown that CT Dual Energy a sensitivity of 75 to 90% and a specificity between 83 and 93%, respectively [9]. This type of examination, therefore, represents an excellent alternative for the diagnosis of gout and in particular, in the case of clinical doubts or inconclusive microscopic analysis.

The abundant consumption of drinks, given the high-fructose content, may have helped to maintain the hyperuricemia and played a role in causing acute attacks through urea fluctuations [10, 11].

Another useful starting point in clinical practice is the uric acid levels were normal; this indicates how important are the uric acid fluctuations in blood rather than the peak in parallel with acute attacks of gout [7].

At last, a brief mention of therapy. Regarding the acute attack, you should first use AINS or colchicine and, in case of monoarticular attack, also corticosteroid infiltrations. Because of the failure benefit of AINS, the failure tolerance of colchicine and polyarticular localization, we have resorted to prednisone starting with a dosage of 20 mg to scale gradually down. Febuxostat treatment has been kept, and because of the poor therapeutic effects, we decide to use anakinra, an inhibitor of interleukin 1, which led to total remission. The total duration of the gout flare was 6 months.

3. Take Home Message

Summarizing, the key points are:

(i) Gout can occur in a generalized and systematic way and affect any joint [1]

(ii) Dual-Energy CT or ultrasound scan are the best functional tests chosen in cases of doubt or for special localizations of gout [5, 7]

(iii) The abuse of carbonated soft drinks, rich in fructose, is a risk factor comparable with beer for gout [10, 11]

(iv) Normal uric acid levels do not exclude a gouty attack [5, 7]

References

[1] P. Towiwat, A. Chhana, and N. Dalbeth, "The anatomical pathology of gout: a systematic literature review," *BMC Musculoskeletal Disorders*, vol. 20, no. 1, p. 140, 2019.

[2] Kidney Disease: Improving Global Outcomes (KDIGO), "KDIGO clinical practice guide-line for the evaluation and management of chronic kidney disease," *Kidney International Supplements*, vol. 3, pp. 1–150, 2013.

[3] F. Persson and P. Rossing, "Diagnosis of diabetic kidney disease: state of the art and future perspective," *Kidney International Supplements*, vol. 8, no. 1, pp. 2–7, 2018.

[4] D. J. Hunter and D. T. Felson, "Osteoarthritis," *BMJ*, vol. 332, no. 7542, pp. 639–642, 2006.

[5] M. C. Hochberg, E. M. Gravallese, A. J. Silman, J. S. Smolen, M. E. Weinblatt, and M. H. Weisman, *Rheumatology*, Elsevier, Amsterdam, Netherlands, 2018.

[6] http://journals.plos.org/plosmedicine/article.

[7] P. Richette, M. Doherty, E. Pascual et al., "2018 updated European League against Rheumatism evidence-based recommendations for the diagnosis of gout," *Annals of the Rheumatic Diseases*, vol. 79, no. 1, pp. 31–38, 2019.

[8] H. M. Janssens, J. Fransen, E. H. van de Lisdonk, P. M. van Riel, C. van Weel, and M. Janssen, "A diagnostic rule for acute gouty Arthritis in primary care without joint fluid analy-sis," *Archives of Internal Medicine*, vol. 170, no. 13, pp. 1120–1126, 2010.

[9] T. R. C. Johnson, C. Fink, S. O. Schönberg, and M. F. Rei-ser, *Dual Energy CT in Clinical Practice*, Springer, Berlin, Germany, 2011.

[10] H. K. Choi and G. Curhan, "Soft drinks, fructose consumption, and the risk of gout in men: prospective cohort study," *BMJ*, vol. 336, no. 7639, pp. 309–312, 2008.

[11] J. W. J. Choi, E. S. Ford, X. Gao, and H. K. Choi, "Sugar-sweetened soft drinks, diet soft drinks, and serum uric acid level: the third national health and nutrition examination survey," *Arthritis & Rheumatism*, vol. 59, no. 1, pp. 109–116, 2008.

38

Acute Stroke due to Vertebral Artery Dissection in Giant Cell Arteritis

Marlene Marte Furment,[1] Sandra Antigua Jimenez,[2] and Sangeetha Pabolu[3]

[1]*Internal Medicine Department, Saint Peter's University Hospital/Rutgers Robert Wood Johnson Medical School Program, New Brunswick, NJ, USA*
[2]*Department of Health Sciences, Instituto Tecnologico de Santo Domingo, Santo Domingo, Dominican Republic*
[3]*Rheumatology Department, Saint Peter's University Hospital/Rutgers Robert Wood Johnson Medical School Program, New Brunswick, NJ, USA*

Correspondence should be addressed to Marlene Marte Furment; mmartefurment@saintpetersuh.com

Academic Editor: Gregory J. Tsay

The diagnosis of giant cell arteritis (GCA) when presenting with atypical features such as stroke is very challenging. Only 0.17% of first-ever strokes are caused by GCA, a life-threatening condition when left untreated. Very few cases have been reported on giant cell arteritis leading to acute stroke due to vertebral artery dissection. We present a case of a 76-year-old female with no medical history who presented with sudden onset right visual loss and left hemiparesis. She had been initially treated for acute stroke and upon further workup was found to have left vertebral artery dissection. She had erythrocyte sedimentation rate (ESR) of 71 mm/h, and bilateral temporal artery biopsy was consistent with giant cell arteritis. Patient received high doses of methylprednisolone which resolved her hemiparesis, but her vision loss did not improve. Stroke in the presence of significant involvement of vertebral arteries should raise suspicion of GCA especially if classic symptoms preceded stroke event. High clinical suspicion is required to prevent delay in diagnosis and treatment.

1. Introduction

Giant cell arteritis (GCA) is a granulomatous inflammatory disease of medium and large vessels. It is the most frequent primary systemic vasculitis in patients over 50 years of age. It is more common in women, and genetic predisposition has been associated with this disease [1]. Classic GCA symptoms that represent cranial involvement include temporal headache, jaw and tongue claudication, trismus, diplopia, and sudden vision loss [1]. In addition, large vessel involvement of GCA has systemic manifestations such as limb claudication. We discuss a rare case of GCA presenting with left hemiparesis and right monocular visual loss from left vertebral artery dissection.

2. Case Presentation

A 76-year-old right-handed, Caucasian female with no significant personal history presented to the emergency room for acute onset left facial numbness, difficulty speaking, and left upper and left lower extremities weakness associated with difficulty in ambulation. She also developed painless sudden onset right eye blindness. Prior to presentation, she had 3 weeks of bilateral ear pain that was worse when eating, with no ear secretions, fevers, or hearing loss. She had visited an urgent care facility where she was treated as external otitis media with topical antibiotics and oral NSAIDs without improvement of symptoms. She subsequently developed pain over her temples and frontal scalp. Patient referred generalized myalgia and fatigue for a year which she attributed to stress without associated stiffness or pain on the shoulder or hip girdles.

On admission, her vital signs were significant for blood pressure of 169/67 mmHg, a regular heart rate of 69, and temperature of 97.3°F. Physical exam was significant for moderate dysarthria and complete right monocular visual loss with otherwise intact cranial nerves I–XIX. She had left hemiparesis with a power of 4/5 left upper and left lower extremities with brisk deep tendon reflexes and normal tone. Right-sided motor strength was normal as well as sensory exam in all four limbs. Plantar reflexes were downgoing bilaterally. Gait ataxia was present. Her National Institutes of Health Stroke (NIHS) Score was 8 points.

Imaging studies were performed and were significant for a head and neck CT angiogram (CTA) that showed significant dissection of the left vertebral artery and moderate long segment stenosis involving the distal right vertebral artery (Figures 1 and 2).

Patient was started on dual antiplatelets therapy with aspirin and clopidogrel for acute stroke management as per neurology recommendations. Her erythrocyte sedimentation rate was elevated at 71 mm/h.

Given high suspicion of giant cell arteritis, she was also treated with 3 days of pulse dose steroid followed by prednisone 1 mg/kg per day not exceeding 60 mg. She underwent bilateral temporal artery biopsy, and pathology report was consistent with giant cell arteritis (Figure 3). Her left hemiparesis resolved within 48 hours of corticosteroid initiation, but visual loss did not improve. She was discharged on slow taper of prednisone starting with 50 mg daily and aspirin 81 mg daily. Upon follow-up of 2 weeks after discharge, she was noted to have intact motor and sensory function in all four extremities, and her ESR went down to 2 mm/h, but her right monocular visual loss was not recovered.

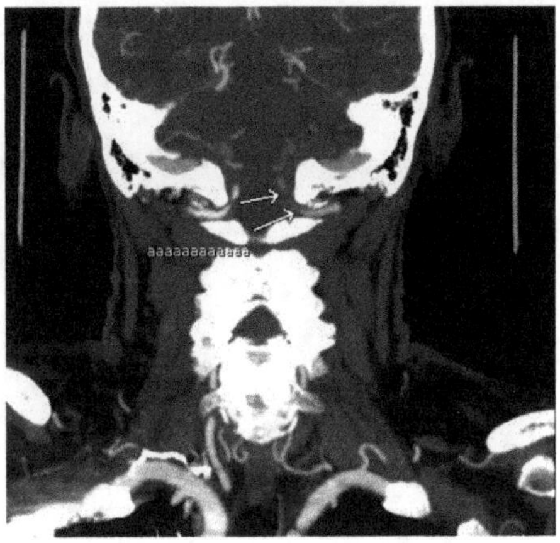

Figure 1: CTA showing left vertebral artery dissection in coronal plane.

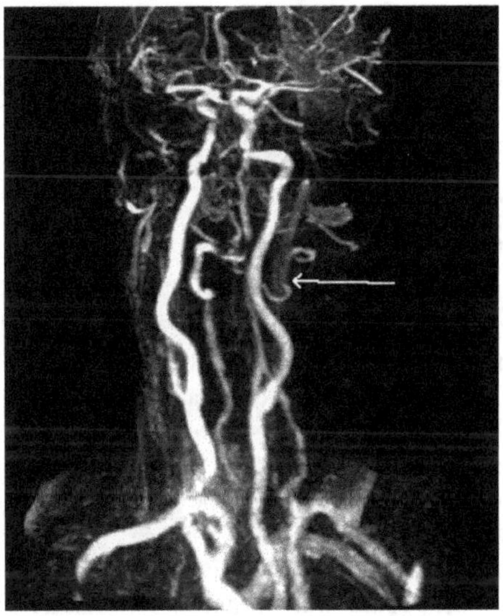

Figure 2: CTA showing left vertebral artery dissection.

3. Discussion

The typical presentation of giant cell arteritis results from vascular inflammation primarily involving external carotid branches including temporal artery and vertebral artery [1, 2]. In early phases, the symptoms can be nonspecific such as malaise, weight loss, and anorexia. Out of all, GCA classic symptoms temporal headache is the most common, and like in our case, it is usually preceded by scalp tenderness [3, 4]. Other symptoms of GCA include jaw and tongue claudication, trismus, diplopia, or sudden vision loss [5, 6].

GCA may occur concomitantly in patients with polymyalgia rheumatica presenting with symptoms of pain in shoulders and hip girdles.

The inflammatory characteristic of GCA results in partial or complete occlusion of the arterial lumen, leading to complications such as ischemic transient ischemic attack (TIA), microembolism, and most importantly, acute ischemic optic neuropathy in 15% of patients [3, 4]. Diagnosis is challenging when presenting with atypical features such as stroke as it only occurs in 2–7% of patients with GCA as per the largest population study published so far [7, 8]. An estimated 0.15% of patients with first-ever stroke will be related to GCA [9]. Stroke related to GCA is usually due to vasculitis of extracranial cerebral arteries involving vertebral or internal carotid arteries.

A relevant characteristic of stroke in patients with GCA is that up to 75% of cases will have involvement of vertebrobasilar circulation, contrasted to only 20% in the general stroke population. Typically, vertebral artery abnormalities are usually due to GCA and not atherosclerosis [10].

The chronic inflammatory process may also lead to vertebral artery dissection, as in our patient, with only two other cases documented in literature. Both cases were female patients more than 75 years old that presented similarly with headaches and bitemporal tenderness, complicated with rapid comatose state and subsequently death. In contrast to these patients, our case had unilateral vertebral artery dissection and did not have a fatal outcome. Patient characteristics are summarized in Table 1.

Temporal artery biopsy is the gold standard for diagnosis as it accounts for a high sensitivity and 100% specificity [13]. However, given emergent need of diagnosis, clinical features

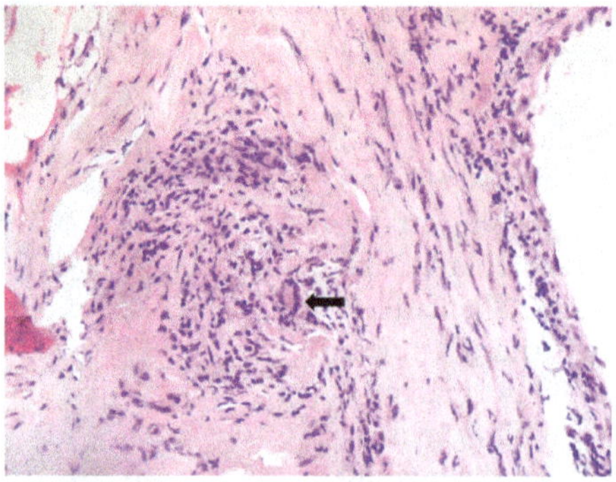

Figure 3: Giant cell indicated in arrow along with granulomatous changes.

Table 1: Comparison of patients' characteristics.

Age	Gender	Clinical findings	ESR	CRP	Radiological findings	Treatment	Outcome	Reference
85	F	Headache and bitemporal tenderness	40 mm/h	Not tested	Not performed	Prednisolone 60 mg/day switched to 5 mg/day after 4 months	Death 9 months after diagnosis	Sheehan et al. [11]
77	F	Right eye blurry vision, bitemporal headache, and jaw claudication	60 mm/h	5.9	CTA with V2-V3 bilateral vertebral artery dissection	Prednisolone 1 g/day	Death 6 days after diagnosis	Proft et al. [12]

are the key to prevent delayed diagnosis and ultimately treatment. For this reason, American College of Rheumatology's (ACR) diagnostic criteria are used. These must include 3 out of 5 between (1) >50 years, (2) new onset headache, (3) temporal artery tenderness to palpation or decreased pulsation, (4) ESR > 50 mm/h, and (5) biopsy proven vasculitis [14].

Meeting the ACR criteria does not necessarily diagnose GCA, as other requirements need to be taken into consideration, being a positive temporal artery biopsy and ESR the main sensitivity and specificity for diagnosis [4]. These criteria have an estimated 93.5% sensitivity and a specificity of 91.2% for the diagnosis of GCA [15]. Temporal artery ultrasound and brain imaging are also emerging as the characteristic "halo sign" also helps to lead to a faster diagnosis.

Systemic glucocorticoids are the cornerstone of treatment and must be started as soon as clinical suspicion is present to decrease the risks of irreversible complications such as vision loss. Hayreh and Zimmerman determined that when glucocorticoids are started before visual involvement, it successfully brings down the risk of visual loss to 1% [16].

When no ischemic events are present, it has been accepted by expert opinion to start prednisone 1 mg/kg (maximum of 60 mg) daily which usually leads to significant symptomatic relief within 48 hours of administration. Inflammatory markers such as ESR also have similar responses.

Although there are no clinical trials or studies available to guide initial dose and tapering dose, high-dose corticosteroids are preferred up to 1000 mg of methylprednisolone daily for three days when ischemic complications such as stroke or vision loss are present [2].

Interferon gamma, interleukin-1 (IL-1), and interleukin-6 (IL-6) pathways are associated with the pathophysiology of GCA. Based on this premise, several studies have been designed to investigate new treatment options. Glucocorticoid-sparing agents such as methotrexate and the IL-6 inhibitor tocilizumab have recently emerged as an alternative for those cases where risks of prednisone use outweigh the benefits. In 2017, the GiACTA trial concluded that the IL-6 inhibitor tocilizumab combined with a course of prednisone taper was more effective than prednisone alone in leading to a sustained remission [17].

On the other hand, Mahr et al. conducted a meta-analysis that concluded that glucocorticoids combined with methotrexate decreases the risk of relapse and reduces the total amount of glucocorticoids needed to achieve clinical response [18].

Other agents such as abatacept, azathioprine, ustekinumab, and cyclophosphamide have been reported to be effective, but formal studies are still needed in literature to prove efficacy.

Moreover, low-dose aspirin in addition to corticosteroids has been reported to decrease the rate of vision loss and stroke during disease course [2].

4. Conclusions

First-ever stroke due to vertebral artery dissection in giant cell arteritis is extremely rare and poses a great challenge for diagnosis. For patients presenting with acute stroke with significant vertebral artery involvement, giant cell arteritis must be considered, especially if classic symptoms precede stroke presentation. Early recognition of GCA helps in providing appropriate and prompt treatment, significantly reducing the risk of irreversible complications. Glucocorticoids remain the cornerstone of management, but other agents such as tocilizumab and methotrexate are being investigated as alternatives. Certainly, more studies are required in order to better understand pathophysiology and management of these complications.

Abbreviations

ACR: American College of Rheumatology
GCA: Giant cell arteritis
ESR: Erythrocyte sedimentation rate
CTA: Computed tomography angiogram
IL-1: Interleukin-1
IL-6: Interleukin-6
GiACTA: Giant cell arteritis actemra (GiACTA) trial.

Authors' Contributions

MMF, SAJ, and SP conceptualized, designed, drafted, and critically revised the manuscript and analyzed and interpreted data. MMF and SP acquired data. All authors have read and approved the manuscript.

References

[1] M. J. Koster, E. L. Matteson, and K. J. Warrington, "Large-vessel giant cell arteritis: diagnosis, monitoring and management," *Rheumatology*, vol. 57, no. 2, pp. ii32–ii42, 2018.

[2] G. Nesher, "The diagnosis and classification of giant cell arteritis," *Journal of Autoimmunity*, vol. 48-49, pp. 73–75, 2014.

[3] D. S. Younger, "Giant cell arteritis," *Neurologic Clinics*, vol. 37, no. 2, pp. 335–344, 2019.

[4] M. Ralli, F. Campo, D. Angeletti et al., "Pathophysiology and therapy of systemic vasculitides," *EXCLI Journal*, vol. 19, pp. 817–854, 2020.

[5] R. Nir-Paz, A. Gross, and T. Chajek-Shaul, "Reduction of jaw opening (trismus) in giant cell arteritis," *Annals of the Rheumatic Diseases*, vol. 61, no. 9, pp. 832-833, 2002.

[6] A. Winkler and D. True, "Giant cell arteritis: 2018 review," *Missouri Medicine*, vol. 115, no. 5, pp. 468–470, 2018, http://www.ncbi.nlm.nih.gov/pubmed/30385998%0Ahttp://www.pubmedcentral.nih.gov/articlerender.fcgi?artid=PMC6205276.

[7] R. J. Caselli, G. G. Hunder, and J. P. Whisnant, "Neurologic disease in biopsy-proven giant cell (temporal) arteritis," *Neurology*, vol. 38, no. 3, p. 352, 1988.

[8] A. Pariente, A. Guédon, S. Alamowitch et al., "Ischemic stroke in giant-cell arteritis: French retrospective study," *Journal of Autoimmunity*, vol. 99, pp. 48–51, 2019.

[9] M. Wiszniewska, G. Devuyst, and J. Bogousslavsky, "Giant cell arteritis as a cause of first-ever stroke," *Cerebrovascular Diseases*, vol. 24, no. 2-3, pp. 226–230, 2007.

[10] J. Zwicker, E. J. Atkins, C. Lum, and M. Sharma, "An atypical presentation of giant cell arteritis," *Canadian Medical Association Journal*, vol. 183, no. 5, pp. E301–E305, 2011.

[11] M. M. Sheehan, C. Keohane, and C. Twomey, "Fatal vertebral giant cell arteritis," *Journal of Clinical Pathology*, vol. 46, no. 12, pp. 1129–1131, 1993.

[12] F. Proft, M. Czihal, J. Remi, G. Fesl, C. Woischke, and H. Schulze Koops, "Fatal spontaneous bilateral vertebral artery dissection in giant cell arteritis (GCA)," *Journal of Vasculitis*, vol. 3, no. 2, pp. 4-5, 2017.

[13] C. Davies and D. May, "The role of temporal artery biopsies in giant cell arteritis," *The Annals of the Royal College of Surgeons of England*, vol. 93, no. 1, pp. 4-5, 2011.

[14] C. Salvarani, C. D. Bella, L. Cimino et al., "Risk factors for severe cranial ischaemic events in an Italian population-based cohort of patients with giant cell arteritis," *Rheumatology*, vol. 48, no. 3, pp. 250–253, 2009.

[15] I. F. Baig, A. Pascoe, A. Kini, and A. G. Lee, "Giant cell arteritis: early diagnosis is key," *Eye and Brain*, vol. 11, pp. 1–12, 2019.

[16] S. S. Hayreh and B. Zimmerman, "Visual deterioration in giant cell arteritis patients while on high doses of corticosteroid therapy," *Ophthalmology*, vol. 110, no. 6, pp. 1204–1215, 2003.

[17] J. H. Stone, K. Tuckwell, S. Dimonaco et al., "Trial of tocilizumab in giant-cell arteritis," *New England Journal of Medicine*, vol. 377, no. 4, pp. 317–328, 2017.

[18] A. D. Mahr, J. A. Jover, R. F. Spiera et al., "Adjunctive methotrexate for treatment of giant cell arteritis: an individual patient data meta-analysis," *Arthritis & Rheumatism*, vol. 56, no. 8, pp. 2789–2797, 2007.

39

A Rare Case of Fatal Hemorrhagic Stroke in a Young Female with Early Mixed Connective Tissue Disease

James R. Agapoff IV

Department of Psychiatry, University of Hawai'i at Mānoa, John A. Burns School of Medicine, Honolulu, HI, USA

Correspondence should be addressed to James R. Agapoff IV; nubis13@gmail.com

Academic Editor: Gregory J. Tsay

Mixed connective tissue disease (MCTD) often presents as a slow progressive illness with low morbidity and mortality. Serious central nervous system disease is uncommon, and fatal outcomes are rarely seen. Here, we report a rare case of fatal hemorrhagic stroke in a 43-year-old female with a rapidly progressive MCTD. She presented to primary care with a history of headaches, visual disturbances, and unprovoked lower extremity swelling and pain. A rheumatological workup showed positive antinuclear (ANA) and ribonucleoprotein (RNP) antibodies. Magnetic resonance imaging (MRI) found a 12 mm hemorrhage along a cortical sulcus of the right frontal lobe, and a follow-up magnetic resonance angiography (MRA) and ophthalmological exam showed no definitive signs of vasculitis. Over the course of her workup, she developed swollen hands, Raynaud's syndrome, myalgias, and synovitis characteristic of evolving MCTD. The patient then began to experience severe headaches over one month. Repeat MRI was ordered, but never completed, and the patient presented to the emergency department (ED) with a severe, right-sided headache, and left-sided visual disturbance. In the ED, she began to display evidence of delirium and seizure activity and became unresponsive. A computerized tomography scan (CT) of the brain showed a right parietal lobe intraparenchymal hemorrhage approximately $5 \times 3 \times 5$ cm in size with secondary mass effect including mid- and hind-brain herniation. Computerized tomography angiography (CTA) of the brain showed signs of large vessel vasculitis. A craniectomy was performed; however, the patient never regained consciousness and died several days later. Vasculitis, while rare in connective tissue diseases, should be aggressively assessed for and managed in patients with any early signs and symptoms of cerebrovascular involvement to prevent fatal outcomes.

1. Introduction

Mixed connective tissue disease (MCTD) is an autoimmune condition characterized by overlapping features of several connective tissue diseases including polymyositis, rheumatoid arthritis, systemic lupus erythematosus, and systemic sclerosis in the presence of high levels of RNP antibodies [1]. Of the diagnostic algorithms available, the Alarcon–Segovia's and Kahn's criteria are considered to have highest sensitivity and specificity [2].

MCTD is a rare disease with incidence rates between 0.2 and 2.1 per 100,000 person-years based on several studies [1, 3, 4]. In one nationwide sample, the prevalence of MCTD was 3.8 (95% CI 3.2 to 4.4) per 100,000 adults, the average age was 37.9 years (95% CI: 35.3 to 40.4 years), and the diagnostic ratio of females to males was 3.3 [3].

Compared to other connective tissue diseases, MCTD is generally considered to have lower morbidity and mortality. In one study, mortality to MCTD did not differ from the general population sampled with a mortality ratio of 1.1 (95% CI, 0.4–2.6) [1]. In another study, 15-year survival rates from diagnosis were 88% [5]. Survival rates may be better considering that it often takes a median time of 3.6 years to make the diagnosis from the onset of first symptoms.

Neurological symptoms are uncommon in MCTD; headache, seizure, encephalopathy, aseptic meningitis, and neuropathy are seen in 10–20% of patients. Reports of immune-mediated central nervous system (CNS) vasculitis seen as the initial presentation of MCTD are uncommon [6–8].

Here, we report on the case of a 43-year-old, healthy Caucasian female, with rapidly progressive MCTD who developed neurological symptoms and later died of hemorrhagic stroke associated with probable CNS vasculitis.

2. Case Presentation

A 43-year-old healthy Caucasian female presented to primary care with short (7–10 days), recurrent flares of lower extremity tenderness, swelling, and redness over several months. She also reported myalgias in the upper back and neck, and a one-year history of headache with transient, reoccurring curtain-like visual disturbances in her right eye that ophthalmology diagnosed as ocular migraines. A rheumatologic workup was initiated. Labs were positive for an elevated sedimentation rate (ESR) 31 mm/H (normal 0–20 mmH), positive antinuclear antibodies (ANA), and an elevated ribonucleoprotein antibodies (RNP) 2.4 AI (reference <1.0 AI). Double-stranded (DS) DNA 1 IU/mL (<4 = Neg), antichromatin (AC), anti-Smith (SM), SM/RNP, and lyme disease antibodies were negative. Based on these results, the patient received a presumptive diagnosis of undifferentiated connective tissue disease (UCTD), started 20 mg of oral prednisone as needed for flares, and referred to rheumatology.

Two months after her initial evaluation, the patient continued to experience episodes or erythema nodosum of the lower extremities. She also began to experience early signs of Raynaud's phenomenon, chest pain, and visual disturbances concerning for amaurosis fugax. A personal symptom journal kept by the patient indicated transient episodes of fatigue and painful hand/finger swelling with petechiae and purpura. Magnetic resonance imaging (MRI) of the brain was ordered, and repeat labs done by rheumatology showed an elevated ESR, 39 mm/H; RNP, 1.8 AI; CRP, 3.7 (normal <0.8 mg/dL); and a negative anti-neutrophil cytoplasmic antibody (ANCA), myeloperoxidase antibodies, proteinase-3 antibodies, and ANA. Complement C3, 118 mg/dL (normal 90–180 mg/dL), and C4, 29 mg/dL (normal 16–47 mg/dL), were within normal limits. The patient was referred for further evaluation at an academic medical center.

The MRI showed a 6 mm lacunar infarct within the left cerebellum and a 12 mm hemorrhage along a cortical sulcus of the right frontal lobe. The findings were noted to be "abnormal" for a woman in her early forties, and a further work was recommended for vasculitis and/or connective tissue disease via magnetic resonance angiography (MRA). The MRA and ophthalmological assessment were unremarkable, and cardiology found no evidence of vascular disease on carotid ultrasound and no evidence of exercise-induced myocardial ischemia on stress echocardiogram.

A second rheumatological consult was completed where concern for possible evolving MCTD was raised; however, the diagnosis of UCTD was retained due to the negative ANA. Seven months following her initial presentation, the patient saw neurology where she reported worsening lightheadedness and 6-7/10 bifrontal/apical headaches lasting hours to days over the previous month. Despite the history of arthralgias/myalgias, purpura, chest pain, evidence of cerebral hemorrhage, and initial labs showing nonspecific inflammation and markers of autoimmunity, vasculitis was considered low on the differential due to a lack of a clear prodromal history and changes in cognition. Similarly, neuro-ophthalmology found no definite retinal vasculitis and believed her homonymous right visual field defect to be associated with the brain lesion previously appreciated on MRI and not amaurosis fugax. A non-emergent repeat MRI with contrast and an MR venogram of the brain were ordered by neurology to rule out thrombosis and evaluate for new lesions.

Approximately two months after her neurology appointment, the patient presented to the emergency room with a severe, right-sided headache with a left-sided visual disturbance. Shortly after arrival, the patient became delirious and exhibited seizure-like activity. A computerized tomography scan (CT) of the brain was conducted that showed a right parietal lobe intraparenchymal hemorrhage approximately 5 × 3 × 5 cm in size with secondary mass effect including mid- and hind-brain herniation (see Figure 1). A CTA showed multifocal narrowing and an abnormal "beaded" contour of the entire cerebral arterial vasculature consistent for vasculitis. Neurosurgical assets were not available, and the patient was transferred to a sister center where craniectomy was performed to evacuate intracerebral hemorrhage and treat intracranial hypertension (see Figure 2). Postoperative prognosis was poor, and palliative measures were initiated. The patient passed away peacefully surrounded by family several days later.

3. Discussion

During the patient's clinical course, the diagnosis of MCTD remained in the differential; however, there was early serological and clinical evidence for this condition. The patient was initially ANA and RNP positive and would experience all of clinical criteria for MCTD, save sclerodactyly, over her clinical course including swollen hands, Raynaud's phenomenon, myalgias, and synovitis [1]. Even though the patient's ANA would later be negative, a positive RNP is often considered diagnostic for MCTD when found in isolation of other biomarkers as seen in this patient [9].

Only 10–20% of patients with MCTD experience neurological manifestations, with few case reports known where neurological symptoms were the presenting symptom [6-8]. [6, 7] Similar to the subject of this report, the patients in these studies presented with severe headaches as a prodrome to an immune-mediated CNS vasculitis. Given the progressive nature of MCTD and the short duration (less than one-year) between the onset of this patient's neurological symptoms and her rheumatologic workup, it is likely that this patient's headaches and visual disturbances were an initial manifestation of MCTD and not an isolated case of ocular migraines.

Vasculitis is rare in connective tissue disease, occurring in less than 10% of patients [10] with central nervous system involvement occurring in a much smaller subgroup [11]. In this patient, early signs of small vessel vasculitis included petechiae and purpura on the hands and lower extremities. Evidence of systemic involvement included persistently

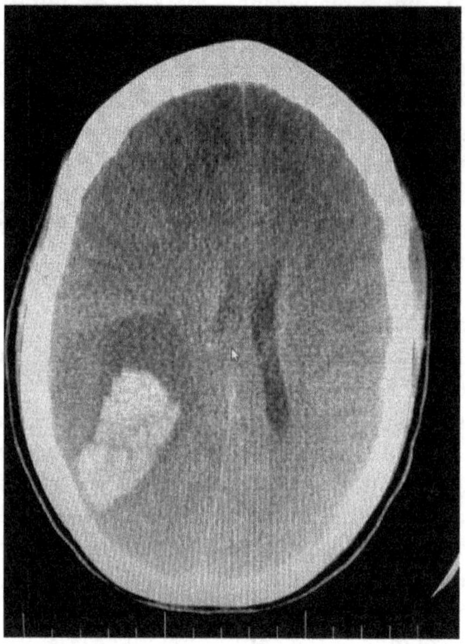

FIGURE 1: Computerized tomography (CT) axial head without contrast showing intraparenchymal hemorrhage and secondary mass effect.

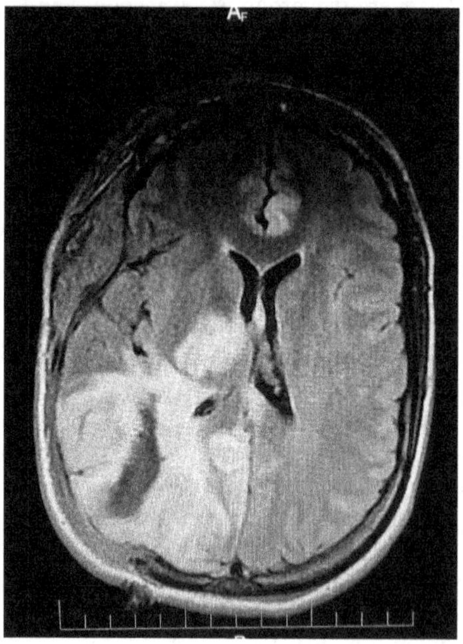

FIGURE 2: Magnetic resonance imaging (MRI) FLAIR axial head without contrast showing intraparenchymal hemorrhage status after craniectomy.

elevated inflammatory biomarkers (CRP and ESR), amaurosis fugax, and cerebrovascular hemorrhaging noted on MRI. Despite these findings, vasculitis remained low on the differential due to lack of a clear prodrome and frank cognitive deficits.

MCTD often presents as a sequential or staggered overlap of SLE, scleroderma, myositis, and rheumatoid arthritis [12]. This nonlinear presentation requires heightened curiosity of potential evolving pathologies where a clear prodrome is not apparent. Throughout her clinical course, the patient reported mental fogginess that might have been interpreted as "cognitive deficits" in a person with lower baseline intelligence and functional status. And, while the initial MRA of the brain did not show any signs of large vessel disease, it did not capture the distal mid-to-small sized vessels of the brain. This incomplete study could not rule out small dissections or other changes that may have informed clinicians about evolving pathologies including systemic vasculitis.

Had the patient's first MRA shown more definitive signs of vasculitis, her report of new and worsening headaches may have prompted her treatment team to pursue a more aggressive assessment of her symptoms. This case illustrates the importance of considering CNS vasculitis in patients with unexplained, progressive neurologic symptoms and adds support to the case reports by Awad, Matsui, and Graf showing MCTD as a possible cause of severe neurological disease [6–8]. Together, these cases illustrate the importance of rapid and assertive assessment and management of neurological symptoms in persons with suspected connective tissue diseases. Awareness of this link may aid in early diagnosis and initiation of appropriate treatments to improve positive outcomes.

Disclosure

The author is an acquaintance of the patient's family.

Acknowledgments

The author would like to thank the family of the patient who supported the publication of the case report.

References

[1] P. Ungprasert, C. S. Crowson, V. R. Chowdhary, F. C. Ernste, K. G. Moder, and E. L. Matteson, "Epidemiology of mixed connective tissue disease, 1985–2014: a population-based study," *Arthritis Care & Research*, vol. 68, no. 12, pp. 1843–1848, 2016.

[2] D. Alarcon-Segovia and M. H. Cardiel, "Comparison between 3 diagnostic criteria for mixed connective tissue disease. Study of 593 patients," *Journal of Rheumatology*, vol. 16, no. 3, pp. 328–334, 1989.

[3] R. Gunnarsson, Ø. Molberg, I.-M. Gilboe, and J. T. Gran, "The prevalence and incidence of mixed connective tissue disease: a national multicentre survey of Norwegian patients," *Annals of the Rheumatic Diseases*, vol. 70, no. 6, pp. 1047–1051, 2011.

[4] O. Kaipiainen-Seppänen and K. Aho, "Incidence of rare systemic rheumatic and connective tissue diseases in Finland," *Journal of Internal Medicine*, vol. 240, no. 2, pp. 81–84, 1996.

[5] A. Hajas, P. Szodoray, B. Nakken, G. Nagy, Z. Szekanecz, and E. Bodolay, "SAT0190 long-term follow-up of 280 patients with mixed connective tissue disease," *Annals of the Rheumatic Diseases*, vol. 72, no. Suppl 3, p. A645, 2013.

[6] A. M. Awad and M. Stevenson, "Isolated central nervous system vasculitis associated with antiribonuclear protein antibody," *Case Reports in Neurological Medicine*, vol. 2011, Article ID 495201, 4 pages, 2011.

[7] H. Matsui, F. Udaka, M. Oda, T. Kubori, K. Nishinaka, and

M. Kameyama, "Encephalopathy and severe neuropathy due to probable systemic vasculitis as an initial manifestation of mixed connective tissue disease," *Neurology India*, vol. 54, no. 1, pp. 83–85, 2006.

[8] W. D. Graf, J. M. Milstein, and D. D. Sherry, "Stroke and mixed connective tissue disease," *Journal of Child Neurology*, vol. 8, no. 3, pp. 256–259, 1993.

[9] Mayo Clinic Laboratories, *Neurology Catalog: RNP Antibodies, IgG, Serum*, Mayo Clinic Laboratories, Rochester, MN, USA, 2021, https://neurology.testcatalog.org/show/RNP.

[10] E. Cozzani, G. Gasparini, M. Papini, M Burlando, F Drago, and A Parodi, "Vasculitis associated with connective tissue diseases," *Giornale italiano di dermatologia e venereologia: organo ufficiale Societa italiana di dermatologia e sifilografia*, vol. 150, no. 2, pp. 221–232, 2015.

[11] A. Sharma, A. Dhooria, A. Aggarwal, M. Rathi, and V. Chandran, "Connective tissue disorder-associated vasculitis," *Current Rheumatology Reports*, vol. 18, no. 6, pp. 31–41, 2016.

[12] P. H. Pepmueller, "Undifferentiated connective tissue disease, mixed connective tissue disease, and overlap syndromes in rheumatology," *Missouri Medicine*, vol. 113, no. 2, pp. 136–140, 2016.

40

Acute Symptomatic Calcific Discitis Mimicking a Septic Spondylodiscitis

Magda Choueiri,[1] **Florent Eymard**,[1] **Sandra Guignard**,[1] **Frédéric Pigneur**,[2] **and Xavier Chevalier**[1]

[1]*Department of Rheumatology, Henri Mondor University Hospital, Paris XII University-UPEC, Créteil, France*
[2]*Department of Radiology, Henri Mondor University Hospital, Paris XII University-UPEC, Créteil, France*

Correspondence should be addressed to Magda Choueiri; magdachoueiri@gmail.com

Academic Editor: Mario Salazar-Paramo

Acute symptomatic calcific discitis is a poorly understood condition that has been mostly reported in children. Cases in adults have been scarcely reported and may mimic an infectious process. Imaging, including computed tomography, can show the disc calcification but might fail to show it because its resorption can occur early after the onset of symptoms. We report the case of an adult patient presenting with severe cervical-dorsal junction pain, fever, high C-reactive protein (CRP) levels, and imaging findings mimicking an infectious spondylodiscitis, including an erosion of the anterior part of the vertebral endplate. However, the patient improved spontaneously and rapidly, with pain and fever disappearing and C-reactive protein (CRP) returning to normal within a week.

1. Introduction

Acute symptomatic calcific discitis (CD) is a rare condition in the adult population, with very few cases reported in the literature [1]. Incident disc calcification is reported in 5% of chest radiographs and 6% of abdominal plain films, as well as in 70% of postmortem adult examinations [2]. However, these calcifications generally remain asymptomatic, but when they do manifest, they can induce acute onset severe spinal pain and stiffness, with imaging features mimicking infectious spondylodiscitis [1–8]. On the other hand, pyogenic spondylodiscitis can be extremely severe and is associated with high mortality rates ranging from 2 to 20% in the literature, which makes it a potentially life-threatening disease [9]. Hence, identifying those cases is crucial, and acknowledging plausible differential diagnosis can be quite helpful.

2. Case Report

A 67-year-old man presented to the emergency department for a two-week debilitating low cervical and high dorsal pain, with fever and asthenia. The pain was severe, throbbing, and occurring in small spontaneously remitting crisis, with an inflammatory pattern. There were no other symptoms, and no clinical signs of infection that could explain his fever. The patient was morbidly obese and nonsmoker and had a history of paroxysmal atrial fibrillation treated with digoxin, a beta-blocker, and warfarin and type II diabetes mellitus for which he was taking glimepiride; on presentation, his blood glucose level was moderately elevated (162 mg/dL, normal lab value (N) < 110 mg/dL) and his latest glycated hemoglobin levels were also slightly increased, reaching 6.8%.

At the emergency department, the patient was afebrile. Upon examination, he had a stiff cervical spine with pain on flexion. Palpation of his spine showed exquisite pain at the levels of C7 and T1. The remaining physical examination revealed no abnormalities including a normal neurologic state and a normal cardiac auscultation.

Laboratory evaluation showed a very high CRP level (306 mg/L, with N < 5 mg/L) and an increased erythrocyte sedimentation rate (68 mm after 1 hour, with N < 21 mm). His blood count and liver and renal function tests were

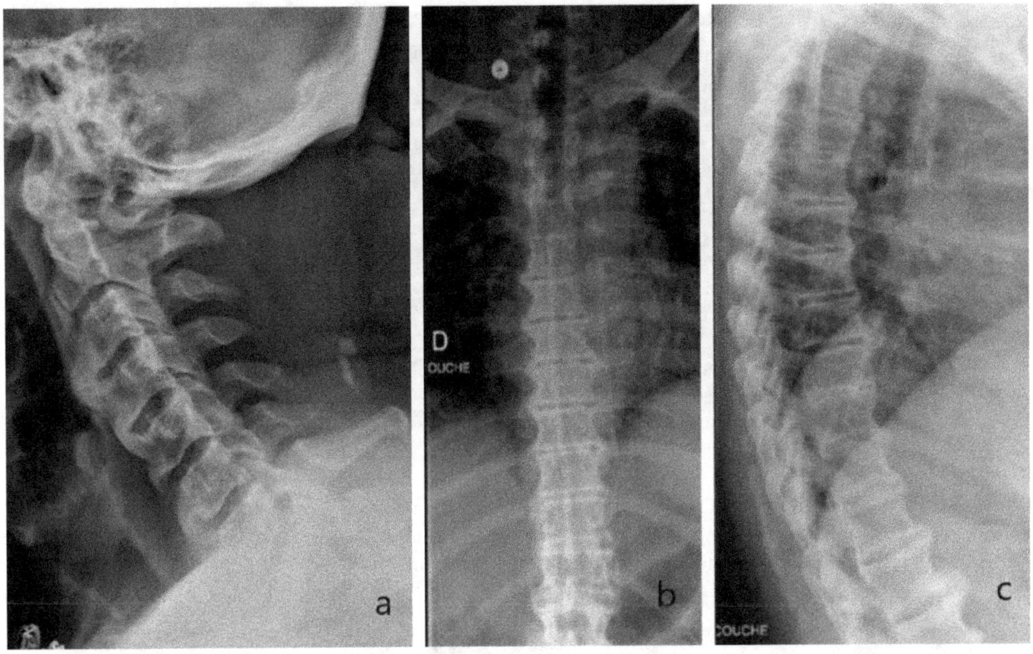

FIGURE 1: Plain radiographs of cervical spine, lateral view (a), and dorsal spine, anteroposterior (b) and lateral (c) views. Findings suggestive of diffuse idiopathic skeletal hyperostosis (DISH or Forestier's Disease) were noted, especially on dorsal spine X-rays. Calcification of intervertebral discs was not seen.

normal. Chest X-ray revealed no abnormalities. Standard radiographs of the spine showed signs of diffuse idiopathic skeletal hyperostosis (DISH) with pseudoankylosis of the dorsal spine (Figure 1). No clear image of intervertebral calcific deposition was detected at this point.

Owing to the strong suspicion of infectious spondylodiscitis, a magnetic resonance imaging (MRI) of the spine was performed (Figure 2) and showed inflammatory changes of both C7 and T1 vertebral bodies, with hyperintense signal on T2 and low signal intensity on T1 sequences, considerably enhancing after gadolinium injection. The intervertebral C7-T1 disc showed no T2 hypersignal and no enhancement following contrast injection. A computed tomography (CT) of the spine (Figure 3) showed erosions on the anterior aspects of the lower vertebral endplate of C7 and the upper vertebral endplate of T1 with a calcification located in between, at the anterior part of the C7-T1 intervertebral disc. Calcifications were noted in the adjacent disc spaces of the dorsal spines.

An echocardiography showed no sign of endocarditis. Urine and blood cultures, Wright serology, *Bartonella*, Q fever, hepatitis B and C, and HIV serologies were all negative. Three additional sets of blood cultures were taken during the first 24 hours of hospitalization and were also negative. Radiographs of the knees, the wrists, the shoulders, and the pelvis showed no signs of calcium pyrophosphate deposition.

A disco-vertebral biopsy was programmed, but it had to be delayed because the patient was taking warfarin for atrial fibrillation. In the meantime, since he remained stable, he received no antibiotics; no specific treatments, such as corticosteroids, were started. He was only prescribed analgesics and bed rest. Surprisingly, he started feeling better and his fever disappeared after a couple of days. His pain progressively decreased and had completely vanished a week later. His spine had retrieved a normal and painless mobility. Furthermore, his CRP levels dramatically dropped to 21 mg/L five days later and reached 14 mg/L seven days after his first consultation to the emergency department (vs. 306 mg/L on admission, $N < 5$ mg/L). No additional procedures were performed, and the patient was discharged.

This spectacular improvement in both clinical signs and biologic tests definitively ruled out the possibility of an infectious process. The diagnosis of acute symptomatic calcific discitis was made, accounting the acute clinical presentation and good evolution, along with the presence of calcifications in the several disc spaces of the dorsal spine.

3. Discussion

Although it has been frequently reported in children, acute symptomatic CD is a rare condition in the adult population, with no more than 10 cases reported in the literature [1].

The real etiology of CD remains unclear, with multiple possible theories. The most common hypothesis is the presence of a vascular insult, which could eventually lead to discal calcification by interrupting blood supply to the nucleus pulposus [10]. Repeated microtrauma might additionally play a role in this poorly understood process [1, 11]. Disc calcifications have also been observed in ankylosis of the spine.

Of note, conditions and metabolic diseases have been associated with intervertebral disc calcification, especially calcium pyrophosphate dihydrate deposition. These include hyperparathyroidism, hemochromatosis, ochronosis, amyloidosis, acromegaly, and poliomyelitis [12]. However, in

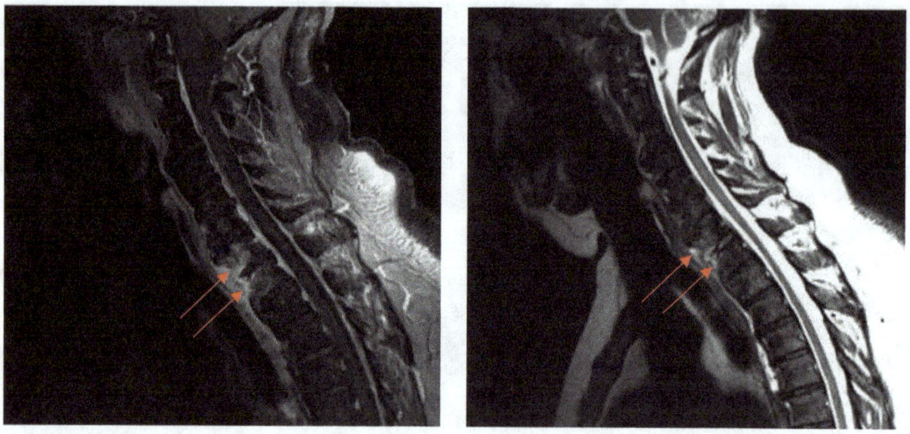

(a) (b)

FIGURE 2: MRI of the cervico-dorsal junction, T1-weighted post-gadolinium injection (a) and T2-weighted (b) sequences, showing enhancement in C7 and T1 vertebral bodies after injection, and hyperintense signal on T2 sequence (arrows). The intervertebral C7-T1 disc does not show any T2 hypersignal or enhancement following contrast injection.

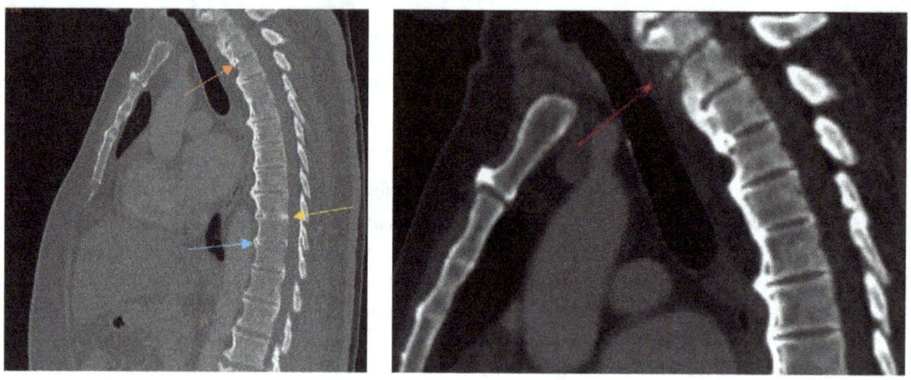

(a) (b)

FIGURE 3: CT scan of the cervical and dorsal spine showing erosions on the anterior aspects of the lower vertebral endplate of C7 and the upper vertebral end-plate of T1 with a calcification located in between, at the anterior part of the C7-T1 intervertebral disc ((b) red arrow). (a) Calcifications were also present in the T2-T3 (orange arrow), T9-T10 (yellow arrow), and T10-T11 (blue arrow) intervertebral discs.

these cases, calcification usually involves several levels, including at least the annulus fibrosus. This contrasts with idiopathic CD which only affects the nucleus pulposus and where no underlying systemic condition is usually found [1].

Interestingly, most case reports of CD occurring in adults show that the commonest locations of CD were the middle and lower thoracic spine, while the cervical localization is more frequently encountered in children. Indeed, among the few reported cases in adults, nine were located between T6 and T12 [1, 13], one was in C2-C3 [7], and one was in L4-L5 [14]. Our case is the first reported CD to occur in the cervico-thoracic junction in an adult patient. Another difference is the predominance of CD in boys contrasting with the adult population where it seems to occur more commonly in women [1]. Moreover, unlike adults, in whom no preceding event has been reported, children with CD often have a prior history of trauma (up to one third of cases) [14] or infection (15% of cases) [1, 15].

Fever and biologic signs of inflammation are usually absent in the few adult patients in whom CD has been reported. On the other hand, in the pediatric population, CD may present with fever and laboratory signs of inflammation (especially high CRP levels), which are detected in up to 15% of children with CD [2].

Hence, our case is the first report of acute symptomatic calcific discitis associated with fever and biological signs of inflammation.

Notably, in its early stages, CD may not be visible on radiographs and may only manifest with disc swelling on MRI [16]. This is often associated with diffuse reactive edema on adjacent vertebral endplates. Additionally, contrast enhancement of the vertebral body is possible, due to the inflammatory response secondary to CD. This finding might be mistakenly attributed to an infectious lesion. To avoid this confusion, a CT scan should be performed to detect the calcification within the disc [1, 5].

Eventually, both pediatric and adult patients presenting with acute symptomatic calcific discitis will usually have a complete resolution of symptoms with conservative medical treatment, including analgesics and bed rest. Radiographic regression of the disc calcification, however, can remain incomplete, especially in adults [1].

4. Conclusion

Idiopathic calcific discitis is a rare cause of neck or back pain in adults. Our case shows that CD can even be associated with systemic signs of inflammation, including fever and increased CRP levels. The diagnosis of acute symptomatic CD must be recognized early enough to avoid disco-vertebral biopsy and subsequent antibiotics which are useless in this aseptic condition. Symptoms due to CD tend to resolve spontaneously with rest and analgesics after few days or weeks.

References

[1] A. Shah, R. Botchu, M. F. Grainger, A. M. Davies, and S. L. James, "Acute symptomatic calcific discitis in adults: a case report and review of literature," *Skeletal Radiology*, vol. 44, no. 12, pp. 1819–1824, 2015.

[2] M. H. Nogueira-Barbosa, C. F. P. da Silva Herrero, W. Pasqualini, and H. L. A. Defino, "Calcific discitis in an adult patient with intravertebral migration and spontaneous remission," *Clinical Neurology and Neurosurgery*, vol. 42, no. 8, pp. 1161–1164, 2013.

[3] D. M. Smith, "Acute back pain associated with a calcified Schmorl's node: a case report," *Clinical Orthopaedics and Related Research*, vol. 117, pp. 193–196, 1976.

[4] L. E. Lipson and M. O'Connell, "Case 37-1991," *The New England Journal of Medicine*, vol. 325, no. 11, pp. 794–799, 1991.

[5] M. A. Rodacki, C. E. S. Castro, and D. S. Castro, "Diffuse vertebral body edema due to calcified intraspongious disk herniation," *Neuroradiology*, vol. 47, no. 5, pp. 316–321, 2005.

[6] J. Bazzi, J. R. Dimar, and S. D. Glassman, "Acute calcific discitis in adults," *American Journal of Orthopedics (Belle Mead, N.J.)*, vol. 31, no. 3, pp. 141–145, 2002.

[7] N. Azizaddini, S. Arefanian, N. Redjal, B. P. Walcott, and R. Mollahoseini, "Adult acute calcific discitis confined to the nucleus pulposus in the cervical spine: case report," *Journal of Neurosurgery: Spine*, vol. 19, no. 2, pp. 170–173, 2013.

[8] M. Piccirilli, G. Lapadula, F. Caporlingua, S. Martini, and A. Santoro, "Spontaneous regression of a thoracic calcified disc herniation in a young female: a case report and literature review," *Clinical Neurology and Neurosurgery*, vol. 114, no. 6, pp. 779–781, 2012.

[9] D. Li, T. Wong, G. Tsai et al., "Appropriate duration of post-surgical intravenous antibiotic therapy for pyogenic spondylodiscitis," *BMC Infectious Diseases*, vol. 18, no. 1, p. 468, 2018.

[10] L. E. Swischuk, M. Jubang, and S. P. Jadhav, "Calcific discitis in children: vertebral body involvement (possible insight into etiology)," *Emergency Radiology*, vol. 15, no. 6, pp. 427–430, 2008.

[11] G. Beluffi, P. Fiori, and C. Sileo, "Intervertebral disc calcifications in children," *La Radiologia Medica*, vol. 114, no. 2, pp. 331–341, 2009.

[12] M.-M. Lefèvre-Colau, S. Poiraudeau, M.-A. Mayoux-Benhamou, and M. Revel, "Les calcifications discales," *Revue du Rhumatisme*, vol. 67, pp. 276–279, 2000.

[13] N. Xu, F. Wei, X. Liu, L. Jiang, and Z. Liu, "Calcific discitis with giant thoracic disc herniations in adults," *European Spine Journal*, vol. 25, no. S1, pp. 204–208, 2016.

[14] A.-R. Sadek, C. Dare, S. Mcgillion, A. Nader-Sepahi, and V. Skiadas, "Lumbar intravertebral disc herniation secondary to idiopathic calcific discitis," *British Journal of Neurosurgery*, vol. 33, pp. 586–590, 2017.

[15] D. H. Sonnabend, T. K. Taylor, and G. K. Chapman, "Intervertebral disc calcification syndromes in children," *The Journal of Bone and Joint Surgery*, vol. 64, no. 1, pp. 25–31, 1982.

[16] L. E. Swischuk and S. D. Stansberry, "Calcific discitis: MRI changes in discs without visible calcification," *Pediatric Radiology*, vol. 21, no. 5, pp. 365-366, 1991.

Permissions

All chapters in this book were first published by Hindawi Publishing Corporation; hereby published with permission under the Creative Commons Attribution License or equivalent. Every chapter published in this book has been scrutinized by our experts. Their significance has been extensively debated. The topics covered herein carry significant findings which will fuel the growth of the discipline. They may even be implemented as practical applications or may be referred to as a beginning point for another development.

The contributors of this book come from diverse backgrounds, making this book a truly international effort. This book will bring forth new frontiers with its revolutionizing research information and detailed analysis of the nascent developments around the world.

We would like to thank all the contributing authors for lending their expertise to make the book truly unique. They have played a crucial role in the development of this book. Without their invaluable contributions this book wouldn't have been possible. They have made vital efforts to compile up to date information on the varied aspects of this subject to make this book a valuable addition to the collection of many professionals and students.

This book was conceptualized with the vision of imparting up-to-date information and advanced data in this field. To ensure the same, a matchless editorial board was set up. Every individual on the board went through rigorous rounds of assessment to prove their worth. After which they invested a large part of their time researching and compiling the most relevant data for our readers.

The editorial board has been involved in producing this book since its inception. They have spent rigorous hours researching and exploring the diverse topics which have resulted in the successful publishing of this book. They have passed on their knowledge of decades through this book. To expedite this challenging task, the publisher supported the team at every step. A small team of assistant editors was also appointed to further simplify the editing procedure and attain best results for the readers.

Apart from the editorial board, the designing team has also invested a significant amount of their time in understanding the subject and creating the most relevant covers. They scrutinized every image to scout for the most suitable representation of the subject and create an appropriate cover for the book.

The publishing team has been an ardent support to the editorial, designing and production team. Their endless efforts to recruit the best for this project, has resulted in the accomplishment of this book. They are a veteran in the field of academics and their pool of knowledge is as vast as their experience in printing. Their expertise and guidance has proved useful at every step. Their uncompromising quality standards have made this book an exceptional effort. Their encouragement from time to time has been an inspiration for everyone.

The publisher and the editorial board hope that this book will prove to be a valuable piece of knowledge for researchers, students, practitioners and scholars across the globe.

List of Contributors

Lina Bayazeed and Jubran Alqanatish
King Saud Bin Abdulaziz University for Health Sciences, Riyadh 14611, Saudi Arabia
King Abdullah International Medical Research Center (KAIMRC), Riyadh 14611, Saudi Arabia
King Abdullah Specialist Children's Hospital, Riyadh 14611, Saudi Arabia

Alaa Felimban, Abdulsalam Alsaiad and Fahd Alsufiani
King Saud Bin Abdulaziz University for Health Sciences, Riyadh 14611, Saudi Arabia
King Abdullah International Medical Research Center (KAIMRC), Riyadh 14611, Saudi Arabia
King Abdulaziz Medical City (National Guard Health Affairs), Riyadh 14611, Saudi Arabia

Benedicta Nnodum and Lauren Dudley
Berkshire Medical Center, Pittsfield, MA, USA

Yusho Ishii, Hiroshi Fujii, Tsuyoshi Shirai, Yosuke Hoshi, Yoko Fujita, Yuko Shirota and Hideo Harigae
Department of Hematology and Rheumatology, Tohoku University Graduate School of Medicine, Aoba-ku, Sendai, Japan

Koichiro Sugimura and Hiroaki Shimokawa
Department of Cardiovascular Medicine, Tohoku University Graduate School of Medicine, Aoba-ku, Sendai, Japan

Tomonori Ishii
Clinical Research, Innovation and Education Center, Tohoku University Hospital, Sendai, Miyagi, Japan

Aureliano Pistone and Muhammad Soyfoo
Department of Rheumatology, Cliniques Universitaires de Bruxelles - H^opital Erasme, Universit´e Libre de Bruxelles (ULB), Bruxelles, Belgium

Syoko Tsubouchi, Takahiro Mizuuchi, Yusuke Yamamoto, Daiki Fujimori, Kayo Ishii, Mayu Tago, Eri Kato, Hiroaki Mori, Haeru Hayashi, Koichiro Tahara and Tetsuji Sawada
Department of Rheumatology, Tokyo Medical University Hospital, Shinjuku, Tokyo, Japan

Jaspreet Kaler, Myint Thway, Karishma Ramsubeik and Gurjit Kaeley
Department of Rheumatology, University of Florida Health, 653 W 8th Street, Jacksonville, 32209 Florida, USA

Liam M. Clifford
Department of General Medicine, Gosford Hospital, Gosford, NSW, Australia

Jamma Li and Suran L. Fernando
Department of Clinical Immunology and Allergy, Royal North Shore Hospital, Sydney, NSW, Australia
Immunorheumatology Laboratory, New South Wales Health Pathology, Royal North Shore Hospital, Sydney, NSW, Australia
University of Sydney, Sydney, NSW, Australia

Christopher J. Renaud
Department of Anatomical Pathology, Royal North Shore Hospital, Sydney, NSW, Australia

Bicky Thapa and Raunak Nair
Department of Internal Medicine, Cleveland Clinic Fairview Hospital, Cleveland, Ohio, USA

Asad Ali
Neurological Institute, Taussig Center Institute, Cleveland Clinic Foundation, Cleveland, Ohio, USA

Rishik Vashisht
Respiratory Institute, Cleveland Clinic Foundation, Cleveland, Ohio, USA

Cassandra Calabrese
Department of Rheumatic & Immunologic Disease, Cleveland Clinic Foundation, Cleveland, Ohio, USA

Gina Ferrero, Marissa Karpoff, Pamela Traisak, David Feinstein and Hala Eid
Cooper University Hospital, Camden, NJ, USA

Kate Chernow
Einstein Medical Center Montgomery, East Norriton, PA, USA
Abington Lansdale Hospital, Lansdale, PA, USA

Anne D. D. Joseph, Jebananthy Anandaselvam Pradeepan and Thirunavukarasu Kumanan
University Medical Unit, Teaching Hospital Jaffna, Jaffna, Sri Lanka

Muthusamy Malaravan
Department of Ophthalmology, Teaching Hospital Jaffna, Jaffna, Sri Lanka

Shigeto Kobayashi and Issei Kida
Department of Internal Medicine and Rheumatology, Juntendo University Koshigaya Hospital, Koshigaya, Saitama 343-0032, Japan

Yuuki Makiyama
Department of Otolaryngology, Yokohama City Minato Red Cross Hospital, Yokohama, Kanagawa 231-8682, Japan

Yoshinori Taniguchi
Department of Endocrinology, Metabolism,Nephrology and Rheumatology, Kochi Medical School Hospital, Kochi University, Nankoku, Kochi 783-8505, Japan

Kurisu Tada and Naoto Tamura
Department of Internal Medicine and Rheumatology, Juntendo University School of Medicine, Tokyo 13-8421, Japan

Taketoshi Nonaka, Makoto Harada, Tohru Ichikawa and Mamoru Kobayashi
Department of Nephrology, Nagano Red Cross Hospital, 5-22-1 Wakasato, Nagano 380-8582, Japan

Masahiko Sumi
Department of Hematology, Nagano Red Cross Hospital, 5-22-1 Wakasato, Nagano 380-8582, Japan

Wataru Ishii
Department of Rheumatology, Nagano Red Cross Hospital, 5-22-1 Wakasato, Nagano 380-8582, Japan

Bernard Ofoe Tetteh
Rheumatology Unit, Department of Internal Medicine and Therapeutics, Korle-Bu Teaching Hospital, Accra, Ghana

Florence-Barbara Yebuah
Ophthalmology Department, Korle-Bu Teaching Hospital, Accra, Ghana

Maame-Boatemaa Amissah-Arthur and Dzifa Dey
Rheumatology Unit, Department of Internal Medicine and erapeutics, Korle-Bu Teaching Hospital, Accra, Ghana
Rheumatology Unit, Department of Internal Medicine and erapeutics, University of Ghana Medical School, Accra, Ghana

Shigekazu Kurihara, Tohru Ichikawa and Mamoru Kobayashi
Department of Nephrology, Nagano Red Cross Hospital, 5-22-1 Wakasato, Nagano 380-8582, Japan

Makoto Harada
Department of Nephrology, Nagano Red Cross Hospital, 5-22-1 Wakasato, Nagano 380-8582, Japan
Department of Nephrology, Shinshu University School of Medicine, 3-1-1 Asahi, Matsumoto 390-8621, Japan

Takashi Ehara
Graduate School of Health Sciences, Matsumoto University, 2095-1 Niimura, Matsumoto 390-1241, Japan

Christine Loftis and Rosa White
University of Texas at Rio Grande Valley, Internal Medicine Department- Doctor Hospital at Renaissance, 5423 S McColl Rd, Edinburg, TX 78539, USA

Emilia C. Dulgheru
Rheumatology Institute-Doctor Hospital at Renaissance, Edinburg, TX 78539, USA

Sukhraj Singh, Zareen Vaghaiwall and Karishma Ramsubeik
Division of Rheumatology, Department of Medicine, University of Florida Health Jacksonville, Jacksonville, FL, USA

Nisha Chowdhury and Swetha Nuthulaganti
Division of Internal Medicine, Department of Medicine, University of Florida Health Jacksonville, Jacksonville, FL, USA

Sandra Sheffield
Division of Internal Medicine, Department of Medicine, University of Florida Health Jacksonville, Jacksonville, FL, USA
Department of Medicine, University of Florida Health, 653 W 8th Street, Jacksonville, 32209 Florida, USA

Bayanne Olabi
NHS Lothian, Department of Dermatology, Lauriston Building, Lauriston Place, Edinburgh EH3 9EN, UK
Rheumatology Section, Imperial College Healthcare NHS Trust, Hammersmith Hospital, Du Cane Road, London W12 0HS, UK

Justin C. Mason and Ziad Farah
Rheumatology Section, Imperial College Healthcare NHS Trust, Hammersmith Hospital, Du Cane Road, London W12 0HS, UK

Indrit Greca, Jihad Ben Gabr, Stephanie Bryant and Dan Zaccarini
SUNY Upstate University Hospital, Syracuse, NY-13210, USA

M. Moshkbar
Pediatric Department, Bouali Children's Hospital, Ardabil University of Medical Sciences (ARUMS), Ardabil, Iran

Andras Perl
SUNY Upstate University Hospital, Syracuse, NY-13210, USA
Departments of Medicine, Microbiology and Immunology, Biochemistry and Molecular Biology, State University of New York, UMU, College of Medicine, New York, USA

Farhad Salehzadeh
Professor in Pediatric Rheumatology, Pediatric Department, Bouali Children's Hospital, Ardabil University of Medical Sciences (ARUMS), Ardabil, Iran

A. Enteshary
Assistant Professor of Rheumatology, Internal Medicine Department, Imam Khomeini Hospital, Ardabil University of Medical Sciences (ARUMS), Ardabil, Iran

Soichiro Obata, Misaki Toda and Shigeru Aoki
Perinatal Center for Maternity and Neonates, Yokohama City University Medical Center, Yokohama, Japan

Koji Kobayashi
Center for Rheumatic Disease, Yokohama City University Medical Center, Yokohama, Japan

Etsuko Miyagi
Department of Obstetrics and Gynecology, Yokohama City University Hospital, Yokohama, Japan

Soo Choi, Natalie Voskanian and Katherine H.Y. Nguyen
University of California, San Diego, CA, USA

Jeffrey Ramos
Scripps Memorial Hospital, San Diego, CA, USA

Georgio Medawar
Internal Medicine Department, St George Hospital University Medical Center and the University of Balamand, Beirut, Lebanon

Joseph Chahrouri
Internal Medicine Department, St George Hospital University Medical Center and the University of Balamand, Beirut, Lebanon
Rheumatology Division, St George Hospital University Medical Center and the University of Balamand, Beirut, Lebanon

Rabih Said
Internal Medicine Department, St George Hospital University Medical Center and the University of Balamand, Beirut, Lebanon
Hematology/Oncology Division, St George Hospital University Medical Center and the University of Balamand, Beirut, Lebanon

Jozélio Freire De Carvalho
Institute for Health Sciences from Federal University of Bahia, Salvador, Bahia, Brazil

Antoniella Fernanda Mendanha Sousa
INPOS, Goiania-GO, Brazil

Rouhin Sen
University of Colorado Denver, Division of Rheumatology, Barbara Davis Center, Mail Stop B115, 1775 Aurora Court, Aurora 80045, Colorado, USA

Kathleen Borghoff
University of Nebraska Medical Center, Division of Diabetes, Endocrinology, and Metabolism, 984130 Nebraska Medical Center, Omaha 68198, NE, USA

Kirk W. Foster and Stanley J. Radio
University of Nebraska Medical Center, Department of Pathology and Microbiology, 985900 Nebraska Medical Center,Omaha 68198, NE, USA

Alan Erickson and Michelene Hearth-Holmes
University of Nebraska Medical Center, Division of Rheumatology, 986270 Nebraska Medical Center, Omaha 68198, NE, USA

Alexis Ziebelman
Department of Medicine "B", Sheba Medical Center, Tel-Hashomer, Ramat Gan, Israel
Sackler Faculty of Medicine, Tel Aviv University, Tel-Aviv, Israel

Shir Raibman-Spector
Sackler Faculty of Medicine, Tel Aviv University, Tel-Aviv, Israel
Department of Medicine "E", Sheba Medical Center, Tel-Hashomer, Ramat Gan, Israel

Omer Gendelman
Department of Medicine "B", Sheba Medical Center, Tel-Hashomer, Ramat Gan, Israel
Sackler Faculty of Medicine, Tel Aviv University, Tel-Aviv, Israel
Rheumatology Unit, Sheba Medical Center, Tel-Hashomer, Ramat Gan, Israel

Ahmed Alhazmi and Rola Yousef Hassan
Department of Medicine, Division of Rheumatology, King Fahad Armed Forces Hospital, Jeddah, Saudi Arabia

Mohamed Moulaye Cheikh
Doctor Soliman Fakeeh Hospital, Jeddah, Saudi Arabia

Anwar I. Joudeh and Salah Mahdi
Department of Internal Medicine, Al-Khor Hospital, Hamad Medical Corporation, Doha, Postcode 3050, Qatar

Mhd Kutaiba Albuni and Sara Seife Hassen
Department of Internal Medicine, Hamad General Hospital, Hamad Medical Corporation, Doha, Postcode 3050, Qatar

Phool Iqbal
Department of Internal Medicine, Hamad General Hospital, Hamad Medical Corporation, Doha, Postcode 3050, Qatar
Department of Critical Care, Hamad General Hospital, Hamad Medical Corporation, Doha, Postcode 3050, Qatar

Elsaid Mohamed Aziz Bedair
Department of Radiology, Al-Khor Hospital, Hamad Medical Corporation, Doha, Postcode 3050, Qatar

Yusuke Ohkubo, Shin-ichiro Ohmura, Ryuhei Ishihara and Toshiaki Miyamoto
Department of Rheumatology, Seirei Hamamatsu General Hospital, Hamamatsu, Shizuoka, Japan

Davisson J. Wriston
Department of Internal Medicine, Geisinger Medical Center, Danville, Pennsylvania, USA

Evan R. Norfolk and Lindsay M. Smith
Department of Nephrology, Geisinger Medical Center, Danville, Pennsylvania, USA

Guoli Chen
Department of Pathology, Geisinger Medical Center, Danville, Pennsylvania, USA

David H. Bulbin
Department of Rheumatology, Geisinger Medical Center, Danville, Pennsylvania, USA

Mehrin Jawaid, Yael Ross and Mohammad Kamran
WellStar Kennestone Regional Medical Center, Marietta, GA 30060, USA

Sukesh Sukumaran
Division of Rheumatology, Department of Pediatrics, Valley Children's Hospital, Madera, CA, USA

Vini Vijayan
Division of Infectious Diseases, Department of Pediatrics, Valley Children's Hospital, Madera, CA, USA

Jordan T. Jones
Department of Pediatrics, Children's Mercy Kansas City, Kansas, MO, USA
University of Missouri-Kansas City School of Medicine, Kansas, MO, USA
University of Kansas School of Medicine, Kansas, KS, USA

Masatoshi Kawataka, Toshiki Kido, Reina Tsuda, Takafumi Onose, Ryoko Asano, Miho Yamazaki, Naonori Sugishita, Hiroyuki Hounoki, Koichiro Shinoda and Kazuyuki Tobe
First Department of Internal Medicine, University of Toyama, Toyama, Japan

Toshiko Kakiuchi
Department of Diagnostic Pathology, University of Toyama, Toyama, Japan

Wasundara Wathurapatha, B. G. A. Rathnamali and Upul Dissanayake
National Hospital of Sri Lanka, Colombo, Sri Lanka

Khalid S. Alshahrani and Abdulellah M. Almohaya
Internal Medicine Department, Ad-Diriyah Hospital, Ministry of Health, Riyadh, Saudi Arabia

Rayan S. Hussein
Department of Medicine, University of Medical Sciences and Technology, Khartoum, Sudan

Rania H. Ali
Department of Medicine, Alzaiem Alazhari University, Khartoum, Sudan

Heather Bukiri
Department of Rheumatology, Virginia Mason Medical Center, Seattle, WA, USA

Steven M. Ruhoy
Department of Pathology, Virginia Mason Medical Center, Seattle, WA, USA

Jane H. Buckner
Department of Rheumatology, Virginia Mason Medical Center, Seattle, WA, USA
Translational Research Program, Benaroya Research Institute at Virginia Mason, Seattle, WA, USA

M. M. Fedeli
Department of Internal Medicine, Ospedale La Carit`a, Locarno, Switzerland

M. Vecchi
Centro Medico, Chiasso, Switzerland

P. Rodoni Cassis
Centro Medico, Chiasso, Switzerland
Department of Radiology, Clinica Sant'Anna, Lugano-Sorengo, Switzerland
Department of Radiology, Clinica Ars Medica, Gravesano, Switzerland

Marlene Marte Furment
Internal Medicine Department, Saint Peter's University Hospital/Rutgers Robert Wood Johnson Medical School Program, New Brunswick, NJ, USA

Sandra Antigua Jimenez
Department of Health Sciences, Instituto Tecnologico de Santo Domingo, Santo Domingo, Dominican Republic

Sangeetha Pabolu
Rheumatology Department, Saint Peter's University Hospital/Rutgers Robert Wood Johnson Medical School Program, New Brunswick, NJ, USA

James R. Agapoff IV
Department of Psychiatry, University of Hawai'i at Mānoa, John A. Burns School of Medicine, Honolulu, HI, USA

Magda Choueiri, Florent Eymard, Sandra Guignard and Xavier Chevalier
Department of Rheumatology, Henri Mondor University Hospital, Paris XII University-UPEC, Créteil, France

Frédéric Pigneur
Department of Radiology, Henri Mondor University Hospital, Paris XII University-UPEC, Créteil, France

Index